Medicines in China's National Health Insurance System

This book conducts systematic research on healthcare medicine management policies of China. In-depth comprehensive research has been carried out, targeting multiple issues of particular importance in healthcare medicine management, such as the purchasing, pricing, payment, usage, and the function of commercial healthcare insurance in medical payment. Policy advice regarding the aforementioned issues has been put forward after the research.

China Development Research Foundation (CDRF) is a public foundation initiated and led by the Development Research Center of the State Council (DRC) on November 27, 1997. Its mission is to advance good governance and public policy to promote economic development and social progress. Financial support for the Foundation is provided by donations from Chinese and international patrons. Funding is used to support policy research, publications, leadership training, development forums, and academic exchanges, as well as rewarding individuals who make great contribution in policy consulting or related areas of academic research and funding other social philanthropic activities that fit with the goal of the foundation.

Routledge Studies on the Chinese Economy

Series Editor:

Peter Nolan

University of Cambridge

Founding Series Editors:

Peter Nolan

University of Cambridge

Dong Fureng

Beijing University

The aim of this series is to publish original, high-quality, research-level work by both new and established scholars in the West and the East, on all aspects of the Chinese economy, including studies of business and economic history.

70 China and the West
Crossroads of Civilisation
Peter Nolan

71 Wind Power in China
Ambiguous winds of Change in China's Energy Market
Julia Kirch Kirkegaard

72 Multinationals, Global Value Chains and Governance
The Mechanics of Power in Inter-firm Relations
Peter Hertenstein

73 China in the Asian Financial Crisis
Peter Nolan

74 China's Commercial Health Insurance
by China Development Research Foundation

75 Finance and the Real Economy
China and the West since the Asian Financial Crisis
Peter Nolan

76 How China Escaped Shock Therapy
The Market Reform Debate
Isabella Weber

77 Medicines in China's National Health Insurance System
China Development Research Foundation

For more information about this series, please visit: www.routledge.com

Medicines in China's National Health Insurance System

China Development
Research Foundation

Routledge
Taylor & Francis Group
LONDON AND NEW YORK

CDRF
中国发展研究基金会
China Development Research
Foundation

First published 2023
by Routledge
4 Park Square, Milton Park, Abingdon, Oxon OX14 4RN

and by Routledge
605 Third Avenue, New York, NY 10158

Routledge is an imprint of the Taylor & Francis Group, an informa business

British Library Cataloguing-in-Publication Data
A catalogue record for this book is available from the British Library

Library of Congress Cataloging-in-Publication Data
A catalog record for this book has been requested

ISBN: 978-1-032-35111-7 (hbk)
ISBN: 978-1-032-35113-1 (pbk)
ISBN: 978-1-003-32534-5 (ebk)

DOI: 10.4324/9781003325345

Typeset in Times New Roman
by Apex CoVantage, LLC

Contents

Figures and tables

Figures

Tables

Appreciation

We wish to express our sincere appreciation to both Chinese and foreign experts of the Project Team for their hard work and tremendous support.

We extend special thanks to:

Foreign experts

Adrian Griffin
Vice President, HTA Policy at Johnson & Johnson

Jie Shen
Founder & Managing Director of Switzerland-based AccessNOW

Neeraj Sood
Vice Dean and Professor at Price School of Public Policy, University of Southern California

Michael Thomas
Global Partner, Pharmaceutical Business at A.T. Kearney

Kevin Haninger
Vice President, International Policy at Pharmaceutical Research and Manufacturers of America (PhRMA)

Jennifer Osika
Assistant Vice President, International Affairs at PhRMA

Linda Distlerath
Assistant Vice President, Global Alliance at PhRMA

Chinese experts

Li Yazi
Director of Research Center for Health and Medical Security, Institute of Medical Information, Chinese Academy of Medical Science

Chen Qiulin
Director of Social Security Research Office, Institute of Population and Labor Economics, and Associate Professor of Chinese Academy of Social Sciences

Wang Zhen
Professor of Institute of Economics, Chinese Academy of Social Sciences

Zhang Yuhui
Vice Director and Professor of China National Health Development Research Center

Yu Baorong
Professor of School of Insurance and Economics, University of International Business and Economics

Lü Lanting
Executive Director of Health Technology Assessment and Medicine Policy Research Center, and Associate Professor of the School of Public Administration and Policy, Renmin University of China

Preface

'Healthcare security' refers to major systemic arrangements that are aimed at improving the welfare of people, preserving and protecting social harmony, and reducing the burden of healthcare costs on people. Given their strong focus on public health, the CPC Central Committee and the State Council have established a system of basic universal coverage in China. Reforms relating to this system have consistently been pushed forward since the start of the New Medical Reform, but particularly since the 18th National Congress of the CPC. Breakthrough progress has been made with respect to achieving affordable healthcare. Nevertheless, the road before us remains a long one, and deepening reform of the healthcare security system remains a heavy responsibility. Inadequate and unequal medical safeguards are becoming ever more apparent given rapid socio-economic change.

In 2018, a film called *Dying to Survive* described the problem of not being able to access cancer medications via the existing healthcare security system. That film remains fresh in our minds. This year, the global spread of the COVID-19 pandemic is threatening the lives and health of people all over the world. The importance and the urgency of setting up a better healthcare security system are obvious. These things only strengthen our resolve to push forward reforms of China's healthcare security system.

The management of drugs that are covered by China's health insurance system is an issue that bridges three different areas: insurance, pharmaceuticals, and medical treatment. It is a determining factor in the success or failure of healthcare reforms. Such reforms have been in the fast track since the establishment of the National Healthcare Security Administration (in 2018), and a series of major policy measures have been passed including reforms to do with 'drug negotiations,' 'centralized procurement with target quantities,' 'payment methods,' and so on. Nevertheless, in actual implementation, these measures have faced multiple challenges. Management of drugs covered by the healthcare system still confronts such problems as irrational pricing mechanisms, as-yet unimproved rules for centralized procurement, long-term price distortion, and improper prescribing of drugs. Standing up to these challenges and resolving these issues is a matter of enormous significance in China right now. Taking action has both theoretical and practical ramifications.

In what follows, the CDRF presents *Medicines in China's National Health Insurance System*. This looks at adjustments to the list of reimbursable drugs under the national healthcare security system, the procurement of such drugs, pricing of drugs, reimbursement systems and usage (prescribing) of drugs, and the role that commercial insurance can also play in paying for drugs. However, this work is merely an exploratory attempt to address the subject. We hope that it will spur others to carry out further research and discussion, including experts, government departments, enterprises, and the public at large. We also hope that the public dissemination of this report will be helpful in pushing forward reform of China's healthcare security system, which was our primary intent in initiating this study.

Lu Mai
Vice Chairman of China Development Research Foundation
and Secretary General of China Development Forum, July 1, 2020

Introduction

China's system of medical safeguards is a major line of defense when it comes to safeguarding the health of the country's people, and it provides major support for the strategic policy of a 'Healthy China.' The country has been confronting highly complex threats to public health in recent years, as multiple factors interact with one another. These include rapid socio-economic development, a relentlessly aging population, and accelerating change in the spectrum of disease. The grim situation has not only exacerbated a swift rise in medical costs, but it has also sparked strong demand for healthcare security. There is still an enormous discrepancy between demand and supply, however, given uneven and inadequate supply of healthcare safeguards and ever-increasing diversification of demand. The sudden outbreak of COVID-19 is also making us profoundly aware of the urgent need to establish and improve upon our healthcare security institutions.

The crux of China's medical safeguards system is the administrative management of drugs that are covered under the system. Improving this system impacts the health and wellbeing of the population, and is intended to realize the policy of a 'Healthy China.' A significant breakthrough in the healthcare security system can be achieved by speeding up the scientifically based adjustments to the list of drugs that the system covers. Such adjustments will help reduce the burden of drug costs on those who are insured, help improve access to innovative drugs, and help guide medical practitioners in the rational and proper use of drugs. It will help curb improper practices. It also will ensure effective implementation of policies relating to procurement, price, payment, and drug usage. It will help ensure that the health insurance funds are operating properly. Since 2009, the government and relevant departments have been highly concerned about reform of the policies that deal with the drugs that are covered under China's medical insurance. They have issued a number of key documents meant to stimulate adjustments to the list of drugs that can be reimbursed under the system, and to ensure that the results are actually implemented.

This is the general context in which we began the work of this report. In 2019, we set up the project team to carry out *Medicines in China's National Health Insurance System*. This team carried out an in-depth, comprehensive study of the subject, including adjustments to the list of covered drugs, procurement of such drugs as well as their pricing and payment and usage, and the role of commercial insurance in paying for drugs. In addition to drawing on a wealth of experience from experts in the field, the team traveled to Germany to conduct surveys and interviews of relevant parties, such as enterprises and hospitals. They gained an abundance of materials and primary data.

After one year of hard work, the expert teams responsible for each of the specific topics completed their reports in outstanding fashion. Those reports are included in this study and are as follows: 'Research on dynamic mechanisms for adjusting China's reimbursable drug list' (Li Yazi); 'Research on drug procurement mechanisms' (Chen Qiulin); 'Research on drug price-formation mechanisms' (Wang Zhen); 'Research on payment for and usage of drugs' (Zhang Yuhui); 'Commercial health insurance in China and its role in the payment of drug costs' (Yu Baorong); and 'Research on drug-pricing mechanisms in other countries' (Lü Lanting).

The team then went on to complete the Summary Report that follows this Introduction, based on the research on specific topics as well as additional supplementary research. This Summary Report describes policy advances to date that relate to the national reimbursable drug list, the current state of affairs, and challenges and problems we now confront. It goes on to propose five key areas that will require coordinated implementation as we adjust the list in the future. The ultimate results of our work, including the Summary Report and the specific topic reports, have been published under the title *Policy Research on Coverage of Medicines under China's National Health Insurance System*.

The smooth completion of this work could not have been accomplished without the wholehearted enthusiasm of the project team, as well as enormous support from the many experts and units who participated. The association known as PhRMA, the Pharmaceutical Research and Manufacturers of America, provided generous financial support for our research. In Germany, the German Ministry of Health, the German Pharmaceutical Research and Manufacturing Association, the company Bayer, and the global management consulting firm A.T. Kearney provided comprehensive and considerate arrangements for the project team during their survey.

Within the project team, Fang Jin, Secretary General of the China Development Research Foundation, provided invaluable advice on structuring the design of the research. Qiu Yue, Director of Research Department 2, was responsible for actual implementation of the project. She worked together with team members Wang Qiguo and Ma Luyan in organizing the structure of topics and completing the preparatory work. Sun Rui, from the publisher Development Research Think Tank (Beijing) Books, Co., Ltd., provided enormous support by ensuring the smooth publication of the work.

We hope that the results of this research will contribute to evidence-based policy in the sphere of China's healthcare security. We hope it will provide scientific backing and helpful reference material with specific regard to the administrative management of drugs. At the same time, we hope and expect that many others will focus on reform of China's healthcare security system. Experts, government departments, enterprises in the health industry and the public at large should work together, through research and discussions, to achieve the goals of the Healthy China 2030 policy.

Fang Jin
Secretary General, China Development Research Foundation
July 1, 2020

Summary report

Policy Research on Coverage of Medicines under China's National Health Insurance System

Wang Qiguo, Qiu Yue
China Development Research Foundation

1 Background, purpose, and significance of the research

The key to China's healthcare security system lies in how China manages drugs that are reimbursed by the system. This key aspect links health insurance, pharmaceuticals, and medical treatment, and not only affects the health and wellbeing of the people but also impacts the realization of the 'Healthy China' strategic policy. The national list of reimbursable drugs has been revised six times since its initial promulgation. Together with constant changes in policies relating to procurement, pricing, payment, and prescribing, these revisions of the list have played an important role in ensuring a number of policy objectives. That is, they have improved the accessibility of innovative drugs, guided medical practitioners toward rational use of medicines and constrained irrational use, and lowered the burden of healthcare costs on people who are insured. They have put reasonable controls on national healthcare expenditures, in order to ensure that the healthcare funds of the country can continue to operate normally.

However, certain problems are becoming more obvious by the day given rapid socio-economic development, a shift in the spectrum of disease, and the intensification of problems of an aging society. Demand for innovative drugs is increasing, improper use of (prescribing of) drugs is ubiquitous, and pressures on the sustainability of the country's health insurance funds are more and more pronounced. We are already faced with an urgent and massive task. That task includes improving policies that govern the administrative management of reimbursable drugs, speeding up scientifically determined adjustments to the reimbursable drug list, and ensuring that we have effective implementation and actual realization of policies that relate to procurement, pricing, payment, and prescribing.

1 A shift in the spectrum of diseases in China, and an increase in malignant cancers have led to a constant increase in the demand for innovative drugs. However, China's system makes affordable access to such drugs fairly difficult.

Global trends indicate that chronic diseases already pose a severe threat to human beings. According to the *2019 World Health Statistics Report*, an estimated 41 million people died of non-communicable diseases in 2016, which represented 71% of total deaths in that year (57 million). Looking at China specifically, the spectrum of disease has experienced a massive transformation given aging of the population, which is gradually intensifying, and industrialization and urbanization, which are ongoing but constantly speeding up. Surveys indicate that chronic diseases leading to death in China already account for 85% of total deaths. They also already account for 70% of the total burden of disease. The direct economic burden caused by chronic diseases comes to 9.73% of China's GDP. Malignant cancers are foremost among chronic fatal diseases. As a severe threat to the health of the people of China, this is the single most important public health issue. In 2015 roughly 3.929 million people developed malignant tumors and 2.338 million people died of malignant tumors, or 23.91% of all causes of death among China's population. In the last ten years, the incidence of malignant cancers has been increasing at a rate of 3.9%. The rate of death from such cancers is increasing at a rate of 2.5%. The cost of treating these cancers every year exceeds RMB 220 billion.

Innovative drugs have brought hope to cancer patients. Data from research in the U.S. indicates that the survival rate of cancer patients has improved by 41% since 1975. Another study attributes the improvement in survival rate to new therapies, including innovative drugs. In China, the five-year survival rate of cancer patients in 2015 was estimated at 36.9%, whereas in the U.S., the survival rate had already reached 70% by 2012. The discrepancy was caused mainly by the lack of effective therapies in China, as well as a different spectrum of types of cancer. China is now experiencing roughly 4 million new cases of cancer per year. If we apply the previous survival rate in China to this figure, and take into account a five-year or even longer delay in having new drugs come to market, this means that roughly 2 million patients are losing the opportunity to be treated with innovative drugs that could possibly extend or even save their lives. Cancer is an enormous problem in China – the country ranks first in the world in both the incidence of the disease and mortality from the disease. The potential demand of cancer patients for innovative drugs is huge.

At the same time, innovative drugs can be effective but require high levels of technology and come at a high price. While they may prolong or even save a patient's life, they do so at an onerous cost. Most drugs that are used to treat cancer, especially newly developed drugs, cost an average of more than RMB 10,000, which directly affects usage by the patient. A major reason for a patient's inability to access new cancer drugs is the fact that patients cannot be reimbursed for such drugs, since the drugs have not been included in the reimbursable drug list. From interviews of patients, we find that even for drugs that are on the list, the non-reimbursable self-pay cost of the treatment is too high. The total out-of-pocket cost for diagnosis and treatment can be up to RMB 140,000. If patients opt for targeted treatment, the total cost to them is roughly RMB 220,000. These two figures are 1.75 and 2.7 times the annual disposable income of the average household, respectively. An additional problem is that it is hard for cancer patients to be reimbursed for outpatient costs as well. Some 49% of interviewees have indicated that they cannot get reimbursed for drugs dispensed at outpatient clinics – a person must be admitted to a hospital in order to be reimbursed. Nearly 30% of people surveyed felt that the way in which prescriptions are limited to hospitals is an (extreme) problem for them. It is hard for people to access innovative drugs in China, to the extent that the increasing demand for such drugs is not being met. (See Figure 0.1.)

2 The irrational usage of (prescribing of) drugs is ubiquitous in China, while the prescribing of 'supplementary drugs' is leading to enormous waste of China's health insurance funds. We urgently need to address mechanisms that allow adjustment of the national list of reimbursable drugs.

International research in the sphere of clinical treatment indicates that the results of 48% of clinical technologies are unclear, 5% are ineffective, 3% are even harmful, 8% have negative results that cancel out the positives, 22% may be beneficial, while only 13% are clearly beneficial. The unnecessary waste caused by unreasonable or irrational treatment technologies is shocking and sad.

In China, statistics indicate that between 20% and 30% of medical funds are wasted by the wanton behavior of medical institutions as they write prescriptions and carry out examinations. Among the reckless behaviors is the writing of prescriptions for supplementary drugs – this is regarded as the real culprit in hollowing out medical security funds.

Supplementary drugs are also known as 'magic medicine.' They are synonymous with the phrase 'safe, but ineffective.' They generally are not backed by evidence-based medical research, and their effectiveness is disputed. Often sold (to prescribers; i.e., hospitals) on the basis of kickbacks, they help increase the burden of medical costs to patients while also leading to irrational spending out of

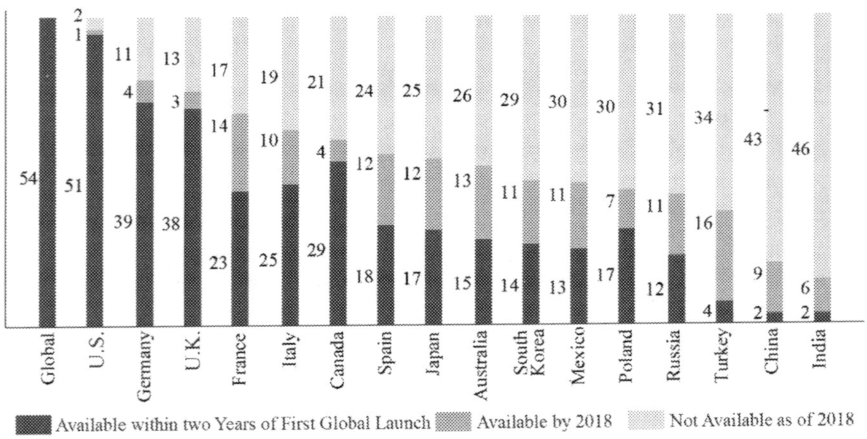

Figure 0.1 Availability in China of Anticancer Drugs in 2018 (Put on the Market in 2013–2017)

Source: IQVIA. 2019. Global Oncology Trends 2019

health insurance funds. Reforming this practice is one of the hardest nuts to crack, however, given that it impacts a multitude of drug companies and is so widely practiced. It is therefore seen as one of the 'deep-water' areas for medical reform.

In July of 2019, the National Health Commission of the PRC and the National Administration of Traditional Chinese Medicine formulated a list called the *First batch of key drugs to be monitored for rational use (including chemical and biological products)*. This was formulated on the basis of recommendations from the same entities at the provincial level. In the course of this most recent revision of the national list of reimbursable drugs, 218 drugs were entered into the list while 154 were taken off, for a net increase of 64 drugs. Roughly one half of the drugs removed from the list had had their licenses revoked by the National Drug Compliance Administration. The rest were mainly found to have low clinical value, were clearly being over-prescribed, and could be substituted with better drugs. Twenty drugs that were major offenders of investigatory controls were removed in this round of revisions. These 'magic medicines' had long been sapping health insurance funds, however. They were able to escape removal from the list up to now, which reflects the fact that the mechanisms for adjusting the list are urgently in need of improvement. Given the speed at which medical technology is improving, and the way in which life-saving drugs are being developed, a great number of drugs are becoming available that can substitute for items on the list. In revising the list, a great deal of work lies ahead.

3 As healthcare costs steadily increase, health insurance funds are under great pressure as they try to maintain positive balances. China urgently needs to put major effort into controlling healthcare expenditures.

Healthcare costs in China have maintained a consistent and rapid increase over many years. Statistics indicate that the total costs of healthcare have gone from RMB 502.6 billion in 2001 to RMB 5.8 trillion in 2018, for a compound annual growth rate of 15.5%. As a percentage of GDP, healthcare costs have gone from 4.58% to 6.4% over the same period. This rapid and ongoing rise in costs presents an enormous challenge to the country's economic growth as well as the healthcare system of the country. Meanwhile, government expenditures on healthcare have also experienced an enormous increase. Public spending has risen from RMB 80.06 billion in 2001 to RMB 1,639.07 billion in 2018. As a percentage of total healthcare spending, these amounts represent an increase from 15.5% in 2001 to 28.3% in 2018 (see Figure 0.2). Over the long run, this rapid increase in government spending on healthcare is putting extreme pressure on public finance. The disparity between the limited funds in the budget that are available for healthcare and the enormous rise in medical costs is quite apparent.

Our research team estimates that the national funds for 'basic insurance,' that is, the pooled funds available for basic healthcare security in the country, will be RMB 2.47 trillion in 2020, RMB 3.6 trillion in 2025, and RMB 4.81 trillion in 2030. Spending out of those funds will be RMB 2.1 trillion, RMB 3 trillion, and RMB 4 trillion. In 2020, China is expected to reach the stage of development

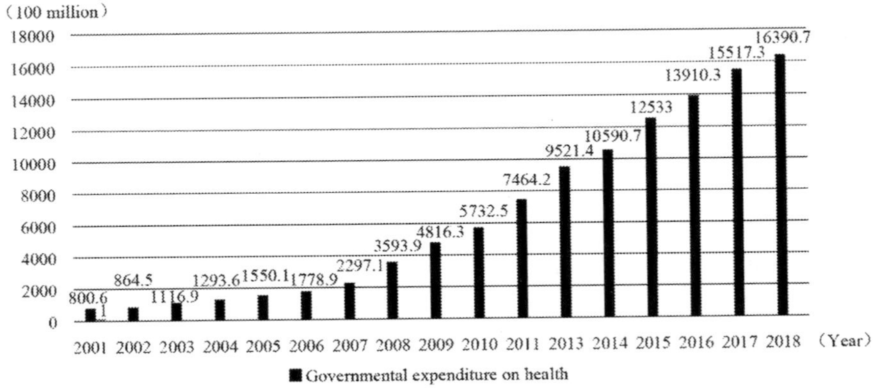

Figure 0.2 Government Spending on Healthcare Costs (2001–2018)

Source: Statistical Bulletin on China's Health Development in 2001–2018

Note: The government expenditure on health in 2012 has not been officially disclosed.

known as a 'moderately prosperous society in an all-round way' (that is, in an inclusive way). This will help improve the actual reimbursement situation as more medical expenses are reimbursed by insurance, given further advances of the basic medical and healthcare security system. As of now, China has not yet set forth a target requirement for actual reimbursement, in terms of a percentage rate. Our research team has used three different levels of hypothetical reimbursement to do its analysis of the funding that will be required and the pressures on raising those funds. If we assume that the level of reimbursement is increased to 60% in the future, then the healthcare security funds will spend RMB 2,3023.39 billion in 2020. This figure will be 93% of all pooled health insurance funds in that year.

Given the previously stated, in 2019 we set up a research team to carry out an in-depth and comprehensive study of the various issues. Those issues included looking at how the national list of reimbursable drugs is revised, how drugs are procured, how their pricing is determined, how drugs are paid for and used, and how commercial health insurance plays a role in paying for them. This team was tasked to carry out 'Policy research into the management of China's national list of reimbursable drugs.' In doing this, the team drew on the wealth of research by experts in the field, it undertook surveys and research in Germany, and it interviewed people in enterprises and hospitals. It analyzed a great volume of statistics and materials to come up with its report.

This *Summary Report* is based on the specific-topic reports and field surveys. It describes progress made to date with respect to policies on administering drugs that are covered under national insurance. It describes the current state of affairs, and discusses challenges and problems we now confront. It goes on to propose five key areas that will require coordinated implementation as we administer reimbursable drugs in the future. We hope that the completion of this report will contribute to science-backed, evidence-based, policy decisions in the sphere of China's administrative management of drugs.

2 Policy considerations and advances

The 'administrative management' of China's national list of reimbursable drugs is a form of systems engineering. It involves a whole series of inter-related subjects that include adjustments to the national list but also the procurement, pricing, payment for, and prescribing of drugs. At the present time, the situation surrounding administrative management of the list is both complex and quite serious. The road before us is long, when it comes to improving the mechanisms that allow for adjusting the list, and improving the mechanisms that relate to procurement, pricing, reimbursement, and usage. The Central Committee of the CPC and the State Council have consistently been highly concerned about these matters and have issued a number of policy documents to address them. They are facing the critical challenge of how to manage drugs, how to improve the accessibility of innovative drugs, and how to help realize the objectives of the Healthy China strategy. In what follows, we therefore use a systems engineering approach in sifting through the policy considerations. (See Appendices 1, 2, 3, and 4.)

Revisions to the reimbursable drug list are of two kinds: allowing drugs in and cutting drugs out. Allowing drugs in is a key step in giving innovative drugs access to the market. Cutting drugs out is a critical way to guide the market in rational use of drugs. Since the National Healthcare Security Administration was established, the main way in which drugs are added to the list is through price negotiation. In October 2018, the National Healthcare Security Administration issued a notice called *Notice on adding seventeen anti-cancer drugs to Category II of China's 'Basic Medical Insurance, Employment Injury Insurance, and Maternity Insurance.'* This inserted the 17 drugs into the reimbursable drug list. As a result, the prices of these drugs fell by an average of 56.7% as compared to the average retail price. Meanwhile, the payment standards (reimbursement prices) for most imported drugs after the price negotiation for their inclusion in the list were an average of 36% lower than prices in surrounding countries or regions.

In August 2019, the National Healthcare Security Administration and the Ministry of Social Security and Human Resources of the PRC issued the list of reimbursable drugs under (three social insurance programs called) the 'national basic medical insurance,' the 'employment injury insurance,' and 'maternity insurance.' This added 218 drugs to the list and took off 154, for a net addition of 64. In November 2019, the National Healthcare Security Administration issued a notice called *Notice of the drugs added after negotiation to Category II of the national drug reimbursement list, employment injury insurance and maternity insurance.* Of 150 drugs that were under negotiation, 97 were successfully added.

In March 2020, the Central Committee of the CPC and the State Council passed an opinion called *Opinion on deepening reform of the medical safeguards system.* This explicitly called for improving the mechanisms for dynamic adjustment of the reimbursable drug list. It added that improving the list should be done within the bounds of funding capabilities, that it should meet the needs of basic medical care of the masses, and that the list may include advanced clinical technology. That is, this *Opinion* noted that treatments and medical consumables with high clinical value and excellent pharmaco-economic evaluations should be covered by basic medical insurance. It recommended standardizing the reimbursement items among medical institutions. It pointed out that both the dynamic adjustment mechanism and the negotiated system of allowing drugs access to the reimbursable list need to be improved. It called for a rational division of the rights and responsibilities of the central and local governments in adjusting the reimbursable list. It said that each separate part of the country is not allowed to formulate its own list or to limit the geographic boundaries within which reimbursement for drugs can take place. The idea behind this was to create a situation in which reimbursement of drugs on the list is national in scope and basically unified. The *Opinion* called for setting up a system of indicators that enables rules to be made for evaluating medical materials and diagnosis and treatment procedures, as well as drugs under the reimbursable list. It called for exit procedures for allowing the removal of drugs and practices. With the publication of this *Opinion*, the process of reforming the mechanisms that allow for revisions of the reimbursable drug list entered a new stage.

Procurement is the key aspect of administering the system that allows drugs to be covered under healthcare insurance. After a series of reforms, the primary method of procurement now involves centralized and quantity-based procurement. In May 2015, the General Office of the State Council issued an opinion called *Guiding opinion on improving the work of centralized drug procurement by government in a pilot program in public hospitals*. This stipulated that an open and transparent multi-party price negotiation should be the basis for drug procurement, in principle done once a year. This should be for patented and/or exclusive drugs. The results of negotiations should be published on the national integrated platform for such information – the national drug-supply safeguards platform. Hospitals should procure drugs based on the results of the negotiations.

In March 2019, the National Healthcare Security Administration issued an opinion called *Opinion on accompanying measures to the pilot program whereby the government organizes centralized procurement of drugs*. This states that the price of drugs with the same name, whether original-research drugs or generic reproductions that have passed a consistency evaluation, should in principle use the same payment standard as drugs that win the centralized purchasing bid. Health insurance funds should settle payments according to this same payment standard (reimbursement price). Policies in recent years have lent greater support to innovative drugs and have notably encouraged research and development of new drugs. They have set up multi-party price negotiation mechanisms that are open and transparent for some patented drugs and exclusive drugs. They give priority to selecting new drugs into the health insurance system that address major diseases and that are major new innovations. From a policy standpoint, these measures have lowered the barriers to entry into the market for innovative drugs.

The *Opinion on deepening reform of the healthcare security system* that the Central Committee of the CPC and the State Council issued in March 2020 explicitly called for deepening reform of the centralized quantity-based system for purchasing drugs and medical materials. It upheld the policy of fully implementing quantity-based centralized purchasing of drugs and medical materials, with price tied to quantity and bidding tied to procurement. It made it clear that the emphasis of reforming drug procurement mechanisms in the future will be on quantity-based centralized procurement.

Price is the core issue in the process of managing drugs that are reimbursed by the health insurance system, and it has been the focal point of multiple rounds of reform. In 2015, seven ministries and commissions including the National Development and Reform Commission jointly issued a policy document called *Various opinions on pushing forward reform of drug pricing*. This completely eliminated the practice of setting prices by administrative fiat. Other than drugs used for narcotics and Class I psychotropic drugs, this stated that (the country now) 'eliminates the setting of drug prices by government so that price-formation should take place mainly through market competition.' In 2016, *Various opinions on further publicizing the lessons learned from deepening reform of drug and healthcare institutions* was promulgated. This made it clear that all public hospitals should stop the practice of adding markups to drugs, should uniformly take into consideration compensation policies set by local government, should adjust price levels properly and accurately, and should adjust prices of medical services in step with one another. The idea was that the country would create room for the dynamic adjustment of healthcare prices by standardizing (regularizing) diagnosis and treatment behaviors and by lowering the fees charged for drugs and materials.

In 2019, the National Healthcare Security Administration set forth an opinion called *Opinion on improving the administrative management of drug prices at the present time*. This adhered to the overall orientation of using the market to regulate drug prices and of having drug prices as determined by the health insurance system play a guiding role in this process. It called for pushing forward a reasonable relationship between target prices and actual prices. It called for implementation of the price of narcotics and Class I psychotropic drugs as per relevant laws. Meanwhile, the *Opinion on deepening reform of the healthcare security system*, presented by the Central Committee of the CPC and the State Council in March 2020, also called for further improvement of the price-formation mechanisms of drugs and medical services. It called for having the market play the dominant role in price-formation of drugs and medical materials, and for setting up a nationwide information-sharing mechanism that would publish transaction prices. It called for controlling the unreasonably high prices of drugs and high-end medical materials. It called for improving the projects aimed at establishing a market-access system for medical services, speeding up projects aimed at reviewing prices of medical services newly added to the reimbursable list, and setting up mechanisms to enable prices to be determined scientifically and in a dynamic fashion. It called for ongoing improvement of the price structure of medical services. It called for establishing mechanisms for monitoring and disclosing indicators that rate the progress of the industry and that provide information on drug prices. It called for setting up a credit evaluation system for bidding and procurement, and it called for improving the systems that relate to price inquiry and negotiation.

Reforming the methods by which insurance reimburses for drugs is also a key component of reforms. This is in order to ensure that the national health insurance policies regarding drug administration are truly being implemented and that drugs are being used properly. In 2016, the Ministry of Human Resources and Social Security promulgated a *Guiding opinion on actively promoting reforms regarding medical treatment, healthcare security (health insurance), and drugs, in which changes in one area affect changes in the others*. This called for

> improving control over 'lump-sum' payments, speeding up use of the method of payment that reimburses for type of illness and number of patients, being proactive in utilizing diagnosis-related groups, exploring a combination of controls over lump-sum and per-item methods, and setting up a composite sort of payment method.

In 2017, the General Office of the State Council issued a *Guiding opinion on going a step further in deepening reform of the payment methods used under basic medical insurance*. This called for

> all-round use of a diversified compound method of payment for healthcare insurance that is centered on payment according to type of illness. Each region selects a certain number of disease categories by which to implement payment by disease type, with some regions carrying out a pilot program of payment by diagnosis-related groups.

In December 2018, the National Healthcare Security Administration issued a notice called *Notice on applying for approval to be included in a national pilot program of payment according to diagnosis related groups*. This proposed speeding up the national-level pilot programs for reimbursement according to diagnosis related groups, and it explored setting up a system for doing this. In March 2020, the *Opinion* of the Central Committee of the CPC and the State Council on *deepening reform of the healthcare security system*, explicitly confirmed the need to carry through with pushing forward reform of reimbursement methods, as well as the need to improve the lump-sum budgeting methods of health insurance funds, to complete the setting up of mechanisms for negotiations between healthcare-security authorized agents and medical institutions, to encourage collective consultation by medical institutions, to formulate aggregate budgets using scientific methods, and to link performance appraisals of the quality of medical care to the results of negotiations. This also encouraged the broad application of big data, it encouraged a diversified and composite method of payment of insurance that is centered on payment by type of illness, and it promoted reimbursement by diagnosis related groups. For long-term hospital stays required by medical rehabilitation or chronic mental illness, the *Opinion* called for payment according to bed-days. For outpatient services involving special chronic disease, it called for payment by headcount.

The *Opinion* also called for exploring separate payments for medical services and drugs. It called for innovative ways to dispense medical services, as appropriate, improvements in how health insurance funds make reimbursements, and improvements in the management mechanisms that govern settlement of payments. It called for exploration into lump-sum or aggregate payment for closely related types of treatment, for strengthening supervisory oversight and assessment procedures, for retaining positive balances and holding them for future use, and for sharing the burden of overspending, within reason. It noted that advance payments to a portion of health insurance funds can be made in certain regions that are so qualified, according to agreed upon terms, in order to alleviate pressures on their finances. That is, managers of the health insurance funds in certain areas can make advances to medical institutions to pay patients who need reimbursing. After a certain amount of policy evolution and policy advances, China has basically formed a healthcare insurance payment system that incorporates diverse health insurance reimbursement methods.

To sum up, a policy structure that governs the administrative management of China's basic healthcare insurance for drugs has taken initial shape. Sifting through existing policy in this way, and summing up the lessons of policies to date, is profoundly significant when it comes to analyzing ongoing problems and recommending reasonable solutions.

3 The current state of implementing policy – a review of the outcomes

1 Negotiations on innovative drugs have achieved remarkable results; mechanisms that allow for adjusting the list of reimbursable drugs are maturing, and health technology assessments are being broadly applied to decision-making.

After the national list of reimbursable drugs was first released in 2000, it went through three cycles of revisions, in 2004, 2009, and 2017. To a certain extent, this irregular pattern of revisions, and the length of time in between revisions, delayed the entry of new drugs into the list. This had an impact on high-priced innovative drugs in particular. Since these drugs were not covered under insurance, they increased the burden of healthcare costs that are born directly by patients and they impacted the willingness of companies to innovate and create new drugs. Because of this, starting in 2017, China began for the first time to incorporate innovative drugs into the list, using a method of negotiated access to the market. This also marked the start of a 'dynamic revision' way of adjusting China's reimbursable drug list. By the end of 2019, the country had carried out three sets of drug negotiations, during which it incorporated 36, 17, and 97 innovative drugs into the list.

By now, the situation is one in which 'routine adjustments' and 'negotiated market access to the list' interact with one another in a coordinated fashion. Mechanisms governing the revisions to the national reimbursable drug list continue to mature. During the revisions of the list in 2019, 148 types of drugs were granted entry to the market through the routine adjustment process. Among these were 47 western drugs and 101 Chinese drugs. A total of 150 drugs were eliminated from the list. Seventy-nine drugs were eliminated through normal procedures, and the rest had their registration numbers revoked by the State Drug Investigation Department. Of the 150 drugs involved in negotiations, 119 were newly discussed while 31 were in a second round of negotiations. Of the 119, 70 were admitted to the list, at prices that were 60.7% lower than before on average. Three therapeutic drugs for treating hepatitis C were reduced in price by more than 85%. Drugs used in treatment of such things as tumors and diabetes were reduced in price by an average of around 65%. Of the 31 drugs involved in second-round negotiations, 27 were admitted to the list at prices that were 26.4% lower than before on average. After these rounds of negotiated entry and conventional adjustment in 2019, the national healthcare reimbursable drug list ultimately included 2,709 different drugs. As compared to the 2017 list, this meant an addition of 218 drugs and elimination of 154 drugs, for a net addition of 64 drugs. After this set of revisions, the capacity of the list to respond to key areas of healthcare security was further enhanced, and the ability of China's 'basic medical security' social insurance program to safeguard the health of people reached a new high point.

One thing that should be emphasized is that such methods as health technology assessments and pharmaco-economic evaluations were already being used on a broad basis in recent years for determining access to the reimbursement list. Since 2017, they have also been used in negotiating prices for innovative drugs. The National Health Commission and the National Healthcare Security Administration jointly recognized that health technology assessments should be used to supplement decision-making on what drugs are allowed entry to China's basic medical insurance reimbursement list. For example, in the revision made to the list in 2017, for the first time China adopted health technology assessments and pharmaco-economic evaluations by analyzing drug data from patients in 600,000 hospitals throughout the country and outpatients from 5.5 million clinics. The results of the analysis were used as technical evidence in determining selections to the list. This

Table 0.1 Categories of Drugs Covered by China's National List of Reimbursable Drugs
Unit: Number of Drugs

Year	*Category I Western Medicine*	*Category II Western Medicine*	*Category I Chinese Patent Medicine*	*Category II Chinese Patent Medicine*	*Total*
2000	327	327	327	327	1488
2004	315	712	135	688	1850
2009	349	791	154	833	2127
2017	402	895	192	1046	2535
2017.7		36 (in negotiation)			2571
2018.9		17 (in negotiation)			2588
2019.8	398	924	242	1079	2643
2019.11	97	2709			

represented a major step forward in going from 'qualitative evaluation done by experts' to 'quantitative evaluation done on the basis of evidence.'

In 2018, the National Healthcare Security Administration added 17 anticancer drugs to the national list of reimbursable drugs. Health technology evaluations based on epidemiological data were used in the course of negotiating. These applied cost-effectiveness and cost-benefit analysis to the drugs in question. Using the same set of data as reference, enterprises could then calculate what they considered to be a 'floor price' for a given drug, and the Health Insurance Bureaus could calculate their 'ceiling price.' Both sides could then carry out negotiations within this price range and could determine the final price as based on the analysis of various parameters.

2 As procurement models have evolved, centralized procurement of drugs has become the dominant method and quantity-quoted procurement has gradually begun to be used.

In the 1980s and 1990s, medical institutions in China basically decided by themselves on what drugs to procure. This led to very high prices with substantial discounts and kickbacks to the buyers. The phenomenon became quite severe as drug procurement became a 'disaster zone of corruption' in medical institutions. The prices of drugs went higher and higher. Because of this, starting at the end of the 1990s, some regions began to experiment with centralized procurement by medical institutions. After 2000, such centralized procurement became the policy on a national basis. The first stage was to conduct centralized procurement at the level of prefectural cities. Market-based procurement was conducted by intermediary institutions. Starting in 2006, centralized procurement of drugs began at the provincial level under a government-guided process. In 2010, as the 'basic drug system' began to be implemented nationwide, China gradually developed a system that is characterized by 1) bidding by manufacturers and a combined bidding-and-procurement process, 2) linking price to quantity, 3) instituting a two-invoice system, and 4) centralized reimbursement. In 2015, the General Office of the State Council issued an opinion called *Opinion on improving the work of centralized procurement of drugs for public hospitals*. This reconfirmed the idea that centralized procurement should be done at the provincial level.

After the National Healthcare Security Administration was established (2018), pilot projects were started in order to carry out procurement at the national level, using quantity-linked bidding. This was an attempt to lower the actual price at which drugs were being procured; that is, prices were meant to be lower by having quantity guarantees take the place of what had been purely price negotiations. In November 2018, the Fifth Meeting of the Central Committee for Deepening Overall Reform was convened. At this meeting, a policy line was approved called *Pilot program on centralized procurement of drugs as organized by the national government*. After this, a document on 'Centralized procurement of drugs by the 4+7 cities' was put forth, with the term 4+7 referring to the four cities under national jurisdiction plus seven provincial capitals. Once this had been approved by the Central Committee for Deepening Overall Reform, the National Healthcare Security Administration organized a pilot program for centralized procurement of drugs. It designated the following cities as pilot-program locations: Beijing, Tianjin, Shanghai, Chongqing and Shenyang, Dalian, Xiamen, Guangzhou, Shenzhen, Chengdu, and Xi'an. It designated 31 kinds of drugs to be used in the pilot program, as defined by specifications. These were generic drugs that were already being produced and that had passed the consistency evaluation. The program then carried out quantity-based procurement.

In September 2019, the National Healthcare Security Administration and eight other government departments issued an opinion called *Opinion on implementing government-led drug procurement and expanding the scope of pilot areas for implementation*. This fully reaffirmed the positive results of centralized quantity-based procurement. It also explicitly stated that the national government formulates basic policies including their scope and requirements, and it organizes the participation of pilot cities. It does this in line with the general idea that it is charge of national organizing, allied procurement, and operation of the procurement platform. Beyond this, it authorizes relevant regions to form alliances of provincial units to carry out the actual procurement – to conduct centralized quantity-based procurement via cross-regional alliances. Following the issuance of the *Opinion on deepening reform of the medical insurance system*, reforms relating to centralized quantity-based procurement have made rapid progress. In the midst of the COVID-19 pandemic, all of the departments concerned with health insurance have been proactive in carrying out centralized procurement of the reagents used to detect the virus. Regions which are qualified to do so have actively carried out centralized quantity-based procurement, which has effectively improved testing capabilities.

3 Explorations into reform of price-formation mechanisms that relate to drug prices are continuing, and pricing mechanisms based on the market are constantly being improved. A series of supportive policy measures has been passed to encourage this process.

Ever since the start of Reform and Opening Up, China has been adjusting the mechanisms that affect drug pricing. It has done this within the overall framework of reforming the institutions that govern drugs and healthcare in the country. To a great extent, drug prices have become the concentrated expression of the many problems in the sphere of medicine, and also the flashpoint of problems. Drug prices are needlessly high. They are divorced from the true value of the drugs. The corrupt and irregular behavior involved in the realm of drug buying and selling has been the cause of repeated efforts to reform the medical/pharmaceutical/healthcare systems. After decades of reform, price-formation mechanisms that apply to China's drugs gradually took shape prior to the 2009 reform called the *New Medical Reform*. At that point, China still maintained a two-track system in which prices set by the government and market-driven prices co-existed.

In the initial period of the New Medical Reform, in 2009, drug-pricing policy still supported the co-existence of these two tracks – administrative determination of prices on the one hand and market negotiation of prices on the other. Drug prices therefore could not accurately reflect the real situation of supply and demand in the market. They could not encourage innovative development of new drugs, and they were not achieving the objective of lowering the actual prices at which drugs were being sold. Given this situation, it was necessary to carry out fundamental reform of drug-pricing mechanisms. In 2015, seven ministries and commissions, including the National Development and Reform Commission, published an opinion called *Opinion on pushing forward reform of drug pricing*. This completely eliminated the setting of prices by administrative fiat. Other than prices of narcotics and Class I psychotropic drugs, it 'eliminated government determination of drug prices, and allowed market competition and the conduct of actual transactions to formulate drug prices.' This then achieved the transition from a two-track pricing system to a system that was primarily market-driven and accomplished by single-price-formation mechanisms.

Taking aim at drug prices that are still fairly high and drug reimbursements that are unreasonable, China has gone on to adopt three other important measures that are in addition to the reforms of price-formation mechanisms. First, given the idea that the reason drug prices are too high is too many links in the distribution chain, one policy orientation has been to reduce and consolidate the various links in the chain. The specific policy measure implements a 'two-invoice system.' Second, given the belief that the fundamental reason drug prices remain high is due to hospitals, this measure has implemented a 'zero-margin system.' Hospitals had been allowed to charge a fixed markup of 15%, which meant that they were motivated to procure and use high-priced drugs, a practice that pushed drug prices even higher. The policy orientation here has been to eliminate the markup that medical institutions charge for drugs. Third, the idea has been that methods for purchasing drugs are 'defective' or contain various drawbacks. These methods do not enjoy the benefits of centralized procurement in helping to push down drug prices, which hurts both the supplier of medical services and the payer who pays for the drugs. The policy measure here has been to reform the drug procurement system by conducting centralized tenders for procurement, in order to force down prices.

4 Reforms have been pushed forward that deal with the ways health insurance is reimbursed. Factors have been loosened that limited the ability of policies to control medical insurance costs and the percentage of drugs in total costs. Measures have constantly been improved that ensure that the drug reimbursement list is actually being followed.

China has implemented a series of reforms of the methods for reimbursing medical insurance costs, in order to achieve cost control and guide the more rational use of drugs. In the early years of Reform and Opening Up, many parts of the country adopted a lump-sum method of management. This was the era of publicly funded medical care, and it was the responsibility of a hospital to manage the total sum of its budget, a system that was meant to control costs. In the 1990s, many regions voluntarily began to explore reform of their own reimbursement methods.

In Shanghai, this resulted in a division of the overall budget into grade levels, and management at each level. In Huai-an, it resulted in budgeting according to type of illness. In Liuzhou, the total budget was divided up into contracted projects and budgeting was done by project; Mudanjiang and Jining had a system of specific fees for specific individual types of illness.

Since the start of the New Medical Reform, China has put major effort into pushing forward a combination of multiple reimbursement methods. A number of pilot projects in various regions have explored practical solutions. The basis of these remains centralized control over the total amounts in medical insurance funds. On that basis, some of the more widely used methods of reimbursement have included payment according to type of illness, according to headcount, and according to bed-days (such reimbursements go to hospitals, not directly to patients). The scope of pilot tests of diagnosis related groups continues to broaden and more innovative pilot programs that explore different reimbursement methods are also continuing as China implements multiple reimbursement methods. The current situation could be summed up as follows:

> China has formed a reimbursement system for basic medical insurance that is based on administrative management of a lump-sum budget, with core mechanisms that allow for negotiated prices and mutually shared risk, with reimbursements [to hospitals] by headcount and by chronic illness at outpatient clinics, and by type of illness for inpatients in hospitals. China is reducing the number of reimbursements it makes for 'projects.' It is promoting reimbursements according to a type-of-illness tally and according to diagnosis-related groups.

Drugs that are being newly added to the list of reimbursable drugs are not included in the controls over lump-sum budgets. This is done in order to avoid the effect that certain controls would have on the admitting of new drugs into the list, such as the percentage-of-drugs requirement in budgetary controls. For example, many provincial governments have petitioned to have the drug-percentage requirement loosened as they negotiate on drug prices. By July 2018, 23 provinces explicitly asked for certain drug negotiations to be outside the scope of the percentage requirement – they asked for these to be calculated separately. After the most recent round of negotiations, the National Healthcare Security Administration and the National Health Commission jointly issued a notice called *Notice on proper implementation of the policies on drugs admitted for reimbursement under the Basic Medical Insurance by negotiation in 2019*. This called for getting drugs that had been negotiated and approved into designated hospitals in a timely fashion. It prohibited any attempt to influence their allocation and use on the grounds of total-budget controls, limits on the number of drugs in the medical institution's drug list, and the drug-percentage requirements. Meanwhile, other areas are exploring ways to make sure policies are actually implemented. For example, in July 2018, the Medical Reform Group of Hunan Province issued a notice saying that the province is starting a 'two-channel model' for buying prescription drugs. This allows patients to have their prescriptions fulfilled at designated hospitals but also designated pharmacies. The drugs they can be reimbursed for include those that were negotiated by the national government for inclusion in the basic medical insurance reimbursable drug list, but also the drugs negotiated by the province for major illness insurance.

5 Commercial health insurance is increasingly being used as a supplement to social insurance, and there is tremendous room for it to play a greater role in the reimbursement of medical costs. In the future, the Million-yuan Medical Insurance program should enable more people to gain access to innovative drugs.

In the decade that has passed since the New Medical Reform began, China has set up a system of basic medical safeguards that covers the entire population. This universal coverage system has two components, the 'medical insurance for urban employees' and the 'basic medical insurance for urban and rural residents.' The (theoretical) reimbursable rate of drugs within the scope of the reimbursable drug list for the former kind of insurance is 85%; for the latter kind it is 75%. The actual amounts applied for and reimbursed under both approach 50%. China's goal of making medical care accessible when needed has basically been achieved.

The cost of treatment for minor illnesses is not substantial and does not affect people's daily lives that much – given the basic medical insurance, costs are manageable using either self-payment or reimbursement by health insurance. However, major illnesses are a different matter. The very high treatment costs for such illnesses pose a real risk to the majority of the population. Reimbursement of these costs through the public health security system comes to less than 50%; commercial insurance presents the possibility of covering the rest. For example, according to reimbursement data of hospitalized patients gathered by Taikang Life Insurance, 51.7% of people that Taikang insures had less than one half of their costs covered by public health insurance. Of this group, only 13.21% applied for reimbursement of more than 70% of their costs from public insurance. (A great deal of medical costs went uninsured.) It is obvious from this example that commercial health insurance can play an enormous role in helping cover medical costs in the future.

The 'Million-yuan Medical Insurance' program was born out of this situation. This is a product that sets out a fairly high self-paid initial amount. Without raising premiums significantly, however, the program increases the leverage of funds and raises the amount available for insurance. It helps supplement the shortfalls of the public health insurance system when it comes to the inability to cover high medical expenses. By the end of the first half of 2019, there were 29 insurance companies selling Million-yuan Medical Insurance products. Some 317 different products were on the market: life insurance companies were selling 40 and property insurance companies were selling 277. The total amount being underwritten brought in RMB 26.1 billion in premium revenue for assuming risk on 47.28 million specific policies. A total of 41.12 million people were investing in this

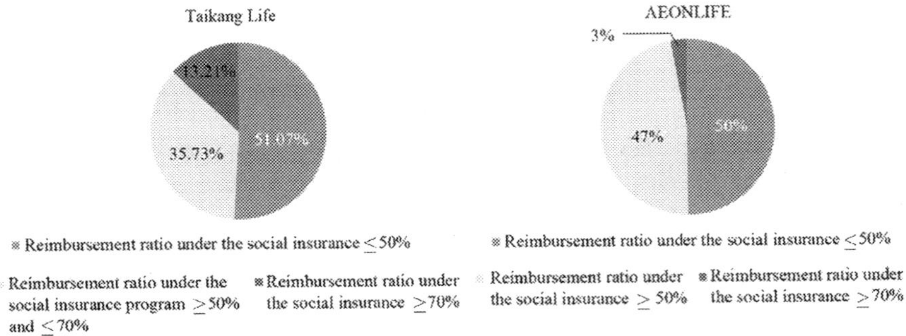

Figure 0.3 Reimbursement of Hospitalization Expenses under the Basic Medical Insurance in 2018, in Percentages (Taikang Life vs AEON LIFE).

Source: 2018 Annual Claims Report of Taikang Life/AEON LIFE

insurance. Reimbursements of RMB 2.9 billion were made to 230,000 beneficiaries, and the per capita reimbursement amount came to RMB 12,600. In terms of large-sum reimbursements, some 234 people received over RMB 500,000 in reimbursements. Among these, the highest reimbursement to a single person was RMB 13,100. Clearly, this form of insurance provides effective security against high-end costs of medical care.

The Million-yuan Medical Insurance is mainly aimed at covering high-end medical costs that are currently paid by the patient. It is purely a safeguards-type product that features low premiums, coverage of high-end costs, and that has a high leverage ratio. It can be effective in addressing the problems of people who want to pay for insurance and want it to cover high-end medical costs. At present, the cost of cancer treatments in China runs between RMB 300,000 and RMB 500,000. If targeted drugs, cell therapy, heavy ion therapy, and other advanced technologies are used, costs can run up to over 1 million yuan. In the United States, the treatment of complex cancers commonly approaches USD 1 million. Within China, costs of intensive cancer treatment in top-tier hospitals come to more than RMB 30,000 per day. For quite awhile to come, medical costs in China are expected to continue their rapid and inexorable rise. 'Medical cost inflation' is going to be hard to resolve in any effective way in the immediate future. Meanwhile, however, Million-yuan Medical Insurance products do provide people with more and better options as they think about how to deal with the cost of hospitals, drugs, and treatment.

4 Problems and challenges to be addressed

China has made a series of advances with regard to its policies on managing drugs that are covered by insurance and in implementing those policies, but the country is still facing a number of challenges. Specifically, these lie in the following areas: mechanisms that allow for adjusting the reimbursable drug list, pricing, payment, and prescribing, and the limited role that commercial insurance is currently playing in insurance reimbursements.

Right now, the length of time in between list adjustments is quite extended. Evaluation mechanisms are inadequate and the process is insufficiently open and transparent. Regulations that govern the purchasing of drugs are imperfect, centralized procurement has been tasked with a rather large number of functions. The process of linking procurement prices with specific quantities should focus on the possibility of various problems arising that need to be dealt with. Distortions in the market prices of drugs have existed for a long time, and paying the prices being required of health insurance funds is leading to financial difficulties. It is hard for new drugs to get into hospitals and be used, given that the cycle for introducing new lists of reimbursable drugs is not only long but faces many restrictions. Not only is there the pervasive problem of getting new drugs into hospitals even if they are on the list, but once drugs do have access to hospitals, there is a problem of their being misused. With respect to commercial insurance, health insurance products are overly homogeneous. Mechanisms that allow them to dovetail with China's basic medical insurance and with hospitals are not well prepared, and the role that these insurance products play in actually paying for drugs is limited.

1 The national drug reimbursement list is subject to long adjustment cycles, defective evaluation mechanisms, and inadequate openness and transparency.

First, China's adjustment cycle is longer than that in developed countries. According to regulations that govern the adjustment procedures in China, in principle the list should be adjusted once every two years. In fact, adjusting the list has taken as long as four to eight years. The list was first promulgated in 2000. Since then, it was adjusted three times, in 2004, 2009, and 2017. Three negotiations have taken place since 2017 – in that year and in 2018 and 2019. Meanwhile, adjustment cycles of reimbursable drug lists in Germany, the United States, Japan, and France do not exceed one year. Comparatively speaking, China's adjustment period is too long, leading to the inability of any drugs at all to either be entered into the list or eliminated from it. This means that new drugs and innovative drugs in particular cannot be added to the list in a timely manner, which makes it hard for them to meet the demand for clinical use. Not only does this increase the cost of healthcare to patients (who must therefore pay for these drugs out of pocket), but it affects the enthusiasm with which companies invest in new drugs. It also means there is no effective response to major national policies that are promoting new and innovative drug programs.

Second, health technology assessments lose a great deal of their significance in China given that the country lacks independent organizations that can carry out drug evaluations, and it lacks the scientific standards by which to evaluate drugs. By now, pharmaco-economic evaluations are being used to a certain degree in the negotiations as one measure of evaluation. Companies that are involved in negotiations must provide the results of such evaluations. However, China has neither clear standards nor designated institutions to conduct evaluations. The model of health technology assessments that is used overseas cannot easily be applied to China without making modifications. China is still in need of a model and evaluation methods that are suited to its own situation. In reality, health technology assessments are in large part conducted either by pharmaceutical companies themselves or by university research entities and consulting companies that have been authorized by the companies. Such entities do not have a sufficient number of employees who are technically qualified, however, and the quality of entities themselves is uneven. In addition, the country lacks a unified framework for assessments, it lacks a system of indicators and standards, all of which means that the assessments handed over by companies cannot easily be compared to one another. This lowers their value when drugs are being evaluated.

Third, the process of adjusting the list does not include the participation of stakeholders. The review and approval process of the list does not accept reports from pharmaceutical companies. Selections for the list and adjustment procedures are basically carried out by an 'adjustment leadership small group.' After being revised, the list is examined and approved by relevant government departments, and the government then publicly issues the revised document. For example, mature standards and rules have not yet been set up in China with respect to such things as the principles governing selection of drugs, the standards, the methods, and the weighting of different indicators. In addition, as a stakeholder, the public at large has little understanding of the subject or of how to participate in the dynamic adjustment of the list. This also increases the costs of trying to gain widespread application of the results of negotiations and actual implementation of the list.

2 Procurement rules need improvement, centralized procurement has been given too many functions, and the problems involved in quantity-based procurement still need to be addressed.

First, the way in which centralized procurement of drugs is organized and the procedures it employs are still inadequately standardized. Administrative (government) interference is too strong. The problem of local protectionism is pronounced. In the course of procuring drugs through centralized procurement, many provincial governments employ administrative fiat to force enterprises to lower prices. They insert conditions into economic and technical indicators that are clearly intended to protect their local pharmaceutical industries. The primary reasons for this fall into two categories. First, (local governments) regard the pharmaceutical industry as a key driver of economic growth and a source of tax revenue. Meanwhile, rule by law is relatively ineffective and self-interest can drive local governments to be unenthusiastic about making sure policy is put into effect. Alternatively, they may want to ensure that policy achieves aims it was not intended to achieve. Second, relevant departments at the central government level have not yet put in place regulatory oversight to enforce market order. There are no effective constraints on the illegal and improper behavior of local governments.

Second, the government has expected too much of the centralized procurement of drugs. At the outset, the implementation of centralized procurement policy goals was a matter of 'regulating the procurement practices of medical institutions.' This sole objective later grew to include

> rectifying the way drugs are circulated [distributed], standardizing drug prices, correcting improper behavior in the buying and selling of drugs, lowering the cost burden of drugs on the public, and eradicating the way in which selling drugs contributes to the bottom line of hospitals.

People put overly high expectations on the roles that centralized procurement of drugs was expected to play. Among these roles, it would be more accurate to say that rectifying the way drugs are circulated and eradicating the way in which drug sales support hospitals are preconditions for the normal and proper procurement of drugs. They are not functions that the centralized procurement of drugs can fulfill. The main reason for this situation is that the distribution of drugs impacts a complex set of interest relationships and requires reform of the links among those relationships, which is in contrast to the straightforward production of drugs. Relatively speaking, it is easier to push forward centralized procurement of drugs than it is to tackle distribution. As a result, centralized procurement of drugs has become a key policy issue 'to grasp' at this present time.

Third, pilot programs that undertake 'quantity-based procurement' are gradually being pushed forward. In this regard, we must fix the roof before it rains, and prepare well in advance for problems that may arise. The National Healthcare Security Administration has promoted a pilot program of quantity-based procurement for the following objectives: to improve procurement mechanisms that pertain to centralized procurement of drugs and price-formation mechanisms that aim to have drug prices that are primarily market-guided, to lower the cost burden of healthcare on the public, to standardize distribution structures that pertain to drugs, and to improve public safety in terms of how drugs are prescribed and used. The pilot program uses the guarantee of ordering a given quantity of a drug, in return for a lower negotiated price for that drug. In the short term, if the order quantity is relatively small, then prices of some drugs may indeed decline. But in the long term, the uncertainties of quantity-based procurement remain to be seen and we should prepare for problems that may arise by focusing on the following key issues.

First, in order to have an accurate forecast of how much of any particular drug will be needed, it is necessary to have a source of accurate data and a proper forecasting method. This is difficult at the outset due to the homogeneity of many drugs and the ease with which one can be substituted for another. This lowers the accuracy of calculations about needed quantity. Second, with respect to guaranteeing a given quantity, China lacks the corresponding supervisory oversight and ways to enforce compliance. Even if a medical institution provides the base figure for a quantity it requires, manufacturers must consolidate demand from various institutions and develop production plans based on those, as well as on the distribution plans formulated by distribution channels. Finally, if drug prices fall drastically for companies who have winning bids, this has a negative impact on the companies. A dramatic decline in prices affects profits, to the extent that some companies may find it hard to keep operating.

3 Price distortion has existed among drug prices for a long time, and the implementation of payment standards (reimbursement standards) remains weak.

First, even though reform of the price-formation mechanisms that apply to drugs continues to move forward, price distortion of drug prices remains an enduring problem. The distortion of drug prices could be called the distillation, or the ultimate manifestation, of all the problems in the health insurance arena. Repeated attempts to change things have been made since the beginning of Reform and Opening Up, but straightening out prices must remain the core focus of reform.

In the 1980s, after China gradually relaxed the controls on drug prices that had been in place under the planned command economy, price-formation mechanisms for drug prices underwent a number of modifications. In the 1980s and 1990s, administratively fixed prices and market-suggested prices co-existed. After 2000, the list of reimbursable drugs under the 'workers and employers medical insurance' list used a 'maximum administrative price limit.' By 2015, all administrative controls over drug prices were lifted. Nevertheless, these changes in pricing mechanisms, together with corresponding changes in policies and administrative control structures, not only did not resolve the problem of drug prices being exorbitantly high, but they did not solve the problem of distorted pricing. Moreover, the changes only stimulated the appearance of even more distortions. Between 1997 and 2013, the government adjusted drug prices downward 32 times. The results of these downward adjustments were that drug prices continued to rise. In addition to reforming price-setting mechanisms, in an attempt to control drug prices the government also passed other related measures, for example controls over the markup rates, rules about price ratio differentials, the 'two-invoice system,' a zero-markup system, government-guided centralized procurement of drugs, and so on. All of these, without exception, failed to get at the root of the problem and did nothing to alleviate the distortion in drug prices.

Second, the implementation of price standards, that is, the prices at which medical insurance reimburses costs, is not happening at sufficient speed. The international practice in setting reference prices for innovative drugs is mainly done through negotiations. In recent years, the use of health technology assessments has been used to determine the clinical value of drugs, and this then becomes the basis for negotiations – this has already become the mainstream method overseas. With respect to generic drugs, reference prices are mainly determined on the basis of market price surveys. The average market price is used to determine the reference price. These methods, however, require certain institutional preconditions.

First, the existing price for drugs cannot incorporate payments made to hospitals and doctors. If prices do incorporate such payments, then you have a condition of 'supporting medical institutions through drugs,' and the market price ceases to be valid. What's more, using such a price may well solidify the practice of charging astronomical prices for drugs. Second, you need a valid market for the supply of medical services and drugs, one that is diversified and competitive. Otherwise, again, it will be hard to prevent opportunistic behavior on the part of hospitals and drug suppliers. Third, you need a sound foundation of health technology assessments, one that can make valid comparative judgments about the clinical value of drugs. Finally, the quality, safety, and clinical results of generic drugs have to be the same as patented drugs. This last point is of ultimate importance when it comes to setting the reference price of generics that can be substituted for patented drugs. China has already begun the process of ensuring that generics are of a consistent quality. However, most generics have not been put through evaluations, and the quality of generics remains uneven. In China today, ensuring that all of these preconditions are met remains a difficult task.

4 It takes too long to actually implement the national list of reimbursable drugs, so that it is hard for new drugs to gain access to hospitals. This phenomenon is fairly universal.

First, not only does implementing the list take too long, but the list faces other constraints. Ever since the national list was first promulgated, during each revision, provinces have all decided to modify it by adding in their own preferences. As a result, each province has its own reimbursable drug list. The list of each province still requires linking up with the healthcare information system of that province and the healthcare information systems of hospitals. In addition there is the problem of delays in uploading to the Internet, so that the release date of products in different provinces is not the same. Generally speaking, the implementation of the new list in provinces lags behind publication of the national list by one to two years. In addition, actual implementation of the reimbursable drug list is limited by the fact that health insurance policies are substantially different in each province. To take the negotiations for the 2017 list as an example: one year after the results of the negotiations were published, six provinces delegated authority to determining regulations on the self-paid percentage to lower levels of government and nine provinces have not released regulations at all on this percentage; 22 provinces and municipalities have explicitly declared that drugs under negotiation should not be included in the percentage that drugs occupy in a total hospital budget; five provinces and municipalities have ruled that drugs under negotiation should not be included in their total budgets for a hospitals' health insurance. A lack of regulations on the percentage of self-pay (out-of-pocket costs) means that patients cannot apply for reimbursement. Meanwhile, blurring the distinction between the total budget and the percentage of the budget that goes for drugs has a tremendously negative impact on the willingness of hospitals to use new drugs included in the list.

Second, it is hard for new drugs that have been added to the national list to find entry into hospitals – this is a universal phenomenon. On the one hand, the policy of 'no markup' has lowered the incentives for hospitals to order new drugs that require higher administrative costs. To take cancer drugs as an example: the zero-markup policy has turned hospitals' pharmacies into a cost center. Some cancer drugs require a chain of frozen transport and cold storage – this takes a relatively large chunk of money out of the budget and increases administrative costs of the warehouse, all of which has to be paid for by the hospital itself. Hospitals understandably are not keen on this. On the other hand, regulations on drug specifications and the mechanisms for making adjustments to the reimbursable drug list are not conducive to enabling new drugs to get into hospitals. Rules that the Ministry of Health issued in 2011 state that top-tier comprehensive hospitals with more than 800 beds shall have no more than 1200 western drugs in their specified 'Supply list of basic drugs' and no more than 300 Chinese patent medicines. Many of these hospitals have already reached their upper limit on these numbers, however, so that adding new drugs means revising their list. Revision of lists in hospitals requires approval of the administrative committee charged with this task, but hospitals have little incentive to take action and there are no relevant mechanisms to force them to do so. Meanwhile, these committees meet rarely in a given year, and when they meet they make relatively few changes to their list. The result is that any given manufacturer of drugs can only get a new drug into a hospital if one of its old drugs is removed.

Third, once drugs do gain entry into hospitals, they are still subject to irrational use. Prescribing inappropriate drugs is the biggest problem in the area of clinical practice. One phenomenon, for example, is the way practitioners of western medicine in hospitals prescribe Chinese patent medicines. Zhang Hongchun, member of the National Committee of the CPPCC, has noted that western medicines (namely, chemical compounds) constitute 75% of the funds paid out of China's healthcare security for drugs, while Chinese patent medicines constitute 25%. Among the Chinese medicines, however, 40% are erroneously prescribed. That is, practitioners are prescribing the wrong medicines for their patients. Further, it was reported that within a three-month span in 2012, Chinese patent medicines accounted for 38% of the prescriptions in the People's Hospital of Sichuan Province, which is a top-tier hospital. More than 95% of these prescriptions were from western-medicine practitioners in all departments. Therefore, in order to ensure that revisions to the reimbursable drug list get implemented, we must strengthen administrative controls over drug prescribing in hospitals.

5 Commercial insurance products are far too similar to one another and they cannot cooperate easily with medical institutions and the basic medical insurance system. The role that commercial insurance can play in paying for drugs is therefore limited.

First, the uniformity of commercial health insurance products means that their use as a supplement to public health insurance is limited. As China's comprehensive health reform continues to enter deeper waters, people are increasingly aware of how health insurance can play a role in their own health. The diversification of demand in the healthcare arena also means that commercial insurance is increasingly important. Nevertheless, actual demand in the commercial health insurance market right now is far below potential demand. One reason for this is that products are too similar to one another and they duplicate too many of the features offered by China's basic health insurance. Commercial health insurance has not yet differentiated its products to align with the actual needs of people and has not sufficiently provided innovative products. It is not meeting the multi-level diversified needs of the public. In addition, even innovative products have a number of problems. For example, the rapid development of the Million-yuan Medical Insurance could meet the demands of a majority of people who become sick, but widespread problems first need to be addressed – false claims of inflated coverage, pricing issues given little basis on which to calculate prices, excessive screening of people who sign up for insurance, and inadequate protection of the rights of consumers. Commercial insurance still has a long way to go.

Second, mechanisms that allow for cooperation between commercial insurance companies and China's basic medical insurance as well as hospitals need fixing. The long-term trend is to have commercial insurance gradually take on the task of managing healthcare in China. However, the unique characteristics of China's healthcare structures leave little room for commercial insurance companies to develop and to provide innovative services. Problems include fairly limited communications between commercial insurance companies and hospitals and doctors. They include the inability of insurance companies and medical institutions to share data. The claims management systems of health insurance companies are inadequately connected via the Internet to the information systems of medical institutions. Operating at a remove from these systems means that companies lack effective supervisory oversight and controls that would enable them to place restrictions on irrational medical costs. As a result, the compensation rates of health insurance companies remain very high.

Third, the general practice is to pay claims based on an invoice. This model is relatively outdated and has limited ability to help control costs. In addition, it makes it impossible to carry out effective control over medical expenditures. Insurance companies can only participate in claims settlement – they have no say over medical services, which means they cannot provide the necessary supervisory oversight. As a result, medical services and insurance services constitute two independent procedures. On the other hand, the 'post facto payment system' makes it hard to provide optimum control over medical costs and moral risk is quite severe. Moreover, China's policies and regulations with respect to a direct claims payment model need improvement, and medical institutions are not inclined to adopt this procedure – their systems and platforms are not set up for direct claims. Yet another model involves pharmacy benefit management providers. As a third party, these providers are expected to initiate price negotiations with drug manufacturers and chain pharmacies. In so doing, they help lower premiums and they help manage the reimbursable drug list while at the same time providing other healthcare management services. Through market-based measures they control drug costs and help coordinate the interests of all stakeholders. However, influenced by an immature insurance industry and by the structures that govern pharmaceuticals and healthcare in China, the role of pharmacy benefit managers has yet to be fully explored.

5 Future orientation and key areas

The reality is that administrative management of China's reimbursable drugs still faces a number of challenges. Given the issues described, we should promote coordinated reform of the 'three medicines': medical treatment, medical insurance, and medicinal drugs.

Such reform involves the following five aspects. 1) Set up mechanisms for adding to and subtracting from the reimbursable drug list that combine periodic revisions and dynamic adjustments. Establish independent health technology assessment institutions and improve the openness and transparency of adjustment procedures. 2) Construct risk-sharing procurement mechanisms whereby price is linked to quantity. Strengthen systems design behind procurement of drugs by taking full advantage of the role of procurement platforms. 3) Speed up reform of insurance reimbursement methods. Formulate science-based payment standards (reimbursement prices) for drugs, set up dynamic links between payment prices and procurement prices. 4) Adhere to the policy of mobilizing reform of the three medicines in coordinated fashion. Increase the degree to which local (provincial) governments enforce policy. Standardize the decision-making behind drug admission to hospital drug lists. Strengthen management that promotes rational use of drugs, push forward reform of the pharmaceutical services charge. 5) Strengthen the links between commercial health insurance and the healthcare insurance system. Ensure that commercial insurance plays a greater role in paying for drugs.

Specifics regarding these five key areas follow.

1 Set up mechanisms for adding to and subtracting from the reimbursable drug list that combine periodic revisions and dynamic adjustments. Establish independent health technology assessment organizations, and improve the openness and transparency of adjustment procedures.

First, set up and improve upon access mechanisms to the reimbursable drug list that combine period adjustments with dynamic adjustments. This involves formulating working guides and technical rules that contribute to the process. It involves strengthening organizational coordination among departments at the national level, in order to join forces behind policy and shorten the timeframe for revising the list. At the same time, we should open a 'green lane' for new drugs as appropriate, and we should set forth specific application procedures that cover screening standards, adjustment cycles, negotiation channels, and exit mechanisms for such things as newly approved drugs, patented drugs, and non-exclusive medicines. We should encourage manufacturing companies to apply to national or provincial-level departments using mandated procedures, and we should encourage the use of generics whenever they can be substituted for patent medicines. Corresponding payment policies should be drawn up in this process. In addition, we should improve upon the mechanisms that allow for removing drugs from the list – this should involve re-examination of drugs on the list at regular intervals. In order to retain drugs that are cost-effective, we should remove drugs that meet removal requirements and replace them with same-class drugs that help conserve any surplus in insurance funds. Funds then can be used to pay for innovative drugs that are both economical and have high clinical value. The aim is to improve the efficiency with which funds are used.

Second, set up independent health technology assessment organizations that maintain an arms-length relationship with stakeholders. Other countries share the following features in how they handle adjustments of their reimbursable drug lists and payment of insurance compensation. First, they use health technology assessments that focus on efficacy, and they tie price to the effectiveness of treatment. Two, they support the substitution of generics for original drugs and they adjust reimbursement accordingly. In China, therefore, in the course of adjusting the list, we must focus on the efficacy of treatment and link price to efficacy. We recommend making full use of health technology assessments: in screening drugs, we must require that the manufacturer supplying the drugs provides accurate data on safety and efficacy as the key indicators for selection. At the same time, it should provide a comparative economic analysis of its drug and similar drugs being produced in China that treat the same disease, or a comparison of non-medicated treatment measures that treat the same disease. This should be regarded as key reference material that helps determine whether or not a drug should be included in the list. The results of such comparative drug cost-benefit analysis will allow for a ranking of drugs. Decisions on whether or not to admit a drug will then depend on its economic as well as therapeutic benefits. We should set up a database of drug economics and an assessment model. We can then develop guidelines for health technology assessments in order to guide practical experience.

Right now, China lacks any intermediary bodies that are completely independent of government and that can represent all stakeholders and mobilize the forces of everyone in coming to objective solutions. The international experience indicates that independence is a crucial part of health technology assessment organizations. Most of the organizations responsible for drug screening have an arms-length relationship with government departments. For example, in England, NICE is an important part of the National Health Service System – it maintains an arms-length relationship with such interest groups as the Department of Health and Social Care and medical service providers. The drug screening evaluations that it prepares are handed directly to the Department of Health. It enjoys its own separate budget. The person in charge of it is appointed by Parliament and is not subject to orders from the Department of Health. In France, the relevant body called HAS, or the French National Authority for Health, has no direct or indirect hierarchical relationship with either the Ministry of Health or the Medical Insurance Fund. It too maintains an arms-length relationship and is directly responsible to the French Congress. In Germany, the equivalent organization is the FJC, which is independent of the central government and the medical insurance fund. Beyond this, however, it is directly responsible to the national health department and is tasked with handling assessments by that department. In Australia, the PBAC (Pharmaceutical Benefits Advisory Commission) directly takes guidance from the national health department's pharmaceutical evaluation board (PEB). This board assists the PBAC in screening evaluations and it then carries out price negotiations with pharmaceutical manufacturers. It also promotes education on health topics.

Given this information, China should gradually take advantage of the capabilities of similar organizations in formulating its own reimbursable drug list. These could include industry associations or other specialist advisory groups. In the course of formulating the list, we should set up mechanisms that incorporate multi-party consultation-based decision-making. Over the long run, we should establish an organization dedicated to health technology assessment. It should maintain relative independence from the central government, medical insurance organs, and the pharmaceutical industry. It should carry out testing and corroboration of the assessment results provided by manufacturers with regard to safety and efficacy indicators. It should carry out evaluations of the economic efficacy of different drugs. The groundwork that it does in screening drugs should be institutionalized and done on an ongoing basis.

Third, we should make full use of the Internet in improving the openness and transparency of list adjustment procedures, and in this regard, we should set up a monitoring mechanism. Specifically, we recommend putting information on the websites of the national reimbursement list of drugs covered by insurance, and other relevant departments. This should be done to publicize list adjustment programs, progress, and results, and we should include useful explanations for the material. The intent is to enable the public to understand as well as monitor the behavior of relevant departments. It is to enable the manufacturers of drugs to be clear about the evidence and processes behind the list selection so that they can guide their research and development in directions that allow for progress. The intent is also to enable hospitals, health insurance organs, and other relevant organs access to information about list adjustments in a timely manner, to facilitate their daily work.

At the same time, we recommend setting up monitoring mechanisms that involve the public at large, and we should draw up supporting documents to follow through on execution. We should make it mandatory for experts who are participating in the screening and selection process to sign a written declaration stating their own interests. They must confirm they are willing to be monitored by all interested parties. At the same time, we should accept opinions, complaints, and charges from all sides and publicize the publicly available channels via which grievances can be expressed. Such channels should include official (government) websites, government WeChat, official Weibo accounts, and so on, and they should include mailing address, telephone, and email addresses. Moreover, as per the requirements of relevant documents that require the acceptance of monitoring, we should make sure complaints are dealt with and responded to in a timely manner.

Australia's experience is worth studying in this regard. The composition of members of the PBAC (Pharmaceutical Benefits Advisory Commission) remained confidential until 1970. Until that time, reasons for decisions on drugs were also not made public. The situation now, however, is that the Australian PBAC carries out revisions of the plan according to a specific law that provides procedures for revising the drug list. This is to ensure strict compliance with all processes and requirements, and to ensure the legality, openness, and transparency of all proceedings. All stakeholders, including government departments, drug companies, medical personnel, and the public at large can read all proceedings on the BS website established by the Ministry of Health (www.pbs.gov.au) and can download the information. This website openly publishes the list of drugs, a guide to the PBPA, information on adjustments made within the list, and information on such things as drug prescribing and reimbursement for drug costs. PBPA's guide has been revised and reissued numerous times – the current version is the fifth edition. The guide specifies the Advisory Commission's responsibilities, work procedures, and meeting times of relevant meetings. It also gives procedures for applying for drug inclusion and advises on deadlines, required documentation, and the various standards used in evaluating evidence.

2 Build risk-sharing procurement mechanisms whereby price is linked to quantity. Strengthen the systems design behind procurement of drugs by taking full advantage of the role of procurement platforms.

First, construct a pricing mechanism that shares risk and is linked to quantity. It is assumed that medicines that are procured will be of guaranteed high quality. Given that premise, the aim of centralized, quantity-based procurement is to lower drug prices as much as possible. A sole focus on low price is insufficient. We must also set up scientific price-formation mechanisms, since excessive emphasis on lowering prices may well lead to the inability to ensure quality. Second, we should allow for reasonable margins, since providing a reasonable profit margin provides the assurance that quantity-based procurement is sustainable. If companies are not paid a reasonable margin, there is always the risk that they may cut off supply. Creating risk-sharing mechanisms, assuming that quantities are actually procured, will help link quantity to pricing. Finally, the link between price and quantity can take many forms – there are various approaches to realizing quantity-based pricing. For example, we may get a commitment from just one, or from two or three suppliers, after confirming a total purchase volume. Each commitment, however, will require a well-defined procurement period.

Second, further strengthen the institutional design of the drug procurement system. We want to avoid monopolies that are the sole winner of bids, and that can lead to all kinds of risk. For drugs that are not supplied by only one manufacturer, therefore, we can consider widening the scope of entry to a reasonable degree. We also want to avoid having too few bid-winning companies, out of the possibility that they may be colluding. The fundamental principle is to maintain a reasonable degree of competition. The idea is to lower and to stabilize prices, within reason, while raising quality, through effective competition. With respect to drugs produced by just one company, we should be explicit about amounts to be purchased and the procurement period while also speeding up the process of substituting in generics, in order to guarantee supply and explore reasonable pricing. The stability of supply should be one of the criteria by which companies are allowed to engage in negotiations – priority of supply should be one of the negotiating conditions. Any company that withdraws from the network, or breaks a contract by cutting supply, must be subject to disciplinary action.

Third, make better use of the role of a procurement platform. A key goal of the next stage is to use a centralized procurement platform to carry out tenders and bidding, price negotiation, procurement, payment, and monitoring. We want to reduce offline transactions as much as possible in order to gather in actual data on drug procurement – this will help lay the foundation for the next round of policy adjustments. Second, we need to improve the professional capabilities of centralized procurement organs. In this regard, we should explore reform of their operating procedures. Right now, most organs responsible for centralized procurement are public (government) entities. They are circumscribed by having to follow the salary system of public employees. It is therefore hard for them to attract high-caliber personnel who can implement professional administrative management. In this regard, we can learn from the example of the Chongqing Municipal Drug Exchange. The 'public institution' nature of this entity has not changed, but it is implementing corporation-type management. This has the potential to draw in outstanding people who can help improve both management skills and technical capacities of the centralized procurement organization.

3 Speed up reform of the fees for pharmaceutical services. Formulate science-based reimbursement standards for drugs, and set up dynamic links between drug reimbursements and procurement prices.

First, we need to speed up reform of the fees for pharmaceutical services. We recommend clarifying and confirming the legal status of pharmacists, including defining their responsibilities, rights, and obligations. Not only will this safeguard their social standing in a legal sense, but it will provide a legal basis for the promotion of pharmaceutical service charges. On this basis, we can start to address the many problems that currently exist in China with respect to pharmacists. These include the lack of explicit job positions and definition of responsibilities, regional gaps in personnel, inadequate training and simplistic knowledge of the subject, narrow scope of defined tasks with respect to clinical medications, insufficient ties to clinical practice, and so on. We should move further in building up the ranks of pharmacists, plan for a rational allocation of pharmacists in different locations, improve the diversified evaluation system, set up a reasonable salary structure for pharmacists, ensure that pharmacist resources are allocated to each level of grassroots medical and healthcare institutions, ensure that on-the-job training is carried out at grassroots-level institutions, and provide opportunities for continuing education. Finally, we should emphasize the role that pharmacists can play in revisions of the reimbursable drug list.

Second, we should push forward a system that allows for separate payment to doctors and to hospitals for their services. Soaring drug prices and excessive prescribing of drugs have been a calamitous problem in the sphere of medicine ever since the beginning of Reform and Opening Up. The distortions in drug prices come from the supply side of medicine and their root cause lies in China's medical and healthcare services system. As noted earlier, China's problems with regard to drug prices lie in the medical system and not in the drugs themselves. It will be impossible to resolve the current problem of 'having drug prices subsidize hospital operations' if we do not set up a separate payments system.

We can learn from the international experience in this regard. In the majority of OECD countries, since the pharmaceutical industry is operated as a separate industry, health insurance (or a different payer) makes separate payments for medical services and for drugs. That is, the payments that health insurance pays out for hospital services, doctors' services, and drugs are all separate. To take the United States as an example: Medicare and Medicaid payments are mainly paid to hospitals on the basis of the type of illness group. Payments to doctors and clinics are, instead, made on the basis of Physician Fee Schedules. Payments for drugs are divided into two categories, those for inpatients and those for outpatients. Insurance pays according to a reimbursement standard that adds a specific markup; hospitals purchase drugs on their own and the drugs that hospitals purchase mainly are acquired through group purchasing organizations (GPOs). The markup involved and the procurement price are lower than the payments received from insurance; the remaining increment constitutes income for hospitals. In 2016, among total medical service fees charged to individuals, healthcare or insurance providers paid out 38% for hospitals, 24% for doctors and clinics, and only 12% for drug prescriptions. (See Figure 0.4.) Prices of drugs in other countries therefore include just the costs of production and distribution, together with profit.

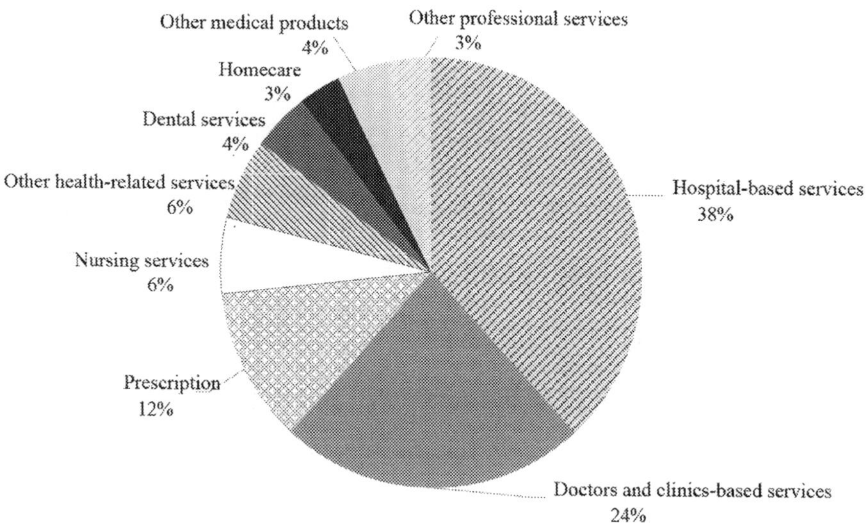

Figure 0.4 Composition of the Sources of Income from Medical Services in the U.S., 2016

Source: Cothran, J., 2018, US health care spending: who pays? California Health Care Foundation, www.chcf.org/publication/us-health-care-spending-who-pays/

Note: Personal medical service charges exclude public health expenses, etc.

Third, we need to formulate scientifically derived reimbursement standards for drugs that are covered by health insurance. Such standards should be separated into two categories: drugs used for inpatients in hospitals and drugs used for outpatients at clinics. First, reimbursements made for drugs used in hospitals should be incorporated in payments made according to type of disease, and a unified payment standard should be adopted. With respect to payment for drugs used by outpatients at clinics, this should be promoted depending on progress in separating medical costs from drug costs, in setting up payment systems for doctors, and in the management of retail pharmacies. Since we have already eliminated the income that hospitals get from a markup on drugs, hospitals are now less eager to have their own in-house pharmacies. This begins to create the conditions for outside sales of prescribed drugs. From the standpoint of healthcare security (medical insurance), we should gradually allow the reimbursement of prescribed drugs that are sold in retail pharmacies. At the same time, we must strengthen supervisory controls over such pharmacies and incorporate them into the functions-monitoring network of medical insurance. We should set up a system of pharmacists and payment to pharmacists under the health insurance system.

At the same time, we need to establish a system that surveys and monitors prices. This can serve as the basis for establishing reimbursement standards for health insurance that are themselves based on price monitoring. The scope of price surveys should not be limited to the mainland but should include major drug markets as well as the Hong Kong, Macao, and Taiwan regions. In the initial period of setting up reimbursement standards, we can set up an external reference-price system that links reimbursement standards with the levels of social and economic development of a given country or region. The price surveying and monitoring system can, at the same time, begin to serve as the basis for price negotiations on drugs and centralized procurement.

Meanwhile, price reform must be coordinated with our current reform of reimbursement methods, reform of public hospitals, and with centralized procurement of drugs. In regions that have already set up payment of insurance to hospitals that is based on type of illness, and where this reform is operating smoothly, we can gradually transition from centralized procurement toward using payment standards for reimbursement by medical insurance. By using tenders and bidding or similar methods, we can first establish and confirm the payment standards for the initial period. At the same time, through reform of the payment methods of medical insurance, as well as reimbursement standards for drugs, we should be able to push forward reform of public hospitals.

4 Adhere to the policy of mobilizing reform of the 'three medicines' in coordinated fashion, that is, medical treatment, medical insurance, and medicines. Increase the degree to which local governments enforce policy. Standardize the decision-making behind drug admission to hospital drug lists. Strengthen management that promotes rational prescribing of drugs, and mobilize reform of the pharmaceutical services charge.

In this arena, we should first strengthen local implementation (of policy) and standardize the evaluation procedures that allow drugs to be prescribed in hospitals, that is, that allow drugs access to reimbursement by medical insurance. After the 2019 adjustments to the national reimbursable drug list were determined, we were able to synchronize the uploading of list adjustments to the Internet at the same time websites at the provincial level uploaded the information. We recommend setting up a schedule for such events that includes the full set of accompanying policies. This would require the passage of detailed rules and regulations within 180 days of starting to implement the new lists, in order to standardize usage of the list. It would also give explicit regulations on such things as the percentage of self-pay costs for innovative drugs, the definition of 'drug percentage,' that is, the percentage of drug costs in hospital costs, controls over the total health insurance budget, the reimbursable drug list for clinics, and so on. To ensure implementation, we recommend that certain indicators be included in the performance appraisals of people who are responsible for health insurance at the provincial level. Those indicators would include speed of implementing the reimbursable drug list and results. Provinces whose work in this regard is not progressing properly will be subject to notifications and criticism.

At the same time, we recommend that drugs that are newly added to the list should not be subject to the limits on specification-based products of a hospital's drugs. We should set up a system that applies to the dynamic adjustment of hospitals' 'basic prescription drug list.' This system should explicitly state that the pharmaceutical committees of hospitals should hold meetings that compare their lists with the national reimbursable drug list and that hospitals should then make timely adjustments of their prescription drug lists. We should look into having the number of actual meetings held and the number of actual drugs that are revised become a part of the performance appraisals of hospitals. Performance in this regard could be linked to government investment in building projects of public hospitals, and public-finance allocations could be adjusted accordingly. Setting up such a guarantee mechanism to ensure the safeguarding of the reimbursable drug list at the hospital level is a way to make sure adjustments to the national list reach the final stage ('the last mile') where list adjustments are actually implemented.

Second, we should strengthen management controls over drug prescriptions to make sure prescribing is reasonable. We can do this via the 'percentage of drugs' requirement, that is, the percentage of a hospital's total budget that is occupied by drugs. We link the target figure for this percentage to performance appraisals. We can carry out investigations of whether or not prescriptions are reasonable by doing both periodic checks and surprise checks. Drug acquisition and prescribing should be an important part of the publicly available information on hospitals. We should strictly enforce regulations that relate to reviewing western-medicine prescriptions and traditional Chinese medicine treatments, with the emphasis being on supervision and controls over the use of antibiotics, supplements, and nutritional medicines. Doctors who are prescribing drugs improperly should not only be subject to public censure but should be subject to measures involving administrative punishment and loss of the authority to write prescriptions. We should strictly control any ad hoc procurement of drugs. Medical institutions that are prescribing drugs properly should be given higher ranking in their performance appraisals, and the results of appraisals should be linked to hiring as well as the performance-related bonuses for the head of the hospital.

Looking at the international experience, developed countries promote reasonable prescribing of drugs by controlling two kinds of mistakes. One results in irrational or unreasonable prescriptions due to the lack of knowledge and capability on the part of the doctor or pharmacist. This is an unintentional form of negligence. The second results from intentional negligence whereby either the doctor or the doctor and pharmacist together, mis-prescribe drugs out of a profit motive – they seek to earn the largest profit from a transaction. Developed countries emphasize interventions that deal with intentional mis-prescribing. They do this by sound management of medical services systems.

First, with respect to medical institutions, we must regard the control of drug costs as a form of cost control. We must force medical institutions to prescribe for the right reasons through such things as strict control over clinical procedures, payment methods, the reimbursable drug list, and so on. Second, we can use rewards and punishments as incentives and constraints on doctors. On the one hand, we can monitor prescriptions, investigate clinical behavior, evaluate unfavorable outcomes, and then punish doctors who break the law through wrongful prescriptions. By making it known that severe cases will have their licenses revoked, we make it so doctors do not dare mis-prescribe drugs. On the other hand, we use such positive incentives as physician's training, bonuses for proper behavior, and so on, to get doctors to not even want to mis-prescribe drugs. Third, by separating (the business of) medicine from (the business of) drugs, we get doctors and pharmacists to constrain one another. The key thing is to separate the interests of the two – once interests are not linked, the income of doctors will be disengaged from income a doctor might formerly have received by prescribing drugs. Such separation is not simply a matter of physically separating pharmacies from hospitals. In cases when unreasonable prescribing of drugs is a matter of ignorance or incompetence, the main solution will be to carry out interventions as hospitals and drugs are being separated from one another. The aim here will be to reduce the probability of improper prescriptions.

Third, we should initiate a 'dual-channel model,' and promote the flow of electronic prescriptions that are fulfilled outside of hospitals. In order to push forward the actual implementation of the reimbursable drug list, and ensure that the benefits of the medical reform reach more patients, we recommend initiating a two-channel model for drugs. Prescriptions would be able to be filled outside of a hospital and patients would be able to get reimbursed by health insurance at designated pharmacies. This model should help alleviate the problems that people are facing in getting access to hospital care, and the difficulties that people who are insured face in buying drugs. At the same time, this model should stimulate (pharmaceutical) companies to be more innovative, which should result in win-win solutions for all sides.

Electronic prescriptions are an important medium for realizing this kind of 'external flow' of prescriptions. Whether seen from the perspective of convenience or security, this is going to become the mainstream way of fulfilling prescriptions. We therefore recommend that China speed up the process of making electronic prescriptions legal, and that we strengthen the access to information among drug companies, hospitals, pharmacies, patients, and the health insurance system. We should bring into effect a prescription-sharing platform that is at the center of externally fulfilled prescriptions. Government should vigorously encourage prescriptions to be fulfilled outside of hospitals, particularly prescriptions for chronic illness, while at the same time it should encourage the development and implementation of an interconnected platform that has standardized rules and procedures. We must ensure that the platform has sufficient inter-operability with respect to supply chains, services, and information technologies. On the other hand, we also need to focus on strengthening supervision and monitoring to make sure prescriptions are authentic, and to ensure their security and controllability.

5 Strengthen the links between commercial health insurance and the (social) health insurance system. Ensure that commercial insurance plays a greater role in paying for drugs.

First, we must clearly define the positioning of commercial insurance with respect to the public healthcare system. At present, the sum of reimbursements paid out by commercial insurance is tiny compared to China's total healthcare costs. Although China's basic health insurance provides extremely broad coverage, in terms of number of people, the amount of coverage per capita is fairly limited. Costs that fall outside the amounts covered under China's basic medical insurance are a substantial burden to those who have to pay for them. What's more, China's healthcare safeguards differ by region and by different income groups. It would be impossible for commercial health insurance to provide coverage for all those who, relatively speaking, already have a low level of coverage under the public health insurance system. At present, commercial insurance is mainly aimed at high-income groups – in that sense, it could be described as embroidering flowers on brocade. Commercial insurance also cannot possibly cover the great majority of urban and rural residents, and serve the function of 'sending them coal in the midst of a snowstorm.' International experience indicates that the positioning of commercial health insurance in other countries is also aimed at high-income groups, and is used as a supplement to public health insurance safeguards. It is not intended to serve a universal role. Even if commercial insurance is fairly widespread, the premiums are generally shared by employers and employees. It can be seen, therefore, that commercial health insurance cannot be a universal choice for the common man in China. If commercial health insurance hopes to gain entry into various markets, it must strengthen the nature of safeguards, have more innovative products and health management features, and must rely on its technology advantage in controlling both risks and costs.

Second, commercial insurance must strengthen its connections to the medical and pharmaceuticals systems. With respect to payments for drugs, generally speaking, a normal family can afford to pay for a hospital stay for a common illness or the fees paid at an outpatient clinic. These are not insurmountable costs. However, families generally lack the deep pockets to pay for the drugs required for more serious illness. Meanwhile, as chronic disease becomes more prevalent and the country becomes an aging society, insurance companies are paying more attention to the equation of 'health insurance + health management.' This model requires corresponding adjustment of various factors – product structure, services model, design of the list of reimbursable drugs, and so on. The key breakthrough areas for commercial health insurance companies will involve high-priced drugs that are outside the scope of normal reimbursement by the health insurance system and safeguards with respect to drugs for chronic illness. Moreover, the role that commercial insurance companies can play is inextricably linked to the integration of the medical system and the industrial chain of pharmaceuticals. First, it should be possible for insurance companies to use their negotiating advantage to control drug costs, and to ensure the supply of drugs to patients. Second, the technical advantages of insurance companies in understanding pricing and risk control should be brought into play. These should be helpful in constructing an information network that is based on policy holders.

As the market for commercial health insurance expands and material circumstances improve, people are becoming ever more aware of insurance. In overall terms, the future of commercial health insurance looks very good. The government is also taking a positive approach to the industry in terms of policy, in order to lower the burden of healthcare costs on people in an effective way. It has extended favorable treatment in the form of lower tax rates and it has loosened policy restrictions in order to stimulate the healthy development of the industry. It is encouraging the creation of an information platform. Provided the platform provides adequate information security, information sharing is generally more efficient than information monopoly. Through the joint efforts of government and all walks of society, the intent is to lower the burden of medical and drug costs on the country's people.

Third, we must put more effort into product innovation. The primary form of healthcare insurance in China today is the 'basic medical insurance' that provides very low coverage but to a broad number of people. The national reimbursable drug list has strict rules about what drugs can be reimbursed and the scope of allowable indications. This social insurance mainly serves the needs of low-income groups and covers basic drugs. Basic medical insurance does not generally reimburse the cost of new medicines – ones that are more effective but have a higher price. Patients either cannot be reimbursed for those or the percentage of reimbursement is low. To a degree, this limits the use of new drugs in clinical practice. It shrinks the market for new drugs. Commercial insurance companies are not limited by either the national reimbursable drug list or national healthcare funds. They represent a supplementary form of medical insurance that can contribute to more widespread use of new drugs. They can be more flexible in their negotiations with drug manufacturers, in the sense that the two parties can come together to jointly set pricing. They can lead the way in helping some high-quality innovative drugs meet the needs of high-end medical services and the drug needs of some portions of China's public. However, at the same time, they must be subject to the macro-economic controls of government and to the guidance of government policies. Different insurance companies should be guided in the direction of developing insurance products for different types of illness. They should avoid taking on overly high risk as a result of moral hazard or adverse selection that might come from their insuring certain innovative drugs that have received preferential treatment.

Appendix 1

Policy statements on the negotiation-based access of drugs

Year	*Document*	*Promulgator*	*Related Policies*
April 2017	*Notice on Soliciting Opinions and Suggestions on Establishing and Improving the Dynamic Adjustment Mechanism for the National Drug Reimbursement List, Employment Injury Insurance and Maternity Insurance*	Ministry of Human Resources and Social Security	Establish a dynamic adjustment mechanism for the NDRL, and adopt different approaches and rules for the newly approved pharmaceuticals, patent drugs, non-exclusive medicines, and non-approved products available on the market.
July 2017	*Notice on Adding 36 Drugs to Category II under the National Drug Reimbursement List, Employment Injury Insurance and Maternity Insurance*	Ministry of Human Resources and Social Security	36 products (including liraglutide injection) were included in the NDRL. The stipulated payment standard is valid until December 31, 2019. Compared with the average retail price in 2016, the decline in the price of drugs in negotiation is 44% at average, and 70% at the maximum.
October 2018	*Notice on Adding 17 Anticancer Drugs to Category II the NDRL of Drugs under Basic Medical Insurance, Employment Injury Insurance and Maternity Insurance*	National Health-care Administration	17 drugs were added to the NDRL and witnessed an average decrease of 56.7% in cost compared with the average retail price, and the payment standard of most drugs imported by negotiation was lower than the market price in the surrounding countries or regions by 36% at average.
August 2019	*Notice on Promulgating the National Drug Reimbursement List, Employment Injury Insurance and Maternity Insurance*	National Health-care Administration, Ministry of Human Resources and Social Security	2,643 products were approved in the conventional adjustment, including 1,322 western drugs and 1,321 Chinese patent medicines (including 93 ethic drugs); 892 traditional Chinese medicines prepared in ready-to-use forms that shall be subject to access management were included in the application scope of national standards, which can be supplemented according to the local procedures. The list includes 398 Category I western medicines and 242 Category I Chinese patent medicines, with a moderate increase in the number of Category I drugs, which testifies to an improvement in health-care security.

November 2019	*Notice on Adding Drugs in Negotiation in 2019 to Category II under the National Drug Reimbursement List, Employment Injury Insurance and Maternity Insurance*	National Health-care Administration, Ministry of Human Resources and Social Security	The negotiation included a total of 150 products, including 119 for the first round and 31 for renewed negotiation. Of the 119 products in the first round negotiation, 70 were passed, so that the average price decreased by 60.7%. Particularly, the average price of three therapeutic drugs for hepatitis C decreased by more than 85%, and that for tumors, diabetes, etc. decreased by approx. 65% at average. Of the 31 products in renewed negotiation, 27 were passed, so that the average price dropped by 26.4%.
March 2020	*Opinions on Deepening the Reform of the Medical Insurance System*	CPC Central Committee, State Council	The dynamic adjustment mechanism on the NDRL of Drugs under Medical Insurance should be improved. Considering the fund affordability, based on the basic medical needs of the public and the progress in clinical technology, the NDRL of Drugs under Medical Insurance should be adjusted and improved to include medical products, diagnosis and treatment items, and medical consumables with high clinical value and excellent economic evaluation to be covered by the basic medical insurance and to standardize the scope of payment for medical service facilities. Both the dynamic adjustment mechanism and the negotiation system of medical insurance access for the NDRL of Drugs under Medical Insurance should be improved. The responsibilities and authorities of the central and local directory adjustment should be rationally divided, and each region should not make its own reimbursement list or adjust limits of payment for medical insurance covered drugs, so as to gradually realize the basic unification of medical insurance coverage nationwide. Evaluation rules and an index system for medical products, diagnosis and treatment items, and medical consumables under coverage should be established, together with a sound exit mechanism.

Appendix 2

Drug circulation and procurement-related policy statements

Year	*Document*	*Promulgator*	*Related Policies*
February 2015	*Guiding Opinions on Improving the Centralized Drug Procurement in Public Hospitals*	General Office of the State Council	Carry out classified procurement according to the guarantee for drug supply based on dual-envelope open bidding, negotiation, direct procurement, designated production, or other methods, so as to expand the functions of the centralized procurement platform at the provincial level, eliminate the practice of profiting from drug-selling for compensation of medical services, and reduce the high prices of drugs and thus the burden of patients.
April 2016	*Notice on Implementing Centralized Procurement of Drugs in Negotiation*	National Health and Family Planning Commission, National Development and Reform Commission, Ministry of Industry and Information Technology, Ministry of Human Resources and Social Security, etc.	Strengthen and expand the centralized procurement of target drugs in negotiation, reduce the excessively high prices and thus the burden of patients. Moreover, the results of price negotiation at the national level shall be released on the centralized procurement platform at the provincial level, and the purchase quantity shall also be included in quotation.
August 2018	*Notice on Initiating Special Centralized Procurement of Anticancer Drugs at the Provincial Level*	National Health-care Administration, National Health Committee	Focus on anticancer drugs, carry out special centralized procurement of drugs for major diseases, reduce the price through quantity-quoted centralized procurement, and thereby alleviate the burden of the massive patients.

January 2019	*Notice on Promulgating the Pilot Program for State-Organized Centralized Procurement and Use of Drugs*	General Office of the State Council	Consolidate the pilot areas into an alliance and encourage the public medical institutions in these areas to implement cross-regional quantity-quoted centralized procurement according to the general idea of state organization, alliance procurement, and platform operation, under which the State shall determine the basic policies, scope, and requirements. On the basis of summarizing and evaluating the pilot work, gradually expand the coverage of centralized procurement and guide the entire society to develop long-term and stable expectations.
February 2020	*Circular on the Second Centralized Procurement and Use of Medical Products of National Organizations*	National Healthcare Security Administration, National Health Commission of the People's Republic of China, National Medical Products Administration, Ministry of Industry and Informatization, Logistic Support Department of the Central Military Commission	Organize alliances should be organized to summarize the demand for centralized procurement and use of medical products; the scope of centralized procurement and use of medical product varieties should be clear; the rules for centralized procurement should be better; the mechanism of national organizations, alliance procurement, and platform operations should be adopted; and the policies and measures on quantity-quoted procurement should be well conducted.
March 2020	*Opinions on Deepening the Reform of the Medical Insurance System*	CPC Central Committee, State Council	The reform of the centralized and quantity-quoted procurement system for medical products and medical consumables should be deepened. The integrated bidding and procurement, quantity-based pricing, and centralized and quantity-quoted procurement of medical products and medical consumables should be developed. Based on the medical insurance payment, a provincial bidding and procurement platform integrating bidding, procurement, trading, settlement, and supervision should be set up, so as to develop regional and national alliance procurement mechanisms to form a supply guarantee with good competition, reasonable prices, and orderly regulation. The direct settlement of medical insurance funds and pharmaceutical enterprises should be advanced, with the improvement of the coordination mechanism between medical insurance payment standards and centralized procurement prices.

Appendix 3

Drug price-related policy statements

Year	*Document*	*Promulgator*	*Related Policies*
November 2015	*Opinions on Promoting the Drug Price Reform*	National Development and Reform Commission and other 6 departments	Administrative pricing shall be completely eliminated, except that of narcotic pharmaceutical and Category I psychotropic drugs, and the transaction prices should be mainly based on market competition.
November 2016	*Several Opinions on Further Promoting the Experiences in Deepening the Reform of the Health-care System*	Leading Team of the State Council for Deepening the Reform of the Health-care System	All public hospitals should call off medicine mark-ups, consider the compensation policies determined by the local government as a whole, accurately calculate price adjustments, and simultaneously adjust the price of medical services. By standardizing medical diagnosis and treatment and reducing the cost of drugs and consumables, make room for the dynamic adjustment of medical service prices. The price adjustment should focus on enhancing the payment of diagnosis and treatment, surgery, nursing, rehabilitation, and traditional Chinese medicine that truly reflect the value of the technical services of medical professionals, reducing the part for the inspection with large-scale medical devices, and ensuring tight bridging with medical insurance payment, hierarchical diagnosis and treatment, cost control, and other policies.
November 2019	*Notice on Several Policies and Measures for Further Deepening the Reform of the Health-care System by Centralized Procurement and Use of Drugs*	Leading Team of the State Council for Deepening the Reform of the Health-care System	Formulate guidance on the dynamic price adjustment for medical services, promote the development of price adjustment rules and procedures in line with the characteristics of the medical industry, and continuously optimize the price comparison in accordance with the principle of 'lump-sum control, structural adjustment, and progressive implementation.' Local governments should reform and improve the pricing procedures of medical services in accordance with pertinent laws and regulations. It is also required to accelerate and improve the price review for newly added medical services, standardize the review process, and promote the development of medical innovation and clinical application.

December 2019	*Opinions on Strengthening Drug Price Administration*	National Health-care Administration	Follow the overall direction in regulating drug prices by the market, give full play to the medical insurance in guiding drug prices, promote the development of a reasonable relationship between the target and actual prices, and implement the administration of the prices of narcotic drugs and Class I psychotropic drugs according to the law.
March 2020	*Opinions on Deepening the Reform of the Medical Insurance System*	CPC Central Committee, State Council	The pricing mechanism of medical services should be improved. A market-oriented pricing mechanism for medical products and medical consumables should be established, and a national mechanism for transaction price information sharing should be put in place. Measures shall be taken to control the prices of medical products and high-value medical consumables. The access system for medical services should be improved to accelerate reviewing the prices of new services. A mechanism for scientific price determination and dynamic adjustment should be established for the constant improvement of the price structure of medical services. A mechanism for monitoring and disclosing medical price information and industrial development index should be established. A system for evaluating drug prices and bidding and procurement credit should be put in use. The system for price inquiry and negotiation needs improvement.

Appendix 4

Drug payment and reimbursement-related policy statements

Year	*Document*	*Promulgator*	*Related Policies*
May 2011	*Opinions on Further Promoting the Medical Insurance Payment Reform*	Ministry of Human Resources and Social Security	Local governments shall determine the lump-sum control indicators under each payment method within the upper limit of expenditures from insurance, which shall be implemented in the designated medical institutions according to their levels, categories, characteristics, workload, among other factors. It is required to strengthen the lump-sum payment control by combining budget management.
November 2012	*Opinions on Implementing Lump Sum Payment Control under the Basic Medical Insurance*	Ministry of Human Resources and Social Security	Conduct lump-sum control over the payment from basic medical insurance in combination with the comprehensive implementation of budget management on basic medical insurance funds, which shall be strengthened in order to reasonably determine the overall objectives of lump-sum control in the regions included in overall planning.
February 2018	*Notice on Promulgating the NDRL of Recommended Diseases for Payment by Disease under Medical Insurance*	Ministry of Human Resources and Social Security	Based on payment by disease, the hospitals shall take the initiative and impose pressure on auxiliary drugs so as to achieve cost control. Reasonably formulate the standards for payment by disease under medical insurance and strengthen account settlement.

November 2018	*Notice on the Allocation and Use of 17 Anticancer Drugs under the Medical Insurance in Negotiation*	National Health Committee	The hospitals shall not intervene with the supply guarantee and use of the target drugs in negotiation on grounds of the lump-sum control over medical expenses and insurance funds, or constraints on the drug ratio or the number of pharmaceutical products. Due efforts shall be made to ensure the reasonable use of target drugs in accordance with the relevant diagnosis and treatment standards and guidelines. The 17 anticancer drugs shall not be subject to any constraints on the drug ratio or lump-sum control over payment from medical insurance funds.
November 2018	*Notice on Implementing the Inclusion of 17 Anticancer Drugs under the Medical Insurance in Negotiation*	National Health Committee	Guarantee the normal supply and availability of target drugs under the NDRL for patients. It is prohibited to intervene with the supply and use of the target drugs in negotiation on grounds of the lump-sum control over expenses and insurance funds, constraints on the drug ratio or the NDRL *of Basic Drugs of Medical Institutions*.
December 2019	*Notice on Implementing the Policies on Drugs Admitted for Reimbursement under Basic Medical Insurance by Negotiation in 2019*	National Health-care Administration, National Health Committee	Six measures are proposed in view of promoting the implementation of the target drugs under medical insurance in negotiation in 2019 (hereinafter referred to as target drugs) as soon as possible and guaranteeing that the majority of insured patients may receive treatment as scheduled.

(*Continued*)

(Continued)

Year	*Document*	*Promulgator*	*Related Policies*
March 2020	*Opinions on Deepening the Reform of the Medical Insurance System*	CPC Central Committee, State Council	The lump-sum budget of the medical insurance fund should be improved; the negotiation mechanism between medical insurance agencies and medical institutions should be improved to encourage the collective consultation among medical institutions and scientifically formulate the total budget, which should be linked with the medical quality and the performance of the agreement. Big data need to be widely applied for the promotion of diverse compound payment methods by disease and the payment by DRGs by diagnosis, in which long-term hospitalization, such as medical rehabilitation and chronic mental illness, shall be paid per bed day and outpatient special chronic diseases paid per capita. We need to explore a separate payment for medical services and medical products. Following the development and innovation of the medical service model, the payment and settlement management mechanism of the medical insurance fund should be improved. We need to explore the lump-sum payment for the medical treatment combination, strengthen supervision and assessment, balance retention and reasonable overspending, and conditional areas may pre-pay part of the medical insurance fund to medical institutions as agreed to alleviate the pressure on their operations.
April 2020	*Interim Measures on Drug Administration of Basic Medical Insurance*	National Healthcare Security Administration	A long-term dynamic adjustment mechanism needs to be established, with the procedures, the payment standards of medical insurance, and the division of responsibilities among the administrative authorities of medical insurance at all levels clearly defined.

Project team members

Project Advisor:
Lu Mai, Vice Chairman and Professor of China Development Research Foundation (CDRF)

Head of Project Team:
Fang Jin, Secretary General and Professor of CDRF

Project Coordinator:
Qiu Yue, Director, Research Dept. 2, and Associate Professor of CDRF

Heads of sub-reports

Chapter 1: Research on dynamic mechanisms for adjusting China's reimbursable drug list

Li Yazi — Director of Research Center for Health and Medical Security, Institute of Medical Information, Chinese Academy of Medical Science

Chapter 2: Research on drug procurement mechanisms

Chen Qiulin — Director of Social Security Research Office, Institute of Population and Labor Economics, and Associate Professor of Chinese Academy of Social Sciences

Chapter 3: Research on drug price-formation mechanisms

Wang Zhen — Professor of Institute of Economics, Chinese Academy of Social Sciences

Chapter 4: Research on payment for and usage of drugs

Zhang Yuhui — Vice Director and Professor of China National Health Development Research Center

Chapter 5: Commercial health insurance in China and its role in the payment of drug costs

Yu Baorong — Professor of School of Insurance and Economics, University of International Business and Economics

Chapter 6: Research on drug-pricing mechanisms in other countries

Lü Lanting	Executive Director of Health Technology Assessment and Medicine Policy Research Center, and Associate Professor of the School of Public Administration and Policy, Renmin University of China

Project officials

Wang Qiguo	Program Manager, Research Dept. 2, and Research Associate of CDRF
Ma Luyan	Deputy Program Manager, Research Dept. 2 of CDRF

1 Research on dynamic mechanisms for adjusting China's reimbursable drug list

Li Yazi and Peng Bo

1 Background to the research

China issued its *Reimbursable Drug List* in response to a number of emerging social issues surrounding medicine and healthcare. Formally called the *National Basic Medical Insurance, Work Injury Insurance, and Maternity Insurance Drug List*, this was aimed at the inability of people to access medical care at a reasonable cost. It was meant to reduce the drug costs of healthcare for people who are covered by social insurance, and to control drug expenditures within reasonable limits; it was intended to guide and constrain medical personnel in how they prescribed drugs, and to enable the healthcare security funds to maintain normal operations; finally, it was meant to further the principle of fairness in how people access health services.

At the present time, the number of drugs included in the reimbursable drug list is gradually increasing, and the list has had a clear and positive impact on lowering the cost of drugs for patients and controlling the cost of what are called 'pharmaceutical fees.' However, a number of problems remain. The formulating and adjusting of the list is done at overly long intervals, standards and procedures used in adjusting are immature, standards and mechanisms for selection of experts need improvement, and public notices regarding updates to the list, as well as feedback, are not transparent; social oversight needs strengthening, and so on. These problems have meant that there is still a tremendous cost burden on patients who have to buy drugs that are not on the list. Meanwhile, drugs that are on the list are often not those for which there is a clinical demand, and innovative drugs have a hard time getting on the list. All of this is not conducive to good health on the part of patients, or to their getting medical treatment when needed. The situation is therefore affecting the harmonious and stable development of society at large.

For these reasons, it is of utmost importance that we set up stable and enduring mechanisms that allow for adjusting the reimbursable drug list so that coverage of drugs and availability of drugs reaches a wider public. This research therefore looks at the current situation and problems with respect to the list and its adjustment mechanisms, it looks at the application of health technology assessments, it compares China's experience with that of other countries, and it comes up with policy recommendations in four specific areas. It presents these in order to invite further discussion.

DOI: 10.4324/9781003325345-1

2 Research objectives and significance

This research was undertaken in order to improve the coverage of and affordability of drugs in China and it was undertaken in order to make China's unique health insurance system one that is more standardized, institutionalized, and more in accordance with the rule of law. The research grapples with clarifying a number of issues in China's current situation with respect to adjustments to the national reimbursable drug list. Those include selection of experts, standards for adjustment, review procedures, public announcements and feedback, social supervision, and so on. It seeks to understand the relevant experience and methodology of other countries as they make dynamic adjustments to their own lists, in order to understand on a more profound level the issues that China faces in adjusting its list. It offers policy recommendations and reference materials with the aim of setting up an enduring and stable set of mechanisms governing list adjustments and, in synchronized steps, enabling the strategic purchase of medical insurance.

3 Research methods

Research methodology included surveying foreign and domestic literature, combing through and organizing policies, and summing up the results. In doing this, this research tried to understand 1) the current situation and the problems of China's adjustment mechanisms of its healthcare security reimbursable drug list, 2) the application of health technology assessments to China's dynamic list adjustments, and 3) how other countries handled the dynamic adjustments to their lists. We also carried out a comparison between domestic and international practices to analyze the causes of relevant problems. After looking at six aspects in particular, we proposed policy recommendations together with supporting evidence for making those recommendations. The six aspects were: the framework within which the list adjustment program takes place, the selection of experts and their working mechanisms, the setting of standards for list adjustment, the design of procedures, public announcements and feedback on updating the list, and social supervision.

4 Research results

4.1 The current situation with respect to China's adjustment mechanisms, and accompanying problems

4.1.1 The basic situation with respect to the healthcare reimbursable drug list

The 'drug list' refers to drugs that are included within the scope of allowable reimbursement under China's (publicly funded) health insurance policies, as well as the medical procedures that may be reimbursed.

4.1.1.1 NUMBER OF DRUGS IN THE REIMBURSABLE DRUG LIST

After first being released in 2000, China's reimbursable drug list (for drugs covered under the country's basic medical insurance) was revised in 2004, 2009, 2017, and 2019, at intervals of four years, five years, eight years, and two years. In 2017, 2018, and 2019, three sets of negotiations were carried out. The total number of drugs on the list has gone from 1,488 in 2000 to 2,709 in 2019 (See Table 1.1.)

4.1.1.2 CONTENTS OF THE LIST

The current list was published in 2019, and is divided into four parts, namely a guide to using the list, western medicine, Chinese patent medicine, and traditional Chinese medicine potions. The western and the Chinese patent medicine parts are in turn divided into two categories, Class A and Class B. When a person with coverage has costs that are in line with the rules of Class A drugs, the total amount can be included within the scope of reimbursable costs, and the funds will be reimbursed according to the prescribed percentage of reimbursement. Costs associated with Class B drugs first have a specified amount deducted from the total before the reimbursable amount is calculated according to prescribed percentages. The deducted amount is considered the self-pay portion of costs.

4.1.1.3 METHODS OF MANAGING 'COMMON-NAME' DRUGS UNDER THE HEALTHCARE SECURITY REIMBURSABLE DRUG LIST

As per the requirements of putting a drug on the market in China, and the management of this process, the western medicines and Chinese patent medicine portions of the reimbursable drug list are described in terms of common-name drugs. Specific companies are not involved or put on the list. Any drug that has the same common name (and dosage type) can be included within the scope of reimbursement, no matter who has produced the drug or what its specifications are.

Table 1.1 Classification of Drugs in China's Reimbursement Drug List

Year	*Class A Western Medicine*	*Class B Western Medicine*	*Class A Chinese Patent Medicine*	*Class B Chinese Patent Medicine*	*Total*
2000	327	327	327	327	1488
2004	315	712	135	688	1850
2009	349	791	154	833	2127
2017	402	895	192	1046	2535
July 2017		36 (negotiation)			2571
August 2018		17 (negotiation)			2588
August 2019	398	924	242	1079	2643
November 2019	398	972	242	1097	2709

4.1.2 The current situation with respect to adjustments of the list

China's medical insurance funds are the largest 'payer' in China's market for pharmaceuticals.

Drugs covered by healthcare security (publicly funded medical insurance) account for over 60% of the drug market in the country. Access to the list of reimbursable drugs is therefore of ultimate importance to the market performance of a drug. The number of drugs on the list is constantly being increased, as well as the types of drugs that can be included. Nevertheless, the relatively long periods in between revisions of the list limit the extent to which new drugs are added, or at least holds back their entry for awhile. This relates especially to high-priced innovative drugs, which adds to the burden of healthcare on the public since these drugs are not reimbursable. This also discourages companies from developing innovative drugs.

Therefore, in order to move a step further in improving the work of adjusting the reimbursable drug list, China's Ministry of Human Resources and Social Security issued a notice on April 18, 2017, called the *Notice on soliciting opinions and suggestions on establishing and improving a dynamic adjustment mechanism for the basic medical insurance, work injury insurance, and maternity insurance drug list*. This was published on the official website of this Ministry. The *Notice* proposed a dynamic adjustment mechanism for the healthcare security reimbursable drug list, but also adopted different methods and rules for the different types of drugs, that is, newly approved drugs, patented drugs, non-exclusive drug types, and drugs already being sold on the market that are not yet included in the list. On April 14, 2017, the same Ministry publicized a list of 44 drugs scheduled to be negotiated, and 36 drugs for which negotiations were successful. These were to be formally included in Class B of the national reimbursable drug list on July 19 of the same year. On August 17, 2018, the National Healthcare Security Administration yet again initiated a special negotiation on anticancer drugs and on October 10 of the same year it negotiated for the inclusion of 17 such drugs into the national healthcare security reimbursable drug list. It also confirmed payment standards (i.e., the reimbursement prices) that healthcare security would pay out on these drugs. On March 13, 2019, the National Healthcare Security Administration's website issued a notice formally soliciting public opinions on the *2019 Work program for adjustments to the national healthcare security reimbursable drug list (*DRAFT *for soliciting opinions)*. In August and November 2019, the National Healthcare Security Administration issued, in sequence, the 'routine' or regular list, and the list of drugs under negotiation to join the list. This revision came two years after the previous revision, called the 2017 edition of the *National basic medical insurance, work injury insurance, and maternity insurance drug list*. This also represented the first time since its establishment that the National Healthcare Security Administration had undertaken a complete revision of the reimbursable drug list. At the same time, the National Healthcare Security Administration announced it would be setting up mechanisms for dynamic adjustment of the list. Among drugs not yet incorporated in the list, the Administration would be taking in more life-saving emergency medicines after full consideration of the ability of the healthcare fund to bear the costs and continue to operate sustainably, and after evaluating clinical demand. At the same time, the Administration would be eliminating those drugs that did not meet the requirements. Meanwhile, it noted that relevant policies relating to the dynamic adjustment process were under study and documents were being formulated.

Other specific contents of the 2019 Work Program were set forth as follows.

4.1.2.1 FRAMEWORK OF THE LIST ADJUSTMENT PROGRAM

The overall framework of this program includes six parts, namely objectives, basic principles, adjustment contents (i.e., the adjustments themselves), organizational form, working procedures, and supervision mechanisms. Among these, the 'adjustment contents' includes drugs that are being excluded as well as those being included. 'Organizational form' includes the structure of the organizations and methods by which experts for organizations are selected.

4.1.2.2 SELECTION OF EXPERTS AND THEIR WORKING MECHANISMS

Expert selection methods Categories include consulting experts, selection experts, measurement experts, and negotiating experts. These categories are filled by people who are mainly clinical practitioners and pharmaceutical experts, although there are also a certain number of experts in medical insurance and in the pharmaco-economic evaluations. The medical insurance experts are responsible for specific tasks in reviewing drugs and the economists are responsible for quantitative measurements relating to drugs under negotiation. Consulting experts and selection experts have no interaction with one another.

1 Consulting experts: around 300 people. These are recommended by academic groups and industry associations, and are characterized by sound judgment and high level of competence and their enthusiasm for and familiarity with the field of healthcare safeguards. This group is composed of scholars who are voluntarily willing to participate in reviewing the list. They are subdivided into two groups, dealing with western and Chinese medicines. They are further divided into several sub-groups including integrated teams and specialty teams. Their primary task is to do data analysis and provide consulting advice on how to categorize drugs. They debate and help determine the key technical points in reviewing drugs, and they set forth opinions on the scope of candidate drugs.
2 Selection experts: around 25,000 people. This group is made up of people from every province (including autonomous regions and directly administered cities), where health insurance departments recommend participants from academic groups and industry associations. The group includes experts from clinical practice and pharmacology, and experts from the government bodies managing the basic medical insurance, from each region and each grade

level of hospital and government organ. Care is taken to include a certain number of experts from grassroots-level medical and healthcare organs. From within this group, a certain number of experts are randomly chosen to carry out consultative surveys and to vote on drug selections from a prepared list of candidates.

3 Measurement experts: around 30 people. These are recommended by the health insurance departments from each area as well as relevant academic groups. They are composed of health insurance administrators and pharmaceutical economists. The group is divided into two sub-groups, one handling calculations to do with the security funds, and one looking at the economics of specific pharmaceuticals. They provide opinions on drugs that are under negotiation from two different standpoints, the impact of selections on the fund and the economics of each drug.
4 Negotiation experts: these are composed of people from the institutions actually operating China's national health insurance, as well as representatives of provincial health insurance departments and related experts. They are responsible for on-site negotiations with pharmaceutical companies.

Working mechanisms of experts Experts mainly participate in the processes of review, negotiation, and supervision. In the review stage, some experts are randomly chosen from the library of all experts for the purpose of conducting consulting surveys on healthcare insurance-covered drugs. They then vote on all the drugs and give opinions and recommendations. After that, consultancy experts decide upon technical parameters by which to carry out reviews. They then carry out reviews according to these parameters as well as the results of consultancy surveys. They determine which drugs to admit to the list of candidate drugs, and which to eliminate. After this, experts from each region and each discipline are randomly selected to vote on candidate drugs. Finally, through voting and according to the number of types of drugs to be in the final list, consultancy experts determine the drugs that are to be added to, or eliminated from, the reimbursable list of drugs. In the negotiation stage, measurement experts calculate impacts on healthcare funds as well as the economics of each drug; negotiation experts and companies then conduct negotiations to determine the unified payment standard (reimbursement price) that is to be applied to each drug as well as administrative management policies. With respect to supervision, experts improve supervisory management over all experts by setting up systems for defining responsibilities, avoiding private interest, and accountability. The entire review and selection process is recorded to ensure that experts put forward independent and fair opinions.

4.1.2.3 FORMULATING THE STANDARDS FOR ADJUSTING THE LIST

This process includes five main areas: principles behind adjusting the list, scope of adjustments, key emphasis of adjustments, standards for base-level data, and methodological basis for adjustments.

Adjustment principles: 1) maintaining the health of the insured is regarded as the starting point. Assuming the health insurance funds can afford the costs, adjustments should be done that emphasize clinical value, make up for existing shortcomings in safeguards, and improve the results of safeguards. Adjustments should modify the scope of the list in ways that can better meet the clinical drug needs of people who are insured and that serve to protect the health-related rights and interests of the entire body of those who are insured. 2) Any adjustments should hold firmly to defining the insurance coverage as 'basic.' They should be positioned in line with the level of China's socio-economic development, should take into consideration not only the ability of health insurance funds to bear the costs but also the needs of insured people and their ability to bear the costs of unincluded drugs in the reimbursable drug list. Adjustments should hold firmly to the positioning of China's 'basic medical insurance.' That means ensuring that the scope of safeguards is matched to the ability to pay for safeguards, not only that 'all efforts be made' but that 'efforts result in achieving what is doable.' 3) The expert reviewing system must be open, fair, and just. The drug list should be determined through standardized and scientific procedures and administrative departments are not allowed to interfere with the results. The adjustment program should consider opinions from all sides and carry out its review procedures in a standardized and open manner. This includes maintaining strict discipline and voluntarily accepting discipline inspections by supervisory authorities and the public. This is in order to ensure that the process is open, fair, and just. 4) Adjusting the list should hold firmly to the principle of 'overall consideration.' This means taking into account the benefits of both western and Chinese medicine and setting up targeted review methods that are in line with the basic theory of each one. It includes overall consideration of the quantities, rate of increase, and overall structure of western and Chinese medicine in the drug list. Adjustments should take into overall consideration theories and regulations that pertain to clinical drugs, as well as the policy requirements of departments that handle the regulatory management of drugs, public health, and traditional Chinese medicine.

Adjustment contents: this pertains to three aspects, namely type of drugs being adjusted, scope (which applies to the time of listing), and adjustment direction (which refers to whether a drug is being included in or eliminated from the list). Adjustments to the list involve the inclusion or elimination of three types of medicine: western medicine, Chinese patent medicine, and Chinese decoctions, which are medicines to be infused in liquids. The National Medical Products Administration supervises and grants permits for drugs to be sold on the market – all drugs under consideration for the list use information from this Administration as the basis for decisions. Adjustments to the list are not to accept applications or recommendations from pharmaceutical companies; no 'review fees' or other forms of payment are to be accepted. Adjustments to the list are managed on the basis of common names of drugs; that is, specific companies are not under consideration. 1) Any inclusions in the list of western drugs and Chinese patent drugs must have been registered on the market-approved list of the National Medical Products Administration prior to the date December 31, 2018. Priority consideration should be given to 'national essential drugs,' cancer drugs and drugs for rare diseases, drugs used for chronic disease, drugs for diseases of children, and drugs for use in emergency situations. Categories of drugs should be drawn up that are based on sphere of medical treatment, usage of drugs, primary function, and so on, and teams of experts should be organized to review each category. Drugs in each category should then be analyzed and compared according to the principles of pharmaco-economics. Priority selections in each category should be based on full and sufficient evidence of clinical necessity, safety and effectiveness, and reasonable price. Drugs are admitted to the list through two methods, routine admittance and negotiated admittance. Routine admittance is granted to drugs that meet preconditions of safety and effectiveness standards and that also have prices (cost) equal to or lower than existing drugs on the list. Drugs with relatively high prices, or that would have a considerable impact on healthcare security funds, and that are patented and exclusively controlled by one company, must go through a negotiated method of entry (the determination of exclusive drug status is to be made one day prior to the selection vote). 2) The same rules for admittance to the list apply to Chinese medicines that are infused in liquids. At the national level of adjustments to the reimbursable drug list, only such medicines that meet national pharmaceutical standards are allowed for consideration. 3) Any drugs that are already on the list but that are now found to be forbidden by national drug regulatory authorities must be removed from the list. This applies to drugs that are forbidden to be produced or sold or used. In addition, any drugs that experts review and find not in compliance with healthcare security requirements and conditions are to be removed from the list using specified procedures. For example, this would include common-name generic drugs whose approval certificate numbers have been canceled and imports whose 'imported drug registration certificate' has been revoked by the drug regulatory authorities. Such drugs can be removed from the list directly. The exclusion of other drugs should go through strict expert-review procedures. As an example, if experts feel that the clinical value of a drug is inadequate and the drug can be substituted for by something better, then that drug may be eliminated after review. 4) The guide to the reimbursable drug list should be drawn up at the same time as the list is adjusted that standardizes names on the list and the form that dosages take, in addition to methods of managing the use of the list. At appropriate times, the A and B categories of the list should be adjusted, as well as the overall category structure of the list and any accompanying notes. As A and B categories are revised, priority should be given to essential drugs (basic drugs). 5) In line with the fundamental principle of focusing on the 'security' function of the medical security system, and the basic principles of medicine as set forth in China's basic medical insurance, some drugs cannot be included within the scope of the list. They include drugs that serve a bolstering function (tonics), drugs made from nationally endangered animals and plants, public health medicines such as preventive vaccines and contraceptives, drugs used for weight loss, beauty products, drugs used to give up smoking, and so on. Some of these are used to improve quality of life, and some are used as a preventative, while others lie within the scope of public healthcare security. None of these falls within the scope of adjustments to the list. As for over-the-counter non-prescription drugs, these are generally not reimbursable in any country using national insurance. In this particular revision of the list, in principle such drugs (some are already in the list) will not be increased in the list.

Key focus of adjustments: 1) this current revision of the list gives priority to essential drugs in China that are not covered by China's basic medical insurance, to drugs used for major illness such as cancers and rare diseases, to such chronic diseases as high blood pressure and diabetes, to drugs for children's diseases and to drugs used for emergency purposes. 2) As per the positioning (definition) of the safeguard functions of China's basic medical insurance system, some drugs cannot be incorporated into the list: for example, those include 'bolstering' drugs used as a tonic, drugs that incorporate ingredients from China's endangered wild animals and plant materials, preventive vaccines and drugs used to prevent conception (contraceptives) (all of these are public health medicines), drugs used for weight loss, beauty, giving up cigarettes, and so on. Some of these are meant to improve quality of life and others are used as preventative measures. Some are within the scope of public healthcare safeguards. None is included in the scope of this round of list revisions. As for over-the-counter non-prescription drugs, internationally, these are generally not reimbursable using national insurance. In this particular revision of the list, in principle such drugs (some are already in the list) will not be increased.

Standards for basic data: the basis for 'basic information' as used in the list revision is the same information as that provided to China's National Medical Products Administration in granting approval for market listing. With respect to carrying out reviews, the process does not accept applications from companies or any recommendations and (nobody involved) may accept 'review fees' or any other form of payment. With respect to inclusion in the category of 'negotiated drugs,' drug companies must provide materials as requested.

Evidence required for adjustments: this has two categories – the evidence required for drug selections and the evidence required for drug negotiations. The former is made up of the 'key technical points' covered in reviews as formulated by consulting experts, the results of consulting surveys done by the medical insurance, and the results of votes cast by selection experts. The latter is made up analysis of the impact of a given drug on the medical insurance budget, and health technology assessments. Health technology assessments incorporate information on the economics of drugs as well as data from evidence-based medical studies.

4.1.2.4 DESIGN OF THE PROCEDURES FOR ADJUSTING THE LIST

Organizational structure: this includes the working group, the experts group, the negotiation group, and the supervision group.

1. Working group: prior to and including in 2017, adjustments to the reimbursable drug list were led by the Ministry of Human Resources and Social Security. This set up a steering group under which an office did the drafting of the plan for adjusting the list. Since 2018, the work of adjusting the list has been led by

the National Healthcare Security Administration. This meets together with other bodies to development the adjustment plan and to determine principles and procedures and coordinate policy issues. The other bodies are the Ministry of Industry and Information Technology, the Ministry of Finance, the Ministry of Human Resources and Social Security, the China National Health Development Research Center, and the National Administration of Traditional Chinese Medicine. A working group has been set up under the National Healthcare Security Administration to handle daily work.

2. Expert group: experts are divided into four categories – consulting experts, selection experts, measurement experts, and negotiating experts. Drawn mainly from the fields of clinical practice and pharmacology, they also include some experts in medical insurance and the economics of pharmaceuticals. The different categories are responsible for specific work in their respective fields. The consulting experts do not have any interaction with the selection experts.

3. Negotiating group: this group of people is drawn from representatives of the organizations actually handling China's national medical insurance – representatives of provincial departments of medical insurance, and related experts. They are organized into a group that carries out actual on-site negotiations. Those drugs that are successfully negotiated are entered into the scope of the reimbursable drug list and are then subject to a nationally applicable unified payment standard (reimbursement price). They also are then subject to administrative management policies.

4. Supervision group: this is set up under the Discipline Inspection Commission directly under the National Healthcare Security Administration. The group supervises the whole process of adjustment and accepts complaints and reports from the public.

Adjustment procedures: 1) the National Healthcare Security Administration sets up a working group and drafts a work plan. It solicits opinions from representatives of all relevant entities, including government departments, provincial medical insurance departments, relevant academic associations, medical institutions, medical personnel, drug manufacturing and distributing companies, and the public in general. 2) As per prescribed procedures, the working group then sets up a bank of experts, it sets up a database of the basic statistics, and it sets forth regulations on confidentiality and 'clean government.' 3) The working group carries out a 'consulting survey' of drugs used under medical insurance. It then carries out a random selection of a certain number of experts from within the bank of experts and these conduct a vote that covers all the drugs under consideration. Opinions and recommendations are solicited in the process. 4) The consulting experts determine the key technology aspects they will be focusing on in choosing drugs, and they then divide up into disciplines to carry out selections that are based on these aspects. They determine a list of the candidate drugs that will be further voted on to decide whether to enter them into or eliminate them from the list. 5) A group of experts is randomly chosen according to geographic location and discipline, and this group then votes on the candidate drugs. 6) Based on the results of (this second) vote, a list of selected drugs is drawn up for inclusion or exclusion in the list. Depending on the drug itself, each drug is categorized as either 'routine entry' or 'negotiated entry.' At this point, the group also proposes administrative management measures with respect to drugs that may require more stringent management. 7) The list of routine-entry drugs and negotiated-entry drugs is published. 8) For negotiated drugs, a set of required information is drawn up that is based on solicited opinions, and companies are asked to provide materials that cover the requested information. After this, experts carry out pharmaco-economic evaluations of the drug as well as evaluations of the capacity of China's insurance funds to cover the costs of the drug. Depending on the results of these evaluations, and the negotiations with companies, a nationally unified payment standard (reimbursement price) is determined as well as administrative management policies. 9) The Medical Insurance Bureau issues a document that formally places drugs on the list of drugs that can be reimbursed under China's health insurance system. Simultaneously, it sets out regulations on the administrative management of each drug to ensure that implementation is done properly.

The process of adjusting the list is divided into a sequence of periods. Those periods and the actions that apply to each period are as follows.

The periods correspond to five stages: preparation, review, publication of the 'routine entry' list, negotiations, publication of the negotiated access list.

First, preparation (January through March 2019): draft a work plan and solicit opinions from relevant departments and the public. Departments include the Ministry of Industry and Information Technology, the Ministry of Finance, the Ministry of Human Resources and Social Security, the National Health Commission, the National Medical Products Administration, and the National Administration of Traditional Chinese Medicine. Construct a working organization and a bank of reviewing experts, set up a database of base-line statistics, formulate regulations that cover confidentiality and clean-government considerations.

Second, review stage (April to July 2019): 1) Do a consulting survey of medications covered by medical insurance. Make a random selection of a certain number of experts from the entire bank of selection experts, and have this group carry out a vote on all drugs (and dosage type) in order to understand the drug needs of the country on a national level. Regions to be represented in the vote cannot be in less than two-thirds of all provinces. No fewer than 30% of experts who are voting must be drawn from medical institutions that are at or below Grade Two in China's hospital ranking. In principle, each 'drug group' should be composed of at least 50 experts. 2) Determine the list of drug candidates. The consulting experts debate and then determine the key technical issues to be used in determining drug review procedures. They divide into groups by discipline to carry out reviews and determine a list of candidate drugs to be considered for inclusion into and elimination from the list (this list includes negotiated drugs). Their determinations are made according to the key technical issues and also the results of the consulting surveys of medicines covered by medical insurance. Consulting experts are asked to give serious consideration to drugs that are not on the list of basic medicines in the 2018 list of reimbursable drugs. 3) Selection experts vote. Those voting are chosen randomly from among the bank of all selection experts by level and grade. They are also randomly chosen according to their geographic region, type of medical institution and the grade (hospital ranking) of that institution, and their discipline, and they are put into review groups for different categories of drugs. Again, regions to be represented in the vote cannot be in less than two-thirds of all provinces. No fewer than 30% of experts who are voting must be drawn from medical institutions that are at or below Grade Two in China's hospital ranking. In principle, each 'drug group' should be composed of at least 50 experts. 4) Determine the list of drugs to be included into the list or eliminated from it. Depending on the results of the vote of selection experts, consulting experts determine the number of drugs to be added and the name list of drugs to be added to the reimbursable list (including by negotiation) and they discuss those drugs that require more stringent management and research how to implement such management. 5) With regard to negotiated drugs, solicit the opinions of companies that produce the list of candidate drugs for this category, and determine their intentions with respect to negotiations.

Third, publishing the routine-entry list. The next stage deals with issuing the list of drugs that gain routine access to the list (July 2019): draft a notification regarding the list of names of drugs to be negotiated and the printed list of reimbursable drugs. Ask for opinions with respect to this draft from relevant departments, and also report on the status of list adjustments. Print up the new edition of the drug list and make public the name list of drugs to be negotiated.

Fourth, negotiation (August to September 2019): ask companies to provide the requested material for negotiations, in the prescribed form. Have measurement experts carry out evaluations based on analysis of big data from medical insurance and pharmaco-economic evaluations, and then put forth evaluations. Based on these evaluations, negotiation experts then conduct negotiations with companies. They determine a national unified payment standard for reimbursement of drug costs under medical insurance as well as administrative management policies to be applied to these drugs.

Fifth, publishing the negotiated-access list. The fifth stage is to issue the list of drugs that have gained access to the list through negotiation (September to October 2019). The National Healthcare Security Administration issues a document formally admitting drugs that have come through negotiations successfully into the list of reimbursable drugs. Simultaneously, the Administration sets forth explicit management requirements and implementation procedures.

Negotiated access has been a major innovation in recent years in the way in which drugs are admitted entry to the reimbursable drug list. In 2017, the medical insurance departments granted entry to 36 new drugs via a negotiated process; in 2018 the figure was 17 and in 2019 it was 70. Such drugs include liraglutide injection, trastuzumab, lenalidomide, and osimertinib. Negotiated access has played an important role in improving the level of medical safeguards of people who have insurance coverage, and it also has been critical in ensuring the stable operations of the healthcare fund. By summing up the lessons of previous adjustments and building on that foundation, this last adjustment has been able to make further improvements in negotiated access methods. Drugs that have high clinical value but are also very expensive, or patented drugs produced by one company that have a large impact on funds, should only be admitted into the list after both parties reach consensus on a national unified payment standard. The negotiation between companies and negotiation experts follows the standard procedure of having experts review and vote on admittance. This must be done to ensure the security of funds. Also, given the fact that the generic version of some patented drugs may be approved for selling on the market during a list adjustment period, in this last revision of the list, rules were established that said that the approval period for a patented drug would end on the day prior to a selection vote.

4.1.2.5 UPDATING OF THE LIST AND PUBLIC FEEDBACK

The explanatory documentation accompanying the *2019 Work plan for adjusting the national reimbursable drug list* states that procedures should include soliciting the opinions and recommendations of all (government) departments as well as the public at large.

Meanwhile, this last revision of the list strengthened the procedures for conducting a consultation survey of insurance-based prescriptions in order to ensure that adjustments made to the list are open, fair, and transparent. The aim was to better understand the demand for clinical use of drugs and to make sure that the reimbursable list was in sync with that demand. At the same time, the aim was to understand the opinions and recommendations of experts from all geographic regions during the initial review period, so that revisions to the list could be based on a broader, more scientific, and sounder foundation.

4.1.2.6 MECHANISMS FOR SOCIAL SUPERVISION (SUPERVISION BY THE PUBLIC AT LARGE)

Be proactive in accepting supervision from all parties The Discipline Inspection Commission, directly administered by the National Healthcare Security Administration, is responsible for appointing (its own) experts to participate in the entire process of adjusting the reimbursable drug list. Its Work Plan and the Work Procedures include soliciting the opinions and recommendations of others on a broadly defined basis, including from relevant government departments and from the public at large. It also is required to recognize the complaints and reports from all parties.

Improve internal control mechanisms Ensure that the responsibilities of personnel are explicitly defined and that descriptions of each position (job posting) are clear. Improve the systemic measures that pertain to confidentiality, avoiding conflict of interest, and accountability. Ensure that the work of adjusting the list is fair, secure, and orderly.

Strengthen supervision over experts Set up systems relating to experts' responsibilities, avoidance of conflict of interest, and accountability; ensure that all review and selection procedures are recorded, in order to ensure that experts provide review opinions that are independent and fair.

All personnel involved and all experts are to sign confidentiality agreements and clean-government agreements, and experts are also to sign statements confirming they have no prior conflict of interest.

4.1.3 Ongoing problems with the mechanisms that pertain to adjustments of the national reimbursable drug list

1 The list is not adjusted at regular intervals, efficiency is relatively low when it is adjusted, and the work suffers from a lack of official procedural guidelines as well as any technical rules that govern reviews

In principle, the list is to be adjusted every two years, according to the 'Measures for adjusting the list.' In reality, adjustments to the list have taken as long as four to eight years. This means that no drug can be added to or eliminated from the list during this period – new drugs and innovative drugs in particular cannot access the list in a timely manner, which makes it hard to satisfy the clinical demand for such drugs. This then adds to the cost burden of patients (who must pay for unlisted drugs out of pocket). This also affects the enthusiasm of drug companies to invest in developing innovative drugs and it means that there is no effective linkage between companies and government policies that support major new drug projects.

The list is adjusted in a top-down manner by internal institutions within government. The process requires that each drug undergo re-evaluation – given the (large) number of and types of drugs, and the fact that there are a limited number of participating experts, this puts an extremely heavy workload on the experts. At the same time, there are no official guidelines for working procedures and no technical rules and regulations to go by – such things would include drug application procedures, drug selection standards, evaluation methods, and review and approval procedures. Most of the personnel of relevant institutions are working ad hoc and doing their regular jobs at the same time. Not only are many different government departments involved but they are only loosely related to one another. This adds to the workload.

2 Manpower in administrative departments is limited which requires the adoption of a top-down process in adjusting the list. This limits the enthusiasm of drug manufacturers.

Selection departments are the starting point of adjusting the list. Since manpower in these departments is limited, the departments must of necessity adopt a top-down method since a bottom-up method would lead to a massive workload. Drug manufacturers can only take a passive role in the process of revising and updating the list, which in turn limits their active participation to a certain degree. Not only do they wait passively for the list to be revised, but they may miss out on the protection period that applies to their new drugs. This is detrimental to creating a virtuous circle in the development of innovative new drugs.

3 The selection of drugs lacks quantitative indicators by which drugs can be evaluated in an objective way. This makes it easy for selections to be influenced by the objective opinions of review experts.

Selection principles by which China selects drugs for inclusion in the reimbursable drug list do not include quantified indicators and a systematic structure for evaluating drugs. This means that the operability of the process, the ability to have it function outside of the subjective opinions of experts, is poor. Experts must rely on their own experience in coming up with their assessments. The results of such assessments are therefore not backed by solid evidence. The majority of medical data regarding treatments that resulted from the 2017 list adjustment has now been applied to the process of drug selection and some indicators have been provided regarding drug safety and effectiveness. Nevertheless, the process is still insufficiently objective. It still relies on the practical experience of experts and the results of group discussions. The application and review stage of revising the list is also overly subjective, which increases the possibility of rent-seeking behavior between companies and review experts as companies make their applications.

4 The composition of experts who participate in drug selection needs improvement, and there are not enough seasoned experts to do health technology assessments

Drug admittance to and elimination from the list requires consideration of such things as clinical attributes of a given drug, medical demand, level of medical insurance, economic conditions, and government healthcare policies. At the current stage, selection experts involved in the revising of China's reimbursable drug list are drawn at random from among experts that China's medical insurance departments and human resources and social security departments recommend. Most of these people are from hospitals and grassroots health institutions, involved in clinical practice and pharmacology. Only some are experts in public health, medical insurance accounting, pharmaco-economic evaluations, and health technology assessments. In China, the number of people in these latter disciplines is limited. Capabilities vary from high to low. Although all experts work according to a unified set of measurement principles and key technical parameters, and the results are fairly scientific, China still lacks a way to re-evaluate results and there is still room for improvement in terms of the scientific nature of results.

5 Price-negotiation mechanisms with respect to innovative drugs still need improvement

National-level government departments have carried out several rounds of price negotiations for drugs, but they have not yet made public any rules and regulations governing such negotiations, nor any management methods. Individual provinces have explored using various mechanisms in negotiations and have even set up their own individual negotiating plans for negotiated drugs on the reimbursable drug list. The basis of negotiations has different emphases in different provinces, however, which impacts the soundness and scientific nature of negotiation results. It also prolongs the waiting time for innovative drugs to gain access to the list. At the same time, China's information-sharing mechanisms need improvement. In many cases, the statistics that are put forward for certain indicators are sourced from different databases and vary substantially. This makes it hard to carry out logical reviews and cross-verifications. Meanwhile, some R&D companies try to hike up prices for their drugs by reporting false information on costs. This inserts a 'results bias' into negotiations and directly influences the soundness of results.

6 Mechanisms for removing a drug from the list still need improvement

The 2009 reimbursable list explicitly stated that drugs that meet 'drug elimination requirements' must be removed from the list. However, no specific regulations have been issued with respect to such removal. The direct impact of this is that many drugs are not in fact removed from the list in a timely manner, even though they have low clinical value, are not economical, and are not representative of what should be on the list. This wastes limited medical insurance funds.

7 Adjustment mechanisms are not sufficiently transparent, and participation by the public at large is relatively low

The review process for China's national reimbursable drug list does not accept reports from companies. All of the various considerations are still not publicly disclosed, including principles behind expert selections, standards, methodology, and the weighting of evaluation indicators. This means that the interests of both companies and the public cannot go through effective channels to understand the 'dynamic revision' processes of coming up with the list. This lowers the degree to which the public participates in adjustments, and it also prevents government departments from soliciting opinions from the various stakeholders involved.

4.2 Research into applying health technology assessments to the dynamic adjustment of the reimbursable drug list

The term 'health technology assessment' refers to a systematic and comprehensive way of evaluating health technologies. It includes technical characteristics, clinical safety aspects, effectiveness and economic aspects, and social receptivity. It incorporates the fields of pharmaceutical economics, healthcare economics, and evidence-based medicine in its methodology. It can play a very substantial role in determining the optimum allocation of medical resources, as well as entry into the drug list, price negotiations for drugs, procurement of healthcare technologies, the formulation of medical and pharmaceutical policies, and control over medical costs.

4.2.1 Spheres in which health technology assessments can be applied

Health technology assessments are a tool for determining healthcare policy. Used throughout the world, they are based on evidence and real-world data. In developed countries, they have long since been applied to such decisions as access to health insurance, price negotiations for drugs, and reimbursement by medical insurance for medical costs (see Table 1.2). In China as well, they are broadly applied to the decisions surrounding access to the reimbursable drug list, together with such other methodologies as pharmaco-economic evaluations. Since 2017, they have also been applied to the sphere of negotiating list prices of innovative drugs. The National Health Commission and the National Healthcare Security Administration have reached consensus on using them in making revisions to the basic medical insurance reimbursable drug list.

4.2.2 Role of health technology assessments

A comparison of the use of health technology assessments in three countries shows the following similarities and dissimilarities. The three countries and their systems are NICE of the U.K. (1999), IQWiG of Germany (2003), and HAS of France (2004).

1 Similarities

1 All three entities are independent public institutions and all are science-oriented
2 All are a component of healthcare reform
3 All are tasked with the same mission: health technology assessments (for drugs and medical equipment), guidance on routine therapies, policy recommendations and evaluations

2 Differences

1 Type of local healthcare service system: there are differences in national healthcare service systems and social insurance systems, and differences in philosophies behind healthcare services
2 Standing within public policy: there are differences in how the three institutions are used for recommendations versus policy decisions, differences in their management and their requirements of scientific evidence.
3 Standing and role in the course of doing economic assessments: there are differences in whether or not they represent a core part of the process or play a supplementary role.

Table 1.2 Scope of the Applicability of Health Technology Assessments in Different Countries

Country	*Drug Registration*	*Drug-Pricing Management*	*Drug Compensation or Co-payment Level*	*Reimbursement List +Positive/ −Negative*	*Formulation of the Diagnosis and Treatment Standards of the Medication List*	*Allocation of Public Health Resources*	*Guidance on the R&D of Market Strategies*
Australia		√	√	+	?	?	
Canada		√	√	−/+	√	?	√
U.K.					√	√	√
Netherlands			√	+		?	√
Portugal			√	+	?	?	√
Finland		√	√	+	?	?	√
America			√	+	?	√	√
Norway			√	+			
Denmark			√				
Ireland			√	+	√	√	?
New Zealand				?			√
Sweden		√	√		√	?	?
Switzerland			√			?	?
France		√	√	+	√	?	
Germany			√	−/+	√	?	

Source: Yang Li, *Specific Role of Pharmacoeconomics in the Implementation of the Medical Reform Program*, China Pharmacy, Issue 8, 2010.

4.2.3 Methods of pharmaco-economic evaluations

Table 1.3 Pharmaco-economics Evaluation Method

	Cost	*Result*	*Analysis Method*
Cost-Minimization Analysis (CMA)	Direct cost and indirect cost Intangible cost and opportunity cost	Assume or verify that the results are the same for all scenarios	Cost analysis
Cost-Effect Analysis (CEA)	Ditto	Intermediate indicators and health indicators	Cost-effect ratio Incremental cost effect
Cost-Utility Analysis (EUA)	Ditto	Quality-adjusted life years (QALYs) Disability adjusted life years (DALYs)	Cost-utility ratio Incremental cost utility
Cost-Benefit Analysis (EBA)	Ditto	Monetary value of the result Human capital approach Willingness-to-pay approach	Net present value approach Benefit-cost ratio Internal-rate-of-return approach

4.2.4 The application of health technology assessments in making adjustments to the reimbursable drug list

China adopted the use of health technology assessments and pharmaco-economic evaluations for the first time in the 2017 edition of the reimbursable drug list. It analyzed 600,000 hospital patients and 5.5 million patients of clinics, all drawn from a nationwide sample. The results of this analysis were used as a form of technical support for selections. This represented a major step forward in China, a transformation from 'evaluations by experts' to 'quantified evaluations supported by evidence.'

In 2018, the National Healthcare Security Administration included 17 cancer drugs on the list to be negotiated for access to the reimbursable drug list. Health technology assessments based on epidemiological data were used to analyze the cost-effectiveness of these drugs, as well as their cost benefit. Using the same data, companies could calculate the floor price of their drug, while the National Healthcare Security Administration could calculate the ceiling price and both could then carry on negotiations within this price range. Final prices were decided using this range for all of the decision parameters. In 2019, the National Healthcare Security Administration admitted 97 drugs into the negotiation process for access to the drug list. Again, health technology assessments based on data reported by companies as well as disease epidemiological data were used to analyze cost-effectiveness and cost benefit. This produced a 'ceiling price' for the purpose of negotiations. Companies then calculated the lowest price they were willing to accept and negotiations were again carried out within the resulting zone. The same zone was used as the basis for analysis of all parameters in coming up with the final price.

However, China was relatively late to using health technology assessments and the country still needs to establish organizations at all government levels to do them. It still needs to improve guidelines for pharmaco-economic evaluations that can guide practice. Therefore, in considering cost-effectiveness and cost-benefit analysis, China still needs to improve in order to apply results to decisions on granting access to the list or eliminating drugs from the list.

4.3 The international experience and international research on dynamic adjustments to reimbursable drug lists

China's 'national reimbursable drug list' refers to the collection of drugs that are covered by insurance under health insurance policies. After going through specific selection procedures, these drugs can be incorporated into the scope of reimbursement. Other countries have various systems for how they select drugs for their own drug lists, but there are some similarities of organizational structure and operating procedures, despite the differences. Specifics are as follows.

4.3.1 Framework for the overall plan for adjusting a list

Given that healthcare resources are limited, the core issue when adjusting a list comes down to controlling medical and healthcare costs while at the same time ensuring quality medical services. This involves deciding how to make sure the overall plan and design of the system results in a process that is scientific and operationally sound, and that in the end it reflects the value of drugs. Without exception, other representative countries put the adjustment plan and the system for making selections in a position of primary importance.

4.3.1.1 THE ADJUSTMENT PLAN

The adjustment plan in other countries mainly includes the following key aspects: setting up the organizations that adjust the list, standards for making decisions about adjusting the list, and procedures for adjusting the list.

1. Designing and setting up the organizations that adjust the list: this has to do with setting up organizations and determining their functions. It includes establishing organizations and determining the methods by which they cooperate with other external organizations (outside government), looking at the sustainability of organizations, and so on. The building of organizations that are specifically aimed at adjusting the list is the very basis of how the adjustment plan is implemented. Such organizations can play three kinds of roles in adjusting the list. The first is to make recommendations and provide opinions on drug selections. The second is to provide the results of drug evaluations. The third is to make direct and final decisions on drugs.

2. Standards for making decisions about adjusting the list: this is the core of the adjustment plan. It addresses both the evidence behind decisions made about the list and the decisions themselves; it involves evidence required for making drug selections (evidence-based medicine, health technology assessments), the question of who provides opinions about drug selection and who makes final decisions, and what methods are adopted to balance the interests of the various stakeholders in order to ensure the fairness of results.

3. Procedures for adjusting the list: these provide 'rules of the game' in coordinating all kinds of competing interests and getting to an accommodation. These procedures are manifested in structural design of the list-adjustment process such that different interest groups constrain one another and balance one another in order to arrive at the goal of being scientific, fair, and standardized. The most critical part in list-adjustment procedures is drug review and selection.

4.3.1.2 TYPES OF HEALTHCARE SECURITY REIMBURSABLE DRUG LISTS

Different countries principally manage two types of lists, positive and negative.

1 The positive list includes drugs that are covered by insurance and are therefore reimbursable. Countries using such lists include China, France, Japan, Australia, and South Korea. France determines whether or not a drug will be included in the list by looking at type of illness and clinical improvement upon treatment (ASMR). In Japan, all prescription drugs can apply to be included within the scope of reimbursement, as per the *Law on Pharmaceuticals* of the Ministry of Health, Labor, and Welfare. Australia has a universal healthcare security system, and as soon as drugs are put on the market, companies can apply to the Pharmaceuticals Profit Examination Organization to have them included in the Pharmaceutical Benefits Scheme (PBS), that is, the reimbursable drug list.

Prior to 2007, South Korea implemented a system that used a negative drug list. Such things as cost-benefit analysis and impact on budget were rarely used as factors in evaluating drugs. The result was that all drugs that were granted authorization by the Food and Drug Examination and Management Administration were reimbursable and medical institutions carried out such reimbursements. This led to a swift increase in the price of drugs. Starting in 2007, South Korea began to implement a positive list system which operated under a 'plan for reasonable spending on drug costs.' Drug manufacturers whose new drugs were granted permission to be sold on the market now had to apply to the Health Insurance Review and Assessment Services Administration (HIRA) with proper documentation on the new drug. Requirements included econometric data on the drug, cost-benefit analysis and impact on budgets. HIRA then evaluated whether or not the drug met reimbursement qualifications. It also carried out negotiations with both the National Health Information System and drug manufacturers in order to determine the reimbursement price.

2 Negative lists include drugs that are ineligible for (or have been stripped of eligibility for) insurance reimbursement. Countries using such lists include England and Germany. In England, drugs on this list are not granted reimbursement status. All drugs that are allowed to be sold in England are, by default, incorporated in England's National Healthcare System (NHS) and enter the system of reimbursements by medical insurance.

3 The United States has adopted a commercial insurance model that is completely market-driven. The country's medical market is highly fragmented, and there is no list of basic medicines that are reimbursable through insurance at the national level. Each insurance company, hospital, or clinic can formulate its own list according to its own local situation in terms of commonly seen types of illness and supply of drugs. Once new drugs have received approval from the Food and Drug Administration (FDA), the entity holding rights to the drug can carry on negotiations with insurance companies to determine the method of reimbursement. Once agreement is reached, the drug can be entered into relevant reimbursement lists.

4.3.2 Selection of experts and working mechanisms

Academic background of experts: review experts in most countries include people in such relevant fields as hospitals, pharmacology, and health economics. They can even include personnel from pharmaceutical companies and also patients. Australia's review experts include clinicians, healthcare economists, and patient representatives. Canada's include pharmaceutical experts, pharmaceutical economists, and government officials. Those in France include representatives of medical institutions, pharmaceutical associations, clinical doctors, representatives of industry associations, and external experts.

4.3.3 Determining the standards by which to make adjustments

4.3.3.1 ADJUSTMENT STANDARDS

The international practice is to use four parameters by which to select and allow for the use of drugs. Those are safety, efficacy, economy, and appropriateness. Generally speaking, a drug must meet three conditions before gaining access to the reimbursable list: clinical effectiveness, reliable quality, and economy. Only drugs that are clearly effective in clinical practice and have reliable quality have the possibility of entry – these are the most basic requirements. Determining which drug manufacturer's drugs gain entry to the list is then a matter of evaluating the economic aspects of a drug. The first two types of evaluation have long since become systematic and standardized and can be determined directly from laboratory statistics. Each country may have its own requirements in terms of size of sample and standards applied to samples, but other than these details, there are no major differences in how technical methods are applied. Economic evaluations are somewhat different, due to the way all countries have come up with new technologies to try to control medical costs that have been going up inexorably in recent years. Assuming reliable quality and clinical effectiveness, cost-benefit analysis is carried out to come up with a comprehensive determination. This provides objective evidence on which to base such things as the list price of drugs, the formulation of the reimbursable drug list, the formulation of drug-use plans by medical institutions, and so on.

4.3.3.2 EVIDENCE BY WHICH TO DETERMINE ADJUSTMENT OF THE LIST

The majority of countries use the results of health technology assessments as the basis by which to adjust their lists.

1 Mandatory implementation of health technology assessments: in Australia and Holland, drugs must undergo health technology assessments before they are admitted to the list. In the U.K. and Switzerland, this is not required.
2 The thoroughness with which health technology assessments must be carried out: Some countries set forth guidelines on this subject, such as France, the U.K., England, and Holland. Others are just now in the process of formulating their guidelines, such as Italy. Still others have merely made recommendations with respect to using health technology assessments, such as Spain.
3 Subjects covered by health technology assessments: the great majority of countries take into consideration the burden of disease, clinical effectiveness, safety, innovative qualities, social benefit, cost-effectiveness, and ethical considerations. The data on these comes mostly from clinical experience, observational studies, and expert opinions.
4 Methodology of health technology assessments: Australia, the U.K., Germany, and France use cost-benefit analysis in economic models to substitute for clinical trials in evaluating and predicting the economic aspects of drugs.

Table 1.4 Classification and Distribution of Pharmaco-economic Guidelines in Various Countries and Regions

	OECD Countries (and Regions)	*Non-OECD Countries (and Regions)*
Recommended guidelines (Published PERecommendations)	U.S.A., Austria, Denmark, Hungary, Italy, and Spain	South Africa, China, and Russia
Official normative guidelines (PEGuidelines)	Mexico, Canada, Belgium, France, Germany, Ireland, the Netherlands, Norway, Portugal, Slovakia, Sweden, and New Zealand	Brazil, Cuba, Taiwan, South Korea, and the Baltic states
Guidelines on application document submission (Submission Guidelines)	Israel, England and Wales, Scotland, Finland, Poland, and Australia	Thailand

4.3.3.3 SETTING PRIORITIES IN THE SEQUENCE OF ADJUSTING THE LIST

Economic evaluations of both drugs and medical technologies must be carried out in order to determine adjustments to the reimbursable drug list. This requires comparing data from clinical trials and laboratory results, which in turn means that the organizations carrying out economic evaluations must determine the priority by which drugs are reviewed. In this regard, basically all countries have determined that decisions cannot be made solely by the organizations conducting pharmacoeconomic evaluations. All such organizations are constrained by outside forces, such as medical and healthcare service providers, government healthcare departments, medical workers, health insurance systems, and patients themselves. All of these interest groups influence the process.

4.3.4 Design of adjustment procedures

4.3.4.1 FRAMEWORK OF INSTITUTIONS (ORGANIZATIONS)

Institutions are set up specifically to handle selection of drugs for the reimbursable drug list; the purpose of designating organizations for drug selection is twofold – to control medical costs and to ensure the quality of medical services. Specific functions must therefore apply to such institutions. In various countries, considerations are as follows.

1. Functions can range from one sole function per organization to multiple functions. In Australia, the functions of the PBAC (Pharmaceutical Benefit Advisory Committee) are relatively singular – the organization is primarily aimed at selecting prescription drugs. In Germany, France, and the U.K., functions are combined. In France, for instance, the National Authority for Health (HAS) handles medical and health technology assessments, the rating of medical institutions, and continuing education of professional physicians. In Germany, the Federal Joint Council (FJC) handles selection of medical and healthcare technologies, evaluations of medical and healthcare quality, and health education. In the United States, the functional scope of organizations is fairly broad and does not put clear emphasis on any one aspect. So long as a drug, a medical device, or a clinical intervention procedure applies for inclusion, it may be included in the relevant list. With respect to work content, there are some differences among the selection institutions of each country but for the most part all undertake the following tasks: health technology assessments, evaluations of the quality of medical services, evaluations of projects to do with disease management, health education, and health initiatives.

2. Selection institutions derive their funding from multiple sources. Virtually all institutions making selection decisions for the reimbursable drug list are nonprofit, and their budgets come from public finance (that is, either directly or indirectly from tax revenue). The expenses of NICE in the U.K. (National Institute for Health and Care Excellence) are paid for out of the Department of Health, which grants it an appropriation of roughly 35 million pounds per year. In Australia, the budget for the PBAC comes from the Department of Health and is roughly 14 million Australian dollars per year. In addition to funds from public finance,

some selection institutions also get funding from public research departments to carry out research on specific topics. There are also other channels of funding. For example, according to the HAS 2007, in 2006, the HAS 2006 received a total of 70 million francs in funding, the structure of which was as follows: 10% allocated from the government, 31% from the social medical insurance fund, 7% from the medical equipment industry, 34% from pharmaceutical companies (in the form of an advertisement tax on drug producers), and 15% from hospitals for carrying out ranking evaluations.

3. Selection institutions are relatively independent. In the great majority of countries, drug selection institutions are independent of governmental administrative departments. For example, NICE in the U.K. creates an evaluation report which it then presents directly to the Department of Health. In France, the HAS has no direct or indirect subordinate relationship with the central government, the Ministry of Health, or the medical insurance fund. It answers directly to the French Parliament. In Germany, the FJC is independent of the central government and medical insurance fund and answers directly to the national healthcare department. In Australia, the PBAC takes guidance directly from the national healthcare department's drug evaluation division (the PEB). The PEB works together with the PBAC in handling drug evaluation procedures and it negotiates prices with drug manufacturers. In addition, it promotes health education by disseminating educational material.

4. Most selection institutions are independent and permanent. The great majority are designated as independent by their governments, including those in Australia, Canada, the U.K., and Holland. In some countries, such as Germany and Switzerland, community groups are established by relevant interest groups, and some of these provide advisory services, such as in France, Germany, and the U.K. Some institutions also provide supervisory and administrative services, as in Sweden and Italy. In Australia, Canada, and the United States, advisory committees are permanent institutions whereas in the U.K. they are ad hoc working groups.

Health technology assessment institutions or healthcare economics evaluation institutions are 1) *models by which institutions carry out evaluations*: England follows a model by which the organization itself makes decisions. In that country, NICE is a one component of the National Healthcare System (NHS). It is supported by funding from the NHS and it makes policy recommendations directly to NHS. Australia follows a model whereby government and the institution negotiate policy. In this case, the evaluation institution makes its own decisions and recommendations and then government makes final decisions based on budgetary considerations, policy priorities, and other considerations. France follows a model in which multiple stakeholders take turns in participating in decision-making. According to a specific order of participation, interest groups take turns in participating in the decision-making process of organizations that assess the pharmaceutical economics of drugs. Germany has a model whereby multiple interest groups jointly participate in decision-making. Relevant interest groups participate in the process of decision-making that is carried out groups that do pharmaco-economic evaluations. These groups undertake cost-benefit analyses of medical treatment and healthcare services. They assess the results of disease management projects and guide recommendations. They also revise and correct clinical practice manuals on a regular basis. 2) *Sources of funding*: the cost of funding organizations that do pharmaco-economic evaluations is less than USD 100 million per year in each of Australia, the U.K., Germany, and France. This amount is hardly worth mentioning, relative to the cost of drugs or healthcare spending every year in each of these countries (it is less than 0.1% of total healthcare spending). Funding comes either from direct government appropriations, or it can be from business income of the organizations themselves.

4.3.4.2 ADJUSTMENT PROCEDURES

There are two main types of decisions made by institutions that select drugs for the reimbursable drug list. In the first, based on the results of evaluations, selection institutions draw up their recommendations in the form of a report which they then submit to bodies that formulate healthcare policies. Ultimate decisions are made by those bodies. Australia, Germany, and France are examples. The second type of decision involves putting recommendations into law – the bodies that formulate healthcare policies enact laws to ensure that the recommendations of selection institutions have statutory validity. England is an example.

As for the ways in which decision makers participate in decision-making, participants include drug manufacturers, medical services providers, patients, compensation entities for medical costs, and all of these can propose their own opinions through a diversity of channels and methods in the course of adjusting the list. After decisions are made on the inclusion of drugs, if there are objections, they can be dealt with via legal measures. There are two main ways by which decision makers participate in decision-making. One is by putting forth their own opinions as members of advisory committees; the other is by taking turns as groups in decision-making processes, such as in France.

How review procedures are initiated: in some countries, drug companies initiate the process by submitting applications. This is the case in the United States, Switzerland, Australia, South Korea, and Holland. In addition, initiation of review procedures can be recommended by patients, insurance organizations, and medical institutions. This is the case in Spain, Canada, the United States, the U.K., and Australia.

The process is highly strict in some countries, such as the United States. In other countries, it is more flexible, such as in Italy and Spain.

Regarding adjustment cycles, in developed countries, it generally takes less than one year for innovative drugs to gain access to a reimbursable drug list once the drug has been released to the market. In the United States and France, for example, it takes around six months for innovative drugs to go from release on the market to entry into the list. In Japan, the time frame is three months, while in Germany and England it is only one month. At the same time, the majority of countries have set up institutions or committees that are specifically tasked with carrying out health technology assessments for the purpose of making adjustments to the list, whether additions or eliminations.

4.3.5 Updating the list and public announcements of any opinions or feedback

4.3.5.1 DEGREE OF TRANSPARENCY OF REVIEW PROCEDURES

The openness of some countries is better than that of others. In countries like the United States, anyone can go on the Internet to make inquiries and track down information. In Germany, Holland, and Switzerland, however, information is not publicly available.

4.3.5.2 RELEASE OF THE RESULTS OF LIST ADJUSTMENT

Australia, Germany, and France place great emphasis on transmitting the results of drug list adjustments. These countries provide the results of adjustments, as well as any underlying health technology assessments and pharmaco-economics evaluations, to all relevant interest groups through effective channels. (Interest groups include medical services providers, medical insurance institutions that compensate requests for reimbursements, as well as patients.) The adjusted list is usually published in handbook form with the primary audience being doctors and patients. These handbooks are used as a practical guide for doctors and as educational health materials for patients. The reasoning behind this is that only when assessment results are understood and accepted by interest groups will new drugs and medical technology be utilized correctly, and only then will healthcare resources be allocated in optimum fashion.

5 Policy recommendations on the dynamic adjustment of China's reimbursable drug list

Dynamic adjustment of China's reimbursable drug list is in early stages, with progress being made in gradual and exploratory steps. Right now, the country has a number of lists that co-exist. What's more, different departments are responsible for selections and adjustments of different lists. Creating a system whereby drugs are selected in a scientific and transparent way, with clearly defined responsibilities of soundly functioning institutions, remains a powerful challenge. This research combines the experience of other countries – organizational structure of adjustment programs, selection of experts and their working mechanisms, standards and procedures for adjusting lists, and analysis of supervisory oversight by the public – with the existing situation within China. In making comparisons, it comes up with several recommendations.

5.1 Framework of the list-adjustment plan

Formulating and maintaining the plan is a form of systems engineering. We recommend setting up comprehensive guidelines and specific technical rules to ensure that the adjustment work is orderly and has rules by which to proceed. Creating a well-designed plan should include at the very least the following six

Table 1.5 How Other Countries Handle Adjustments to their Reimbursable Drug Lists

List Adjustment Framework	Setting of List Adjustment Institutions	It is the foundation for list adjustment, including the building of institutions themselves, their cooperation methods with other external relevant institutions, and their sustainable development. List adjustment institutions may consist of departments putting forward recommendations for the list adjustment and drug selection, departments providing drug assessment results, and departments directly making list adjustment decisions.		
	Standards for the Decision-Making of List Adjustment	They are the core of the list adjustment plan, including the decision-making basis for the list adjustment and parties participating in the decision-making and involving the reference basis for drug selection (evidence-based medicine and HTA), who should provide opinions on drug selection, who should decide drug selection, and how to balance the interests among parties of the list adjustment to ensure the fairness of the adjustment plan.		
	List Adjustment Procedures	The procedures for the list adjustment are the rules for the game in which all interest parties argue against and compromise with each other, which is reflected in how to achieve mutual restriction and balance among interest groups in the setting of the adjustment procedures, so as to achieve the goal of science, fairness, and standardization. The most critical part of the list adjustment procedures is the drug review and selection procedure.		
	Types of National Reimbursement Drug Lists	Positive list	China, France, Japan, Australia, South Korea, Austria, Belgium, Czech, Ireland, Italy, the Netherlands, Poland, Portugal, Sweden, and Norway	
		Negative list	The U.K., Germany, and Greece	
		Positive and negative lists	Canada, Finland, and Hungary	
Expert Selection and Working Mechanism	Academic Background of Experts	Most national drug review experts include experts in relevant fields like hospitals, pharmacy, and health economics, and even patients or personnel of drug manufacturers		
Setting of List Adjustment Standards	Adjustment Standards	Internationally, drugs are selected and used based on their safety, efficacy, economy, and appropriateness.		
	Adjustment Basis	Most countries based the adjustments on the health technology assessment results.		
		Mandatory HTA	Health technology assessment is required.	Australia and the Netherlands
			Health technology assessment is not required.	The U.K. and Switzerland

		Complete HTA guidelines	Complete official guidelines on health technology assessment	France, the U.K., and the Netherlands
			Only recommendations for health technology and economy assessment	Spain and Italy
		HTA assessment contents	Most countries take into account the burden of diseases, clinical efficacy, safety, innovation, social benefits, cost-effectiveness, and ethical issues, and most of the data come from clinical trials, observational studies, and expert opinions.	
		HTA assessment methods	In Australia, the U.K., Germany, and France, cost-benefit analysis in economic models, instead of clinical trials, is used to assess and predict the economy of drugs.	
	Priority of Adjustments	Basically, no pharmaco-economic evaluation organizations in the world can determine the priority mechanism alone. They are inevitably restricted and influenced by external factors, such as healthcare service providers, government health departments, medical workers, health insurance systems, and relevant stakeholders like patients.		
Design of List Adjustment Procedures	Organizational Structure	Special drug list selection institutions and their setting	Scope of functions	With single-tasking function: Australia
				With multi-tasking functions: Germany, France, the U.K., and the U.S.
			Work	Mainly include the assessment of health and medical technologies, the establishment of health and medical quality standards, the improvement of health and medical service quality, the assessment of disease management items, the development of instruction manuals for the practice of physicians, and the carrying-out of health education and health promotion.
			Funding resources	Public finances (or taxes): the U.K. and Australia
				Public finances + research funding: France
			Independence of institutions	Most institutions are at arm's length from government departments: the U.K., France, and Germany
				Institutions directly under government departments: Australia

(*Continued*)

Table 1.5 (Continued)

			Permanent institutions or not	Institutions in most countries are independent institutions designated by governments: Australia, Canada, the U.K., and the Netherlands
				Community institutions established by departments for interest parties: Germany and Switzerland
		Health technology assessment institutions or health economy assessment organizations	Assessment pattern	Organization decision-making: the U.K.
				Government-organization negotiation: Australia
				Multi-interest groups take turns to participate: France
				Multi-interest groups participate jointly: Germany
			Funding	With funding less than USD 100 million (less than 0.1% of the total health spending): Australia, the U.K., Germany, and France
				Funding sources: subsidized directly by the governments or obtained from the self-run businesses of the organizations
	Adjustment Procedures	Decision-making nature of list selection institutions	Selection institutions present the recommendations to the health policy developers to allow the latter to make the final decisions.	Australia, Germany, and France
			Health policy developers, by enacting legislation, ensure the statutory validity of the recommendations of drug list selection institutions for drugs to be included in the list.	The U.K.

		The way the decision-making participants participate in the decision-making	Decision-making participants put forward their own opinions in the decision-making of the list as members of the advisory committees to affect the selection of drugs to be included in the list.	Australia and Germany
			The groups take turns to participate in the decision-making process.	France
		Initiation of the review procedure	Drug manufacturers initiate the application.	The U.S., Switzerland, Australia, South Korea, and the Netherlands
			Patients, insurance agencies, and medical institutions initiate the application.	Spain, Canada, the US, the U.K., and Australia
		Strictness of the review procedure	Strict review procedure	America
			Flexible review procedure	Australia and Spain
		Adjustment cycle	Less than one month	Germany and the U.K.
			One to three months	Japan
			Three to six months	The U.S. and France
List Update and Feedback Suggestion Announcement	Transparency of the Review Procedure	Have a more transparent review procedure, which can be inquired and tracked on the website	America	
		Do not disclose the review procedure to the public	Germany, the Netherlands, and Switzerland	
	Transmission of the List Adjustment Results	Attach importance to the transmission	Australia, Germany, and France	

components: the framework for institutions that are involved, the formation of adjustment standards, the design of adjustment procedures, selection of experts and their working mechanisms (job requirements), list updating and public announcements of feedback and opinions, and recommendations for supervisory oversight by the public.

5.2 Selection of experts and their working mechanisms

We should strengthen the independence and diversity of the experts who review drugs for the list. Review experts should include people from the various spheres involved, including clinical practice, pharmaceuticals, pharmaco-economics, epidemiology, medical insurance, and healthcare policy. Selection of experts is meant to ensure that list adjustment is done scientifically. This includes implementing a system that avoids conflict of interest between experts and companies.

We recommend streamlining the number of people in the group of experts. Right now, this group has upwards of a 1,000 if not over 10,000 people in it. This vast number of people affects efficiency. As appropriate, we should be able to reduce the number.

We should allocate experts in a more scientific way. To ensure rational results of selections, we should allocate personnel according to the weighting of disciplines in a given group. The weighting should reflect the attributes of medicines being considered – if certain characteristics of a given drug are more important, then more experts in that particular field should be assigned to the group.

We recommend establishing sound and comprehensive decision-making mechanisms for selection of drugs in the reimbursable drug list. Consideration should be given to allowing broad participation by a diversity of stakeholders, and to setting up sound channels so that relevant parties can participate in drug selection.

5.3 Setting the standards by which the list is adjusted

We recommend setting up objective, quantified standards that are in line with the selection principles of the reimbursable drug list. The aim is to form an evaluation system that has a full set of sound and objective standards, that diminishes the subjective evaluations of assessment experts, and that enables the results of drug selection to be more scientific and objective.

We should strengthen and optimize the application of such assessment measures as evidence-based medicine, pharmaco-economic evaluations, and health technology assessments. In looking at ways other countries carry out list adjustments, and their systems for reimbursing, we see the following common themes: first, they make use of pharmaco-economic evaluations, focusing on efficacy of treatment, and they link price to efficacy of treatment; second, they encourage the substitution of generics for patented drugs and they draw up insurance payment policies that support this approach. Therefore, as China undertakes its own list adjustment, it should also make full use of clinical evidence-based evaluations and health technology assessments, in order to provide forceful evidence for the safety, treatment results, and economic benefit of drugs. It should focus on efficacy of treatment and should link price to efficacy of treatment.

We should set up a database of medical insurance information that is nationwide in scope, as well as price negotiation mechanisms for drugs that are used nationwide. For those innovative drugs that have good results but are also fairly expensive, we can adopt the method of 'pharmaco-economic evaluation + price negotiation' in allowing access to the list. Medical insurance departments should set up standards for drug access to the list as soon as possible, as well as negotiation procedures, and they should incorporate all relevant stakeholders in the price negotiating mechanisms for innovative drugs. This would include research and development companies, medical insurance departments, consumers, and regulatory departments that deal with pharmaceuticals. Insurance departments should make the process a multi-player game. In each region that carries out centralized pooling of and management of funds for China's 'basic medical insurance,' we should push forward the information technologies of relevant government departments. These would include all entities involved in 'medicine,' that is, medical treatment, medical insurance, and pharmaceuticals, and it would include public health insurance departments. This is to ensure that there is legitimate and reliable data in the course of negotiations on drugs, and to ensure that the results of negotiations are reasonable.

5.4 Design of list adjustment procedures

(We should) improve upon and standardize the procedures by which the drug list is adjusted. Standards in this regard are fairly uniform in other countries, and we should adopt their example. First, the priority in which drugs are evaluated for selection depends on the needs of the public, and reasons for the priorities are given. Second, detailed information on drugs that are to be evaluated is brought well in hand before evaluations take place. Only then, using such material, are drugs evaluated for social and economic impact. Factors used in assessing drugs are then defined and quantified, including safety, efficacy, reliability, economic impact, and social ethics. Finally, a report is prepared and submitted to the selection institution that handles actual selection of drugs for the list.

(We should) set up independent organizations to do economic evaluations of drugs that are independent, specifically designated for the task, and ongoing as standing bodies. These should maintain relative independence from the central government and medical insurance institutions as well as the pharmaceuticals industry. They should be responsible for carrying out the testing of efficacy standards and safety standards of drugs that drug manufacturers provide, and for carrying out evaluations and reviews of the economic benefits of different drugs.

China lacks intermediary institutions that are completely independent of government departments. Such entities can represent all stakeholders in providing objective opinions and can thereby mobilize the energies of all parties. When formulating the reimbursable drug list, therefore, China should make use of the functions of industry associations or relevant advisory groups to improve upon the list-formation process. In this way, it should turn a process of sole-party decision-making into multi-party consultation-based decision-making.

(We should) set up dynamic adjustment mechanisms by establishing institutions that are defined specifically for the task, and we should improve upon the working guidelines and evaluation standards (indicators) that apply to the task. Setting up such specified institutions is the necessary trend of the future and we should put it on the agenda as soon as possible. At the same time, we should make the basic work of drug selecting more systematic and routine.

(We should) look into setting up dynamic adjustment mechanisms that combine a top-down and bottom-up process, and in doing this we should encourage drug manufacturers to submit applications to national or provincial-level departments according to specified rules and procedures.

(We should) strengthen coordination among national departments and unite forces behind policies so as to shorten the intervals between list adjustments. We can set up different reporting procedures for newly admitted drugs, patented drugs, and non-exclusive drugs, as well as different selection criteria, adjustment periods, negotiating paths, and elimination mechanisms for each of these categories. As appropriate, we can open a 'green channel' for innovative drugs. We should encourage the use of generics as substitutes for patented drugs, and draw up corresponding reimbursement policies.

(We should) improve upon the implementation rules for eliminating drugs from the list, which would include carrying out re-evaluation of drugs on the list at regular intervals. It would include retaining drugs that are cost-effective and eliminating those that meet elimination requirements. The budgetary funds that would have been used for reimbursing for such drugs should be used to pay for innovative drugs that have high clinical value and are also economical, in order to improve the overall efficiency with which medical insurance funds are used.

5.5 Updating the list and public announcements with regard to feedback and recommendations

(We should) make full use of the Internet to improve the openness and transparency of list-adjustment procedures by setting up Internet-based supervisory mechanisms. We recommend taking advantage of the experience of the WHO and Australia in this regard. This means publishing information on the websites of relevant departments, such as the National Health Administration. Such information would include the names of experts involved and the basis for evaluations at each stage of the adjustment process. It would give detailed explanations for decisions on admittance to the list and elimination from the list, including the evaluation results from evidence-based medicine and economic evaluations of drugs. In allowing the public to understand and also oversee the adjustment process of the list, and in allowing drug manufacturers to be clear about why and how adjustments are made, China can guide research and development of drugs in the right direction. This will also allow hospitals and medical insurance institutions access to adjustment information in a timely manner, which will facilitate their daily work.

5.6 Recommendations on social supervision

'Social supervision' comes from multiple parties, including internal experts (those within government), the public at large, government departments, academia, drug manufacturers, and medical insurance processing and management departments. We recommend setting up sound mechanisms for social supervision, formulating written material that describes how to proceed, making it mandatory for selection experts to sign a declaration of personal interest and a confidentiality agreement, and making sure that they accept supervision by all parties. At the same time, we should take in opinions, complaints, and reports from all supervisory parties via channels that are made public via media and that include official websites, WeChat accounts, and microblogs. Publicized channels should include addresses, telephone numbers, and email addresses. In addition, we should process complaints and reports that are received and provide feedback in a timely manner.

Appendix 1

Australia's reimbursable drug list and overview of adjusting the list

1 Background

1.1 Australia's healthcare services system

With a population of 19 million, Australia is a federation composed of six states and two territories. Its main political parties are the Conservative Party and the Labor Party. Its healthcare system derives from a law passed in 1953 called the *National Health Act* and related provisions that govern medical, dental, and pharmaceutical services. The law also sets forth provisions for registering a health fund, nursing homes, and drug benefit plans.

According to Australia's original constitution, the federal government and state governments have a power-sharing arrangement that, at the beginning, did not oblige the federal government to provide healthcare services. These were to be provided by states. With the gradual introduction and improvement of tax transfer systems, the federal government began to provide services jointly with states and the federal government became responsible for community health services, drug services, and subsidies for patients discharged from hospitals. State governments provided the healthcare services and basic infrastructure of hospitals and community healthcare service centers. Lines between the responsibilities of the two became more blurred over time, however.

1.2 Australia's system of medical safeguards

Healthcare safeguards are funded by both government (federal and states) and private medical insurance. The source of government funds for public medical insurance comes from tax income as well as a public health tax. Residents of Australia may purchase private health insurance at their own expense. Generally speaking, the public health tax comes to 2% of all tax revenues. High-income groups are then also taxed another 1%–1.5% if their income goes over a certain figure and they have not purchased private health insurance. This is called the Medicare Levy Surcharge. The specific circumstances are a function of an individual's income, and the Australian government uses this surcharge as a way to encourage high-wealth individuals to purchase private health insurance.

Australia has a mandatory healthcare security system that applies to all citizens of Australia as well as long-term residents, which is similar to that of the U.K. However, in addition to enjoying this national health insurance, some 30% to 40% of the population also purchases private health insurance. People then have the choice of meeting different medical demands with either public insurance alone or both public and private insurance.

The 1953 *National Health Act* set forth some of the legal framework for Australia's universal health insurance system. Under this system, the publicly funded insurance is provided by and governed jointly by both the federal government and states. Medical institutions provide either low-cost or no-cost medical services as stipulated by the universal health insurance. This program began in 1984, and has since grown to play a key role in Australia's overall medical and healthcare system. The universal health insurance includes four components, as follows. 1) Medical Benefits Schedule (MBS): This reimburses for such things as medical services, clinical fees, exams that involve imaging, and case exams. 2) Pharmaceutical Benefits Scheme (PBS): this reimburses for drugs. 3) Contracts between the federal government and state governments that cover insurance responsibilities of the two parties. 4) Single-item subsidies.

1.3 Drug management system

Prior to being sold on the market, any new drug in Australia must be properly registered by the national Therapeutic Goods Administration (TGA). The federal government is in charge of regulating the quality, safety, and effectiveness of drugs that are sold, as per the 1989 revision of the *Therapeutic Goods Act*. The PBS confirms which specific brands have received TGA approval and can be sold on the market.

Australia's system separates out 'drugs' and 'medicine.' Healthcare is quite advanced in the country, there is a fairly high demand for all kinds of drugs, and imports occupy the market for many of these. At the same time, Australia's pharmaceuticals market has one of the highest sales volumes in Asia, and the country's market as a whole ranks 13th in the world.

The Pharmaceutical Benefits Scheme carries out strict regulation of the prices and reimbursement of drugs. As a result, drug prices are fairly low in the country and the per capita cost of drugs is similar to that of Sweden or Holland. Among developed countries, Australia ranks fairly well in this regard. Given policies that encourage low prescription drug prices, generic drugs do not take up a significant part of the market. The government is currently considering legislation to change this and to encourage consumption of generic drugs in order to lower total drug costs. In the future, Australia may change the system of 'reference prices,' to enable access to more innovative drugs. This will have a negative impact on drug companies that hold patents to those drugs that have gone beyond their term of patent protection. Profits of the manufacturers of a large quantity of branded drugs will be noticeably reduced. Competitive pressure will reduce the income of distributors as well, and the government will therefore provide subsidies to retail pharmacies.

In principle, if a drug company receives a registration permit from Australia's Therapeutic Goods Administration, it can then set any selling price it chooses in Australia. The price structure of drugs in Australia is, however, constrained by the prices of Australia's BPS list (Pharmaceutical Benefits Scheme). The PBS controls the wholesale prices of drugs on its list, including the profit of wholesalers. Wholesalers are allowed to charge a differential of up to 7.52% on any drug that has an *ex factory* price that is below AUD 930. They can charge a differential of AUD 69.94 on drugs that are over AUD 930. Meanwhile, pharmacists charge different markups on drugs depending on the wholesale price. They add a markup of 10% on drugs that cost less than AUD 180 from wholesalers. For drugs between AUD 180 and 450, they mark up AUD 18. For drugs between AUD 450 and 1000, they mark up at a rate of 4%. For any drugs over AUD 1000, pharmacists take in a markup of AUD 40. This includes the AUD 5.44 prescription fee charged by pharmacists, in addition to the prescription price of the drug and the wholesaler and pharmacist differentials. Furthermore, there is a fee of AUD 2.71 for any drug classified as hazardous, and a charge of AUD 2.04 for drugs that are prepared on an ad hoc basis by pharmacists.

Both the federal government and the states (territories) of Australia bear responsibility for drug compensation (insurance reimbursements). States (territories) receive funding from the federal government and in turn dispense compensation to public hospitals within their territory. Once a patient is discharged from a hospital, the reimbursement of that patient's drug costs becomes the responsibility of the federal government. To do this, the federal government formulates the Pharmaceutical Benefit Scheme, or PBS, to cover the medicines of patients in community health institutions. The PBS supplies a variety of drugs at no cost to permanent residents of Australia (or it provides subsidies to cover the costs). The charges associated with dispensing the drugs are subsidized by the federal government, and individuals are only required to pay a small portion. The PBS list includes several thousand government-subsidized drugs, and more than 600 of those are updated every year. Meanwhile, Australia is extremely strict in how it monitors PBS drugs, which ensures drug safety.

The Australian government has absolute authority to control over the usage of (prescribing of) drugs in the country. The great majority of prescription medicines are covered by the reimbursement list of the country's universal health insurance. In 2012, 80% of prescription drugs used within Australia were on the reimbursement list; at the community level, 90% of drug prescriptions were on the list. Drugs not on the insurance list hold only a very small portion of the drug market. Australia's government has not made it mandatory for drug manufacturers to apply to join the subsidy system of universal health insurance. Doctors may write prescriptions for any drug outside the system, but since spending on drugs within the system provides pharmacists with subsidies, it is almost impossible for drugs outside the system to be successful in the market. Drug manufacturers therefore do consider applying to have their drugs listed in the PBS reimbursement list. This then means that drug companies must *de facto* negotiate on selling prices with the universal health insurance departments.

In Australia, strict rules apply to who can sell drugs as well as the types of drugs they can sell. When chemical drugs apply for registration, they are put through a stringent categorization process as per requirements of the *Medical Drugs and Narcotic Drugs Act*. Generally speaking, prescription drugs are put into the categories Type 4 or 8, while non-prescription drugs are classified as Type 2 or 3. Within these two, Type 2 drugs can only be sold at pharmacies and must be provided by a pharmacist; Type 3 drugs must also be sold in pharmacies but do not require a pharmacist. In addition, the type of drug determines the kind of advertising that can be done – Type 4 drugs, for example, cannot be advertised directly to the public.

Compensation for drugs involves the following procedure. The patient takes a prescription from his or her doctor to a pharmacist to buy the drug. If the drug is on the PBS list and qualifies for reimbursement, the patient pays a co-pay according to specific conditions. The pharmacist then applies to the PBS for compensation according to the difference between what the patient pays in a co-pay and what the price of the drug is as determined by the health insurance list. In following this procedure, the government has the ability to control compensation costs for drugs from three different angles: 1) the federal government can regulate which drugs qualify for compensation, decide what restrictions to put on the indications for prescribing a drug, and it can set drug prices; 2) the government can fix the difference between the purchase and selling price of drugs; and 3) the government can control the total number of pharmacists, in order to improve the cost-effectiveness of pharmacists' work.

2 An overview of the Pharmaceutical Benefits Scheme (PBS)

2.1 The concept behind the PBS

The Pharmaceutical Benefits Scheme is an insurance program funded by public finance that is comprehensive in nature. It is the core of Australia's policies regarding drugs.

2.2 The purpose and principles behind formulating the PBS list

Purpose of formulating PBS

1) The prices of all drugs on the PBS list are determined by government, and the pricing is generally set at a fairly low level. For this reason, the formulation of the PBS list can control the overall price of drugs and thereby provide the public with reasonably priced, good quality, necessary and effective drugs. 2) Formulating the PBS list ensures the fairness and accessibility of drugs to the public. 3) Pharmacists receive compensation by selling drugs that are on the PBS list.

Principles behind formulating the list

Principles behind formulating the list include to realize effective, safe, fair access to medicines at a cost that is affordable (both to individuals and the community). More specifically, (the PBS list) should ensure the quality and efficacy of drugs, their timely and reliable supply to the people of Australia, at a cost that individuals and society can afford. It should ensure the safety of drug usage (drug prescribing) and should encourage the healthy development of the pharmaceutical industry.

2.3 Funding source of the PBS and reimbursement percentages

The central government pays for the cost of drugs on the PBS list through national tax revenues through a single-cost payment system.

Reimbursement and co-pay percentages: Australia's co-pay model refers to the mechanism by which individuals and public finance jointly pay for drugs on the list. Patients requiring drugs pay a certain amount and the rest is borne by the government in a co-pay system. The percentage of a patient's co-pay mainly depends on the level of the patient's income, followed by the type of illness, brand name of the drug, whether or not the patient is enrolled in the national medical insurance system, the total cost of the drug purchased in one year, and so on. A patient's co-pay for medical fees is fixed and is unrelated to the cost of drugs.

Scope of payment: in 2015, the PBS determined that the maximum co-pay amount (self-pay) that a patient shall pay for any single prescription is AUD 37.7. The PBS reimburses the majority of the cost of a patient's total bill.

2.4 Scope of coverage by the PBS

Groups of people covered: all Australian residents are covered as well as travelers from certain countries.

Types of drugs and number of drugs covered: PBS coverage only applies to prescription drugs. It does not include non-prescription drugs or supplements. However, its coverage does include the main drugs used for clinical purposes. In 2012, the list already had over 2,500 types of prescription drugs (by product name).

Method by which drugs are provided: 1) drugs are provided free of charge to patients in public hospitals who hold a Medicare card. 2) Drugs are provided to patients who see doctors outside of hospitals, through the PBS.

2.5 Government departments related to formulation of the PBS list

Department of Health: this department is under the jurisdiction of the federal government of Australia and is responsible for regulating medical treatment, drugs, and hospital services to ensure that they are both accessible and affordable. At the same time, it is responsible for helping promote public health through advertising and disease prevention activities.

The Therapeutic Goods Administration (TGA): also known as the drug management bureau, this is a division of the Department of Health and is the primary body in charge of handling drugs. It is similar to Australia's Food and Drug Bureau. Before any drug can be sold on the market in Australia, it must be registered by the TGA. The TGA evaluates the drug's qualifications for such registration by looking at treatment effects, quality, safety, and efficacy.

The Australian Drug Evaluation Committee (ADEC): this committee assesses the safety, quality, and efficacy of drugs. Once a drug is approved by the ADEC, it qualifies for registration by the TGA.

The Pharmaceutical Benefits Advisory Committee (PBAC): also known as the Guidance Committee on Drug Reimbursement, the Drug Subsidies Advisory Committee, and the Drug Profits Monitoring Committee, this organization is completely separate from government. Its main task is to carry out the selection of drugs for the PBS list. Specifically, it conducts comprehensive evaluations of drugs that have already been registered by the TGA. It looks at whether or not the drug is cost effective at a certain price level and also within what price range the drug would be cost effective, and it presents its findings to the PBPA (Pharmaceutical Benefits Pricing Authority, see later) for use as reference. It also advises the Minister for Health on inclusion of drugs in the list and it conducts regular reviews of the drugs already on the list. The PBPA has two sub-committees, namely the Drug Utilization Sub-committee (DUSC) and the Economics Sub-committee (ESC). These assist in evaluating drugs. The members of the PBAC include all stakeholders involved in the PBS, including experts from the fields of pharmaceuticals, economics, epidemiology, and medical insurance, as well as representatives of drug manufacturers and patients.

The Pharmaceutical Evaluation Sector (PES): this carries out detailed evaluations of material presented in the course of drug applications. Such material mainly includes abstracts of reports, re-analysis of clinical trial results, and verification of cost factors used in economic evaluations.

The Drug Utilization Sub-committee (DUSC) and the Economics Sub-committee (ESC): the PES provides these committees with detailed evaluations, and these two committees then evaluate every drug application for its comparative clinical effectiveness, quality of data, rationality of assumptions, and economic-evaluation model. They provide the PES with a summary of their findings. Members of the ESC mainly include clinical physicians, epidemiologists, and scholars of healthcare economics. The pharmaceutical industry also has a representative in this committee.

The PBAC Secretariat: this submits all relevant information on drug applications to the PBAC, including the application form submitted by the pharmaceutical company or other applicant, the evaluation of the PES and opinions of the ESC or DUSC, and any supplementary material.

The Pharmaceutical Benefits Pricing Authority: this is an independent, non-governmental organization, whose main functions and responsibilities are formulating and issuing guidelines on pharmaco-economic evaluations, and requiring companies to submit such evaluations when applying for drug listing to the PBS;

formulating wholesale prices at which wholesalers sell to pharmacies; ascertaining whether or not drug prices are reasonable, which includes PBS payment standards and any limiting circumstances, and which includes an annual survey of drug prices already on the PBS list. In order to promote the supply of drugs on the list, the PBPA links prices of drugs with quantity actually sold in adjusting drug prices.

2.6 Management of organizations

The Australian 'pharmaceutical subsidies organization' (the PBS) is based on the 1953 legislation called the National Health Act. It is guided by the provisions of that legislation. The PBAC (Pharmaceutical Benefits Advisory Committee, see earlier) selects drugs for addition to the PBS list and it also reports these selected drugs on up to the Department of Health. The Pharmaceutical Benefits Pricing Authority (PBAC) determines the price of such recommended drugs, and the Department of Health, in line with this price, makes the final decision on putting the drugs on to the list. The Department of Health also makes dynamic adjustments to the list depending on the needs of patients and the cost-effectiveness of the drug.

Two different departments within the Department of Health are responsible for applications to the PBS reimbursable list and for applications to be registered. One is the Administrative Department and the other is the Decision-Making and Consultative Department. Each of these departments is advised by two mutually independent advisory committees, which use completely different evaluation standards for evaluating drugs.

Administrative Department: this is formulated and managed in a unified way by the Australian federal government. Any drugs that are granted admission to the reimbursable drug list must first be recommended by the expert's commission that monitors and examines the profits on pharmaceuticals.

Decision-Making and Consultative Department: comprehensive evaluations on drugs are made by an expert's committee, based on a cost-benefit economic analysis of each drug. The comprehensive evaluation is based on the health needs of different groups of people and not on the health demands of any one person.

Australia also has 'expert review organizations' that are similar to the PBAC and PBPA but that are completely independent of government and instead are organized by all kinds of interest groups. These look at the clinical effectiveness and cost-effectiveness of drugs from an economic standpoint and use the resulting evidence to determine whether or not a drug is qualified to be admitted to the PBS.

Given that guidelines have not yet been issued with respect to pharmacoeconomic evaluations of drugs, the procedure for listing a drug on the PBS is as follows. Pharmaceutical enterprises apply to the PBAC to have their drug listed on the PBS. The PBAC submits its recommendation to the PBPA of the Department of Health. Once that is evaluated, the Department of Health makes a decision based on the information from the PBAC. The PBPA then negotiates with the drug manufacturer on price.

2.7 Length of time it takes to update the list

In terms of selecting new drugs for the list, every year around 40% of new drug applications are admitted to the PBS. The PBS publishes a new edition of the list every quarter. The PBAC does regular reviews of the drugs on the list, and the PBPA reviews prices of drugs on the list once every year.

2.8 The history of the PBS

After World War II, the Australian government hoped to set up some kind of system that would ensure that Australian residents had access to basic (essential) medicines. From the outset, however, the plans stirred up considerable controversy and the first law setting up such a system was found to be unconstitutional by the Australian Supreme Court. Its main opponents were people in the medical profession and it was never passed. The constitution was then revised and in 1947 the second attempt to set up a system was passed. In 1948, the country's Pharmaceutical Benefits System (PBS) formally came into being. The National Health Act of 1953 set up the Pharmaceutical Benefits Advisory Committee (PBAC) as the vehicle for making recommendations to the Department of Health on which drugs to admit to the PBS. The Department of Health then made final decisions. Prior to 1970, the names of people on the PBAC were kept secret, and any reasons they had for not recommending a drug for the list were also not made public.

Meanwhile, the Pharmaceutical Benefits Pricing Authority (PBPA) made corresponding recommendations on drugs, but it did not take costs into account. Prices of drugs on the PBS were determined once negotiations had been carried out between the Department of Health and drug manufacturers. Since these companies were primarily British, the pricing mainly followed British drug prices. As in the U.K., therefore, prices of drugs in Australia rose quite quickly, leading to the establishment in 1963 of Australia's Pharmaceutical Benefits Pricing Bureau (the administrative bureau that sets the price at which drugs will be reimbursed).

A certain amount of reform of the system was carried out in the period between 1987 and 1992. This was due to the efforts of the pharmaceutical industry to make its own views known on pricing and how pricing was affecting the industry, and also due to overall rise in the costs of the PBS. First the National Health Act was revised in such a way as to require the PBAC to take drug costs and clinical effectiveness into account as it made recommendations to the Department of Health. Second, with respect to the composition of the PBAC, the Department of Health appointed scholars to the board who could do cost-benefit analysis. Third, two entities were set up within the PBAC called the Drug Utilization Sub-committee (DUC) and the Economics Sub-committee (ESC) to provide assistance in the process of evaluating drugs. Fourth, a new organization was created called the PBPA which now took the place of the former PBPB in determining the prices at which drugs would be reimbursed. This now took into consideration how pricing of drugs would help the pharmaceutical industry contribute to Australia's economic development.

3 Overview of how adjustments are made to the PBS list

3.1 The framework of Australia's list-adjustment program

At the time of application: when an applicant submits a drug application for entry to the PBS list, the applicant must at the same time submit a report that provides a complete pharmaceutical economic analysis of the drug.

3.2 Design of the procedures by which the list is adjusted (in the case of listing new drugs)

1. R&D procedures for new drugs: from registration of a drug to actual sales, pharmaceutical companies will have participated in most of the process of researching and developing a new drug. This includes theoretical research, pre-clinical research, clinical trials, and so on. On average, such R&D requires at least 12 years and the costs of each drug prior to its being put on the market can come to USD 930 million or more. Only once a company has completed an economic analysis of its drug can the company submit an application.
2. Registration and approval procedures for new drugs of the TGA: before any new drug is put on the market and sold in Australia, either the developer of the drug or the drug manufacturer must apply to the TGA to register the drug and receive a new drug permit. At the same time, the drug must undergo a rigorous classification process as per the *Law on Pharmaceuticals and Narcotics*, in order to determine the target sales audience and advertising methods. To ensure that the quality, safety, and efficacy of a drug meets required standards, the TGA carries out a detailed evaluation of information that the applicant provides on such things as chemical components, pharmacology, toxicology, clinical research, efficacy, and so on. Not only does this help determine whether or not to approve the drug for sale on the market, but it helps decide how to conduct ongoing monitoring and testing once the drug is being sold. The ADEC evaluates the drug for safety, quality, and effectiveness. Once the ADEC grants approval, the TGA then registers the drug. In theory, if a company receives a registration permit from Australia then it can sell its drug for any price it wishes on the market. However, if the company hopes to be a part of Australia's healthcare insurance system and get reimbursements for the drug, then it must also apply to have the drug entered into the reimbursable drug list of the PBS. It must carry on negotiations with the national health insurance departments to determine the actual selling price of the drug in Australia.

The specific procedures for this are as follows. The applicant provides detailed information on such things as the chemical components of products, their pharmacology, toxicology, clinical research results, and drug efficacy, and expert reviewers carry out an initial assessment. An independent commission of experts and the Australian pharmaceuticals review commission (ADEC) then decide whether or not the drug is allowed to be sold on the market. Following that, the ADEC may recommend the product to the Department of Health and Aging. If it is accepted, the product then is registered on the Australian list of medicinal products (this list spells out all of the drugs that are allowed to be sold on the Australian market). Once the new drug enters the market, the Therapeutic Goods Administration (TGA) continues to monitor and evaluate it. In carrying out this series of strict procedures, the Australian government hopes to achieve its primary policy goal, which is to ensure that drugs on the market meet quality standards to acceptable levels, and are safe and effective.

3 PES drug evaluation procedures: Once a drug is allowed to be marketed, its manufacturer or the entity making the application applies to have the drug entered into the PBS list. The applicant or drug manufacturer must now prepare materials as prescribed by a series of comprehensive guidelines (including pharmaceutical economic analysis), and must also submit the application for inclusion into the PBS list (or substitution of this drug for one already on the list) to the Department of Health. Bureaus under the Ministry of Health called PES (Pharmaceutical Evaluation) conduct a detailed examination of technical reports that are included in the drug application. This process mainly involves retrieving and examining summaries of relevant documentation, in order to ascertain whether or not relevant tests have been overlooked, whether the results of analytical experiments need to be redone, to verify numbers used in economic analysis, and so on. Sometimes it is also necessary to run models again to carry out more sensitive analysis and confirm the reliability of test results. The PES then submits its findings to the DUSC and ESC sub-committees under the PBAC.
4 The drug selection process that the PBAC undertakes involving economic analysis: the DUSC and ESC sub-committees use the detailed evaluations submitted by the PES to generate a summary recommendation which they submit to the PBAC Secretariat. This summary recommendation takes into account the comparative clinical results of every drug, the quality of statistics provided in support of the drug, whether or not suppositions are reasonable, what economic modeling says about the drug, and so on. The PBAC Secretariat then reviews the drug according to specific standards and looks at all relevant materials – the PES evaluation and the ESC/DUSC opinion, together with supplementary material provided by the applicant. The review includes various components; in addition to the opinion of the TGA with respect to quality of the product, its safety, and effectiveness, the review also looks at results of pharmaco-economic evaluations, the demand of the market for this kind of drug, and whether or not there should be restrictions on placing the product in the PBS list. Finally, the PBAC submits a recommendation to the Department of Health, and its decision and relevant materials are made public. The results of the PBAC review serve as important

evidence of whether or not the drug should be included in the list, as well as evidence on which the eventual price formulation will be based. If the Department of Health accepts the recommendation of the PBAC, then the PBPA carries out price negotiations with the applicant. The Department of Health makes the final determination as to whether or not the drug will be placed on the PBS list. The Department of Health has the authority to reject the recommendation of the PBAC. However, it cannot add any drugs to the list that have not been through the PBAC recommendation process.

5 Pricing drugs, as mainly based on price negotiations with the PBPA: after the Department of Health agrees to the recommendation of the PBAC, it hands materials to the PBPA and arranges for it to carry out price negotiations on the drug. The PBPA is responsible for negotiating prices of new drugs that are proposed for inclusion on the PBS list. In doing this, it looks at the comparative material on a drug's clinical effectiveness that the applicant has submitted to the PBAC, together with any price-related information (comprehensive cost of the drug, medical service fees, and so on), and it also gives full consideration to the contributions that the pharmaceutical industry has made to Australia's economic growth. Once a relatively low price is confirmed through negotiations between the drug manufacturer and the PBPA Secretariat, the PBPA presents this price to the Department of Health together with (an analysis of) the impact the inclusion of the drug will have on PBS costs. The Department of Health then again makes a decision on whether or not to allow the drug entry into the PBS list.

6 Decision-making by the Department of Health

In determining the final price of a drug, the Australian Department of Health mainly bases its decision on the priced used in pharmaco-economic evaluations. The price is not related to the costs of the drug manufacturer or the availability of a drug or amount of profit it can bring in. Instead, it is closely linked to the clinical effectiveness of the drug. At the same time, the Australian Department of Health uses the advantages of centralized procurement to control the price of new drugs in the process of negotiating for a drug to gain access to the PBS basic (essential) medicines list.

3.3 Determining the standards by which the list is adjusted

3.3.1 PBAC selection standards

The applicant needs to show that there is sufficient evidence to prove its drug is superior to similar drugs in terms of clinical effectiveness, safety, and cost benefit. It needs to show, for example, that the drug may have the same efficacy as other drugs but at a lower cost, that it has better clinical results but can also reduce complication rates and mortality rates, or that it greatly reduces adverse reactions and improves the patient's quality of life.

The PBAC has drawn up an application form that goes through a review of the pharmaco-economic aspects of a drug – this is aimed at facilitating its own economic review. This describes specifically how to address such subjects as the experimental data on a drug, as well as purely economic data. Only when the applicant for a drug has provided detailed experimental data proving the effectiveness of the drug, and has done economic assessments and comparative analysis of one drug with a substitute drug or even other medical therapies, proving the advantages of the drug in economic terms, will the PBAC enter the drug into its recommended list. The costs of manufacturing some drugs are distinctly higher than the alternatives – so only if the clinical effectiveness of such a drug is proven to be clearly superior to alternatives, through the use of experimental data, will such a drug be entered in the reimbursable drug list. The economic efficiency of a drug is one of the key indicators for allowing a drug access to the 'subsidized plan list.'

3.3.2 Negotiation criteria of the PBPA

Selection principles: (select drugs that are) more effective than other drugs of the same type in the list and that are more cost-effective in terms of side effects and safety. In the process of selection, focus more on analyzing the incremental cost-effectiveness of high-value drugs. With respect to the inclusion of high-value drugs, innovative drugs, and rare drugs in the list, however, focus not only on cost-effectiveness and incremental costs as indicators but also look at the public welfare benefits of a given drug as a unique kind of product, look at its clinical effectiveness and the inability of anything else to be a substitute. In order to safeguard patients' access to drugs but also ameliorate pressure on public finance, new drugs have to comply with limited-use principles in the course of selection.

Pharmaco-economic indicators: (these include) cost-benefit analysis and analysis of the effectiveness of incremental costs. The PBPA regulations say that a two-year forecast must be done on the budgetary impact of a given drug being entered into the list. At the same time, a cost-benefit analysis comparing the drug with same-type drugs must be done in order to prove that the new drug does indeed have better cost-effectiveness than one already in the list, and the drug should be looked at in terms of preventive and therapeutic effects in the event of major medical accidents. In addition, the clinical effectiveness and risk-sharing aspects of the drug should be considered.

Australia belongs to the type of country that undertakes 'government-organization negotiation' in resolving issues. When major issues are encountered in the process of setting up the pharmaco-economic evaluation system, the pharmaceutical economic evaluation organizations must hold joint negotiations with the government. Such issues would include, for example, the system of evaluation indicators, mechanisms for setting priorities, whether or not the results of evaluations are valid, and so on. In terms of functions, the pharmaco-economic evaluation organizations in the country are focused purely on the economic evaluation of drugs. They compare drugs in the same class with one another and determine how a drug's indicators relate to those of another drug. Their responsibilities do not include looking at drug pricing or reimbursement percentages. The budget for these organizations comes directly from the Australian government. They make recommendations to the Department of Health on drugs that should be included in the list. Depending on the conditions of public finance and policy priorities, the Department of Health makes the ultimate decision on whether or not to put drugs that have been recommended by evaluation organizations into the PBS list. With respect to the order in which drugs get evaluated, the organization follows the order in which companies submitted applications.

3.3.3 Expert members and the criteria by which experts are chosen

The composition of the PBAC was kept secret until 1970, and reasons for including a drug or not including a drug in the PBS list were also not made public.

The Australian Drug Evaluation Committee (ADEC) is an independent group convened by the Office of the PBAC. The PBAC has two sub-committees that are specifically tasked with conducting reviews. One is the Economics Sub-committee (ESC) and the other is the Drug Utilization Sub-committee (DUSC). The ESC does economic evaluations on all drugs that enter into the drug benefits plan. The DUSC collects and analyzes data on drug use in Australia and compares usage in Australia to that in other countries, and it evaluates potential drug use in the future.

3.4 Disclosure of the list and feedback and opinions

Disclosure of the list: prior to 1970, the composition of members on the PBAC was kept secret, and the reasons for including or not including a drug in the PBS list were also not made public. At present, the PBAC updates the PBS list according to a specific list-procedures law that ensures the strictness, legality, openness and transparency of all proceedings. Any stakeholder can go on the government website for the PBS (www.pbs.gov.au) to download information and understand what is happening – such interested parties include government departments, drug companies, medical personnel, and the public at large. This website makes public the name list of drugs on the PBS list, as well as the PBPA guidelines, information on drug adjustments in the list, and information on drug usage and reimbursement. The PBPA guidelines have been updated several times and are now in their fifth edition. These guidelines make explicit the responsibilities and functions of the PBAC, its working procedures and meeting times, as well as the procedures applicants should follow in making applications. They give deadlines for application procedures, a list of materials required, and the criteria (indicators/standards) that apply to various forms of evidence about the drug.

3.5 Recommendation (of the Australian government) on social supervision

Information on drugs on the list, as well as drugs not on the list, is made available to the public.

4 Pharmaco-economic evaluations

4.1 Guidelines for the pharmaco-economic evaluation of drugs on the PBS list

From October 1991, drug manufacturers were asked to provide a pharmaco-economic analysis of their drug when they applied for it to be on the PBS list. This was to help unify guidelines in Australia, and in 1993 the request became mandatory. Prior to 1993, relevant government departments based their decisions on various aspects of a drug to do with efficacy and therapeutics but did not take economic criteria into sufficient consideration in deciding whether or not to admit it to the reimbursable drug list. This situation changed in 1993. In an application, the applicant now had to submit a full report that analyzed the pharmaco-economics of the drug. This had to include specific data on the advantages of one drug over others in the same class of drugs, together with supporting evidence. For example, one drug might have the same efficacy but lower cost, or one might have stronger clinical results and could also reduce the rate of complications and mortality, or one greatly reduced adverse reactions while also improving quality of life. In November 1995, Australia published a revised second edition of these guidelines but there was still a fairly large gap between research in healthcare economics and the decision makers who decide on healthcare policies. The main reason for this was that the quality of research was not that good while at the same time decision makers' knowledge of healthcare economics was inadequate.

Since Australia formally began to implement pharmaco-economic evaluations in 1993, applications to the PBS list require a shorter time but a smaller percentage are admitted to the list, and the reason relates to the requirement of doing a pharmaco-economic evaluation. By August 2001, the PBS list covered 594 types of prescription drugs (as classified by common/generic name), but 2,448 types of drugs as classified by brand name. Every year, the cost of medicines in Australia continues to rise by around 10%, and medicines constitute roughly 10% of the costs of healthcare in general. If the incremental cost of a drug per life year exceeds AUD 76,000, it is difficult for that drug to get into the reimbursement list. Conversely, if the incremental cost of a drug per year of life is less than AUD 42,000, then it is hard for that drug to be rejected by the list. If a drug manufacturer or a company can produce evidence that a given drug not only has the same efficacy but is not more expensive than a drug of the same class already on the list, then that drug will be added to the list.

1 Initial stage: 1987–1994

In 1987, Australia began departmental revisions of the laws and regulations to do with providing pharmaco-economic evaluations in the course of applying for a drug to be on the PBS list. This was done in order to control the overall rise in costs of drugs on the list. In the revision to do with the National Health Act, for example, the PBAC was required to consider the costs and efficacy of drugs when it recommended any drug to the Ministry of Health. The first actual guidelines to do with pharmaco-economic evaluations were drafted in 1991. These were formally approved in August 1992, and they began to be implemented formally in January of 1993. In the intervening period, 1991–1992, producing a report on pharmaco-economics was not mandatory but drug manufacturers were encouraged to submit such reports. Once formal implementation started in 1993, in applying for inclusion of their drug in the PBS list, pharmaceutical companies were required to provide materials that met the stipulations of the pharmaco-economic guidelines.

In 1993, the PBAC established a committee called the Economic Sub-committee (ESC), based on the existing Drug Utilization Sub-committee (DUC). Its purpose was to assist in evaluating data on the cost-effectiveness of drugs. The members of this Economic Sub-committee mainly consisted of clinical practitioners, epidemiologists, and scholars in the field of healthcare economics. The pharmaceutical industry also had one representative on the committee.

Various problems emerged as Australia suddenly began implementing its pharmaco-economic evaluation guidelines. First, the pharmaceutical industry lacked the capacity to provide sufficient information as per requirements of the guidelines. Second, it lacked information on cost-effectiveness, although this improved once the government published a manual that defined costs. Third, both the pharmaceuticals industry and the Department of Health were somewhat lacking in qualified experts in the field of healthcare economics.

2 Consolidation stage: 1995

Between 1992 and 1995, both the pharmaceutical industry and the Department of Health gradually gained experience in the economic evaluation of drugs, but they also became more opposed to one another as a result of this. In November 1995, the second edition of the pharmaco-economic evaluation guidelines began to be implemented, after having solicited the opinions of the pharmaceutical industry. This edition put particular emphasis on randomized controlled clinical trials (especially matched controlled trials), and it did not encourage such methods as simple observation or use of experts. The second edition asked companies to do a systematic review of all bio-medical literature in order to distinguish among different kinds of randomized clinical trials and to select the most appropriate. It required them to evaluate the quality of such trials and, where possible, to carry out summary analysis of the data. Since the data was mainly collected in the course of doing clinical trials, the second edition also emphasized the need to provide the source of the data. The revision of the second edition came about because of way the guidelines were being implemented. The PBAC realized the bias that came from over-reliance on observation data, and recognized the difficulty in making valid judgments due to over-reliance on clinical opinions and assumptions.

However, the second edition also did not provide an adequate description of the methods of economic analysis, and this was because decision-makers felt that clinical evaluations were of primary importance. This was contrary to the experience of many countries that were setting up such guidelines at the same time – the way Canada revised its guidelines is a particularly good example. Because of this, Australia came under considerable criticism from pharmaceutical companies. The criticism reflected the fact that members of the committee placed more emphasis on trials as the basis of economic evaluations. This was their experience and their bias.

A new problem emerged in 1995. The Department of Health had an extremely limited number of people handling applications from drug manufacturers (only four people), and as the number of applications increased and also became more complex, the daily work load became too heavy. This led directly to the creation of the first outside evaluating body in the country, which was set up within Newcastle University and was called the Newcastle Evaluation Group (NEG). The Group was mainly composed of scientific personnel in the University, and included experts in the fields of clinical pharmacology, pharmaceuticals, epidemiology, and bio-statistics.

3 Assessment and revision stage: 1996 to now (2002)

Once the second edition was published, a number of articles reviewed it from different angles and this marked the start of a systematic process of reviewing Australia's guidelines. At the same time, given the thoroughness of the evaluations, including technical procedures and processes, small revisions were made in the second edition in the following years. In April of 2000, for example, a revision emphasized that the methodology behind all clinical randomized trials and finding methods for randomized clinical trials had to be spelled out. By around 2002 or 2003, the government is expected to publish the third edition of the pharmaco-economic evaluation guidelines.

4.2 The influence of the pharmaco-economic evaluation guidelines on the PBS list

Before the introduction of the pharmaco-economic evaluation guidelines, the procedures for listing a drug on the PBS were as follows: the drug manufacturer applied to the PBAC, and the PBAC submitted recommendations to the Department of Health and the PBPA (the Pharmaceutical Benefits Pricing Authority, which handles reimbursement pricing). The Department of Health then again made a determination based on the PBAC's opinion and the PBPA carried on price negotiations with the drug manufacturer to determine the drug's price.

If drug manufacturers wanted their drugs to be listed in the PBS list, they had to prepare material according to a series of comprehensive guidelines (including pharmaco-economic evaluation guidelines) and then had to submit an application to the Department of Health for either adding their drug to the PBS list or having their drug substituted for one already on the list. The Pharmaceutical Evaluation

Sector (PES), a department within the Department of Health, carried out a detailed review of the technical aspects in the application, including a literature review to determine whether or not any relevant trials had been neglected. It would re-analyze test results and double check the costs of any factors used in the economic evaluation. At times, it might also redo the modeling to see if the degree of sensitivity analysis produced sufficiently reliable results. The PES detailed evaluation and the application of the drug manufacturer would then be submitted to the Economic Sub-committee (ESC). The ESC would do a summary opinion covering all aspects of the application, including comparative clinical results, data quality, reasonableness of assumptions, and economic evaluation modeling. It would then report back up to the PBAC.

The PBAC would prepare a recommendation to the federal government's Department of Health, based on the ESC opinion as well as results of its own discussions, and the federal Department of Health would then decide on whether or not to include the drug within the scope of the PBS reimbursement list. As it made its recommendation, the PBAC not only had to take into consideration comparative costs and benefits of different drugs but also the market demand for a new drug, the importance of treating a particular illness, and its prevalence. Of course, it also had to do its best to avoid any unfairness in the accessibility of the drug, that is, its affordability to the general public.

Finally came price determination. As the PBAC made its recommendation to the Department of Health, it also would provide the PBPA with comparative material on drugs with similar therapeutics. The PBPA would then negotiate with the drug manufacturer on price, and would provide the results to the Department of Health together with an assessment of the impact of the results on PBS costs. In this way, the price of the drug was related to its clinical effectiveness and not related to the production costs of the drug or its availability or its profitability.

It generally took 32 weeks for a drug to be listed on the PBS, starting from the time of application. Within this period, 11 weeks were required for the stage between application and the time the ESC submitted its recommendation to the PBAC. The rest of the time was mainly spent on managing the whole process, on price negotiation, and on preparing for the public release of the catalogue of prescription drugs. In most cases, the economic evaluation of a drug was carried on at the very last stage, simultaneously with the registration of the drug, in order to avoid further delays.

4.3 Features of the pharmaco-economic evaluation guidelines of the PBS

Australia's pharmaco-economic evaluation guidelines standardized the way drug companies apply to the PBAC. For that reason, they are, *de facto*, the PBAC's guidelines. The PBAC has authority over the guidelines and the authority to interpret them within reason. From an overall perspective, the second edition of the guidelines included the following points.

1 Design of experiments

The first edition of the guidelines had no specific limitations on how data should be collected. This led to a certain bias when data was gathered. In the second edition, therefore, paired random clinical trials were recommended as the first option, after which came two random trials but both with the same controls; the third option was non-random clinical trials. Naturally, any application could include multiple levels of data sources.

Paired random clinical trials are recommended as the best option since such trials have a randomization process that eliminates bias and 'noise' in the data. It helps avoid uncertainty in clinical evaluations and economic evaluations. Under certain circumstances in which this option is not possible, the guidelines state that two random clinical trials but with the same controls are a second-best option. Obviously, prior to evaluating two different drugs, the comparability of these two random clinical trial methods should also be analyzed.

Without random clinical trials, it becomes fairly difficult to draw distinctions between two different drugs. In this case, it is possible to adopt non-random clinical trial methods. Such methods include the traditional epidemiological research approach (such as cohort studies, or case control studies), or the design of quasi-experiments (such as pre- and post-control studies and quasi-target studies). Finally, in situations in which there is no data whatsoever, the only recourse is to use the opinions of experts.

2 Analytical methods

The second edition of the guidelines put particular emphasis on the analytical method called 'Intention to Treat.' This is a kind of analytical method that includes all of the resources that are allocated to a specific treatment, whether or not the treatment has adopted a prescription system, and whether or not it has adopted the entire follow-up process of research. This method includes all follow-up projects in predicting possible outcomes when data has defective values.

3 Measurement of results

In looking at the measurement of results, the second edition of the guidelines puts somewhat more emphasis on the 'patient-relevant outcome.' The concept of patient-relevant outcomes has broad implications and can include all health outcomes that are meaningful to the patient, all resources for ongoing treatment of the patient's illness, and all intangible and indirect outcomes and outcomes. The most commonly observed patient-relevant outcomes include preliminary clinical outcomes, quality of life or utility measures, and economic inputs and outputs.

4 Economic evaluation methods

The most controversial aspect of the second edition is its requirement to have two kinds of economic evaluation, that is, a preliminary evaluation based on clinical trials, and an economic modeling evaluation based on model simulation. The PBCA advocates the first type of evaluation for the following two reasons: 1) the use of economic evaluations involves cause-and-effect relationships. For that reason, it is best to minimize bias (systemic error) and chance (random error) as much as possible in the research process. A well-designed random trial can achieve this objective. In contrast, in modeling-type evaluations, it is impossible to minimize bias. A model can only provide judgments that are objective and clear with respect to the model's original assumptions. 2) Advocating for preliminary evaluations that are based on evidence is one way to help decision makers transition from empirically supported decisions to evidence-based decisions.

5 Management of drug prescribing (drug usage)

Australia has formulated an appropriate strategy for managing drug use. It has also established a National Prescribing Service, the NPS, which provides health education to the public as well as training on how to prescribe drugs to doctors, in order to standardize their prescribing behavior.

2 Research on drug procurement mechanisms

Chen Qiulin

In his book *Managing the Myths of Healthcare*, the leading management scholar Henry Mintzberg noted that the one consensus reached globally on the subject of healthcare is that all healthcare systems are failing. The treatment of diseases is a success in the majority of developed countries, and it frequently is quite a notable success. The problem is that it is too expensive. People are not willing to pay for it. The problem therefore is that the headaches of healthcare systems lie in their successes and not their failures. One of the most important achievements, and one of the most troubling to doctors and the medical field in general, has to do with the innovations and advances of drugs. Drug innovations and advances enable more effective treatment, but they also cause medical costs to soar. How best to procure and pay for these successful drugs has become a key task for medical reform.

Managing the procurement of drugs is a form of systems engineering. Sound management of the supply of medicines is the key factor in providing patients with medical services that are effective and that they can afford. According to the definition of the World Health Organization, management of the supply of medicines involves a whole system encompassing the selection of drugs, their procurement, their prescribing and delivery, and relevant managerial support for these processes. Managing the supply of medicines is linked to ensuring that the medical system can obtain drugs that meet quality requirements and are reasonable in cost, as well as to ensuring that drugs are used rationally.

Pharmaceutical procurement includes the management of such processes as tenders and bids, delivery, storage, and quality control. Drugs are not like consumer goods in the normal sense. As a result, their procurement is also not like buying normal products. One of the most complex tasks in China's reform of its medical system therefore involves exploring new ways for the country to handle the procurement of drugs (Figure 2.1).

The inability to access affordable healthcare has long been recognized as a socio-economic problem of great concern to the public. Not only are people in China aware of this but the problem has also aroused a high degree of concern on the part of the government. One of the main reasons for this problem is the exorbitant cost of drugs, together with the irregular ways in which drugs are prescribed. Given that the public and the government are increasingly concerned about high drug prices, the problem has become the core focus of reform in the sphere of

DOI: 10.4324/9781003325345-2

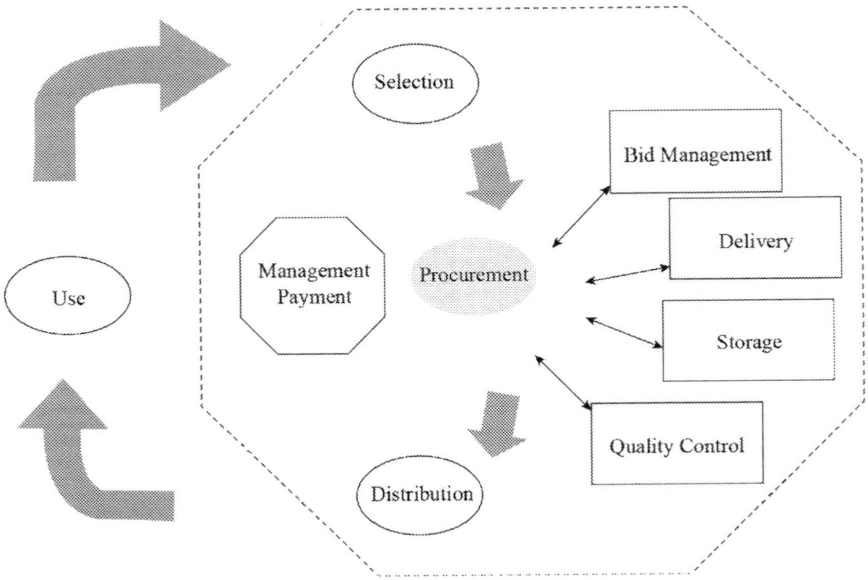

Figure 2.1 Pharmaceutical Procurement Flow Chart

drugs. China is not yet a major force in the research and development of drugs, nor is it a force in drug production, but China's market is enormous and the amount of drugs used in the country is huge – in theory, prices should not be as high as they are. The most important policy in reforming China's drug procurement mechanisms therefore relates to centralized procurement. For now, and on into the future, the government intends to adhere firmly to this policy of centralized procurement.

This research will first look at the history of China's drug procurement mechanisms and ongoing trends, and then will analyze both the theory and actual reality behind how the government is currently deepening reform of procurement mechanisms. It will look at features of the new practice of tying procurement pricing to quantity ordered, together with its accomplishments as well as challenges. In comparing China's experience to that in some other countries, it will propose recommendations for pushing forward reform of the procurement system.

1 How the pharmaceutical procurement mechanism developed in China, and future trends

1.1 Evolution of the mechanism

After New China was founded, the country formed a three-tiered healthcare services network that operated in both cities and the countryside through publicly supported medical and healthcare institutions. The functions of prevention, medical services, and healthcare maintenance were united in one body in each locality. This system provided basic medical services and public healthcare services that were either free or low-cost. It effectively addressed the problems of the country – lack of medical care and scarce medicines in what, objectively, was a low-productivity situation with little in the way of material goods. It satisfied basic medical needs of the great mass of people. Medicines used in this system, in government-run medical and healthcare institutions, were purchased through the method known as 'centralized purchasing and centralized selling.' This meant centralized production at a designated place, centralized purchasing, and centralized distribution. Prices of drugs were controlled in a centralized manner by Material Goods Pricing Departments.

After Reform and Opening Up began, as the planned economy transitioned toward becoming a market economy, medical and healthcare institutions also began to reform their various systems, including management structures, operating mechanisms, and even ownership structures. In line with these changes, the mechanisms used for procuring drugs were forced to reform as well. Since the start of Reform and Opening Up, reforms related to drug procurement have mainly been through the following four stages. The first was characterized by hospitals mainly buying their own drugs in a decentralized self-determined manner. The second experimented with centralized procurement through tenders and bidding at the level of prefectural cities. The third experimented with centralized procurement through tenders and bidding at the level of provinces, and the fourth stage experimented with centralized tenders and negotiated-procurement that was (is) handled at the level of the national government.

1.1.1 First stage (prior to 2000): mainly decentralized procurement of medicines by hospitals

Before 2000, the main practice was for hospitals to procure drugs on their own in a decentralized way. Government policies mainly focused on standardizing and rectifying market competition. Starting in the early 1990s, however, some cities and provinces voluntarily began to experiment with centralized procurement. In 1993, for example, Henan province took the lead in carrying out such centralized drug procurement through a method of designated procurement locations. It selected seven specific drug manufacturers to serve as designated procurement enterprises. This was the earliest attempt of China's public hospitals to shift from decentralized to centralized procurement – a kind of joint procurement through designated locations. In 1998, the city of Zhenjiang in Jiangsu province implemented a centralized supply of drugs to the medical clinics (infirmaries) of both enterprises and public institutions. It authorized the municipal pharmaceutical group to serve as supplier of the drugs, with the (government's) medical insurance bureau and pharmaceutical group together settling accounts for the drug expenses. A certain amount of centrally controlled quota was deducted from the fund of each clinic (infirmary). At the end of the year, the difference between wholesale and retail prices and the unused margins (discounts) was fully refunded depending on quantity of drugs used.

1.1.2 Second stage (2000–2008): explorations in centralized procurement through tenders and bidding by the governments of prefectural-level cities

Starting in 2000, some regions began centralized procurement of drugs using prefectural-level cities as the organizing unit, and using third-party institutions as the service providers. Some regions even began procuring through an alliance of municipalities. In February 2000, the *Guiding Opinion on reform of the urban medical, pharmaceuticals, and healthcare systems* put forth a 'basic framework' for centralized procurement of drugs using tenders and bidding. In 2001, the Ministry of Health released two documents, one after the other, for standardizing work procedures. These actions then formed the basis for the policy framework for procurement of drugs through centralized bidding, the standardization of work procedures, and the evaluation of bids.

Nevertheless, the institutional platforms used for this new attempt at centralized procurement were generally at the prefectural city or even county level. Bidding procedures were plagued by troublesome formalities and bids were mainly won through knocking down prices. Pharmaceutical companies were outraged and constantly demanded that centralized procurement be stopped. In 2004, the Ministry of Health released *Various regulations on further standardizing the centralized drug bidding and procurement procedures of medical institutions*. This firmed up the policy approach to centralized procurement of drugs. That same year, the National Development and Reform Commission released the *Interim Regulations on the management of prices and fees under centralized bidding and procurement of drugs*. This went a step further in standardizing the process.

In the actual practice of centralized procurement, many policy requirements and designs in the system were not in fact carried out. Examples were the requirement that the buyer specifically define purchase quantities, and the requirement that a medical institution pay within 60 days. Nevertheless, after 2004, a number of local innovations were made in centralized procurement of drugs and some regions started using the provincial government as the unit doing the procurement. Sichuan is one example: in 2004, it set up a center for the supervision and management of centralized bidding, procurement, and exchange of drugs. It led the way in organizing provincial-level institutions to implement online (Internet-based) bidding. In 2005, Shanghai's Minhang District organized joint selection procedures for selecting among drugs that had won tenders in Shanghai. Centralized procurement in this case was at the district level. Secondary price negotiations were carried out on the basis of a commitment to purchase a certain quantity and from one source. This was a fairly early realization of the concept of integrating bidding and procurement and linking price to quantity. In 2007, Guangdong province ruled that all procurement of all drug types and also the entire process of procurement had to be carried out via an Internet-based procurement system. The implementation of this ruling marked the start of online procurement of drugs.

1.1.3 Third stage (2009–2017): explorations in having provincial-level governments guide the process of centralized bidding and procurement of drugs

In 2008, an opinion was issued called the *Opinion on implementing the correction of unsound practices*. This explicitly clarified the basic 'line' (program) on the unified procurement of drugs at the provincial level. The background for this was the desire to push forward the New Medical Reform in an overall way. As a result, centralized bidding and procurement of drugs at the provincial level became the irreversible orientation of reform. In 2015, the General Office of the State Council issued the *Guiding opinion on improving centralized drug procurement in public hospitals*, which began the attempt to procure drugs by category. It set out five types of procurement methods, including procurement through tenders and bids, negotiated procurement, direct procurement by hospitals, the designation of production enterprises, and procurement of special medicines. This marked the basic formation of a systemic framework for procurement of drugs in China that had a more targeted approach.

Once the procurement of bidding at the provincial level was fairly well instituted, many regions started reform initiatives that used different procurement models. They experimented with such measures as a 'double-envelope method' and a 'two-invoice system.' In 2009, for example, Fujian province led the way in popularizing its 'two-invoice system,' and third-party exchanges emerged in the country, with Chongqing City being the most representative example. In August 2010, grassroots medical and healthcare organizations in Anhui province adopted a new method altogether – the double-envelope model of bidding. This was the first time the model had been used in China. Meanwhile, further innovative forms were appearing, such as third-party platform bidding, joint bidding done in concert by different areas, and so on. In March 2010, the Chongqing Medicine Exchange was set up as the first third-party medicine e-trading platform that combines the market and government guidance. On this platform, enterprises and hospitals conduct negotiations in an open and transparent way in reaching agreement on transactions. After 2014, a form of bidding procurement emerged in the country that is done by regions working in alliance with one another – what had been cities working together had now advanced to the stage of provinces working in alliances. One example was the Beijing-Tianjin-Hebei Procurement Alliance; another was 13 provinces who formed an alliance in China's western regions. Yet another new form was cross-regional alliances – in September 2016, Fujian hosted the first joint meeting of such an alliance, with representatives from 15 cities and 28 counties in four provinces – Fujian, Zhejiang, Hebei, and Jiangxi. The Sanming Municipal Health and Family Planning Commission (Medical Reform Office) hosted the initial meeting on the joint price-limited procurement of medicines and materials, at which the Sanming procurement platform was set up.

Despite these advances, long-standing problems persist in the procurement of drugs. One that remains fairly serious is the problem of commercial bribes. In response, the government has issued various documents that emphasize the need to go further in standardizing procurement work. Two of these were the *Notice on further cracking down on commercial bribery in the procurement and sales of pharmaceuticals*, issued by the Ministry of Health in 2010, and *Various opinions on further reforming and improving policies on the production, circulation, and use of medicines*, issued by the General Office of the State Council in 2017.

1.1.4 Fourth stage (since 2018): explorations in government-guided centralized bidding and negotiation-based procurement

The Reform Program addressing reform of State Council institutions was formally announced in March of 2018. As per this Program, responsibilities for drug procurement, including pricing and bidding, are now under the unified control of a new entity called the National Healthcare Security Administration (NHSA). After its establishment, the NHSA launched two key reform measures that have to do with pharmaceutical procurement.

The first involved national-level negotiated procurement. In June 2018, the NHSA initiated negotiations to do with 17 anticancer medicines not currently on the reimbursable drug list. The Administration selected negotiation experts from among the national 'bank' of experts, from such places as Shandong, Yunnan, Beijing, and Jiangsu, as well as representatives of relevant companies. They held negotiations on the 17 drugs. In October 2018, the NHSA issued documentation that allowed the 17 drugs to be incorporated into the scope of reimbursable drug procurement, and the documents also specified the payment (reimbursement) standards. At the same time, the documents ruled that no province (or city or region) could remove these negotiated drugs from the list, that is, the medical insurance departments which handle reimbursements in these places are not allowed to remove the drugs from the list. They also are not allowed to adjust the limits on allowable reimbursement. After holding negotiations with the pharmaceutical companies supplying the drugs, the prices of these 17 medicines dropped substantially. As compared with normal retail prices, the average drop was 56.7%. This initiative expanded the quantity of drugs used and it effectively diminished the cost burden of medicines on the public. It improved the quality of medical care.

The second involved a pilot program to do with centralized procurement that tied price to quantity. The pilot program began in so-called 4+7 cities, that is, 4 under the direct jurisdiction of the national government and 7 other large cities. This marked the beginning of a new pattern of drug procurement in China – details are provided next.

1.2 Remaining problems of policies that address drug procurement mechanisms

Since Reform and Opening Up, but particularly in the past two-plus decades, reforms to do with drug procurement mechanisms have been positive in a number of ways. They have played an important role in lowering the astronomical prices of drugs, in lightening the cost burden of medicine, in ensuring that the medical insurance fund is sustainable, in reducing commercial corruption in the sphere of medicine, and in furthering the healthy growth of a cadre of professionals in the healthcare industry. However, in comparison to the outcry of dismay from the public at large (about healthcare costs), and in contrast to the original expectations of reform, they leave many long-term problems that still need to be tackled. Those are described next.

First, price and quantity were uncoupled from one another. The basic principle behind centralized procurement was that the buyer would be able to gain a greater quantity of goods for a lower per-unit selling price. The purpose of implementing centralized procurement was to have it be beneficial in three separate ways, and the third way was to realize a lower procurement price by taking advantage of economies of scale. In 2004, the Ministry of Health and six other associated ministries and commissions issued regulations called *Various regulations on going a step further in standardizing the centralized procurement of drugs by medical institutions*, which began to quantify procurement amounts. For example, it required that 'in all regions, drugs representing over 80% of drug spending must be entered into the procurement list, and the procurement period is to last no less than one year,' 'only drugs that have successfully won a bidding process can be purchased,' and so on. In 2015, a guiding opinion called the *Guiding opinion on improving centralized drug procurement procedures of public hospitals*, explicitly set forth the principle of 'linking price to quantity, with procurement required to be open and transparent, that it be done by categories (of drugs), and that procurement be integrated with a bidding system.'

Despite these rulings, however, in reality the prevailing practice was to 'procure by price but not by quantity.' There were no concrete measures to ensure that promised quantities actually materialized. It was therefore impossible to have centralized procurement play the role it was intended to play.

Without the assurance of a certain quantity, drug companies were unwilling and also did not dare to bring their prices down. Meanwhile, medical institutions began using large quantities of substitute drugs in order to evade the process of bidding. For drug companies, winning a bid meant losing money. In the course of procuring drugs, medical institutions would find that a secondary bargaining process would in fact result in a price that was lower than the government procurement price. Some regions therefore began to hold such 'secondary bargaining' on the basis of the provincial-level bidding.

Wherever the results of centralized bidding were in fact beneficial, price was always successfully coupled with quantity. One example was Anhui in 2010 – the province launched centralized bidding and procurement of basic (essential) medicines in grassroots-level medical and healthcare institutions. Price was linked to quantity and quantity was announced in advance. Actually getting this quantity was achieved by having one sole winner of a given tender, who was then responsible, or by dividing the province up into two or three sub-regions, each of which also had one sole winner. In 2012, Sanming in Fujian began joint procurement of medicines under a 'sunshine' process that used health insurance payments as the basis of procurement – this program was also based on unified management of

22 public hospitals that were coordinated and managed at the municipal level of government. In 2014, Shanghai initiated and advertised a program of centralized bidding and procurement by medical institutions that tied price to quantity. In this manner, centralized procurement of drugs that tied price to quantity and that was guided by provincial governments became somewhat more systematic.

Second, procurement was in fact decentralized. The second aspect of centralized procurement that was meant to be beneficial was that it was intended to save on the costs of personnel, materials, and finances by allowing government departments to cut back on expenses, and medical institutions and pharmaceutical companies to use less labor. It thereby should effectively lower procurement costs. In the early period, government-guided centralized procurement of drugs was carried out at a fairly low level of government. This changed, as the level went from local governments to provincial-level governments, but drug companies still had to go from one city to another and one province to another to carry out negotiations. On the one hand, this dispersed procurement forces and kept the scale of buying at too low a level, and on the other it meant that buyers had insufficient negotiating power. This was true in areas that had lower populations and few medical resources in particular, where hospitals used relatively less in the way of medicines and held no advantage in price negotiations. Another aspect of all this was that the problems – dispersed and costly bidding procedures and their impact on drug companies – were translated into higher prices for drugs. They therefore became a burden not only to patients but a burden on health insurance. What's more, 'troublesome' procedures in the course of bidding, with various ill-defined intermediary 'fees,' also added to company costs.

Third, quality has been hard to guarantee. The third aspect of centralized bidding that was meant to be beneficial was that it was intended to 'be advantageous in bringing together the collective intelligence of experts in a given province, who could select drugs of outstanding quality and who could guarantee drug safety.' The situation in China, however, is that the pharmaceutical industry is made up of companies that are small, fragmented, and not well regulated. This reality has not fundamentally changed. Quality is erratic, purchasing is overly dispersed, and these things add to the difficulty in ensuring quality control. Trying to balance quality and price has been a contentious part of the discussion ever since the start of centralized procurement of drugs. This has been particularly true since the practice of actual bidding means the lowest price wins the bid – something that has led to serious concerns about the quality of drugs.

Fourth, regulatory oversight has not been strict, and contracts have not been strictly implemented. Hospitals that have not adopted centralized procurement in their purchasing of drugs have not been investigated and punished, which has had a negative impact on centralized procurement in general. The various links in the process of procuring drugs have not been well coordinated, from bidding, to procurement, settling accounts, prescribing of drugs and reimbursement. This means that when hospitals do not acquire drugs according to contractual terms they also do not pay on time, and companies do not supply drugs on time. These things are fairly universal. Not only do they increase the cost of money for companies, but they are a major cause of the ongoing high price of drugs. At the same time, corruption is fairly well enmeshed in the procurement process. Selling is done by 'taking along money' (in the form of kickbacks and commissions). Objectively speaking, there are no effective measures to control this.

1.3 The evolution of China's policies with respect to drug procurement mechanisms

Over the past 20-plus years, exploratory reforms to do with drug procurement have gone through various twists and turns and rounds of adjustment. Nevertheless, the overall trend is fairly clear and includes the following primary aspects.

First, the process is going from dispersed to centralized procurement. It started with hospitals making their own procurement decisions, then went to centralized procurement guided by governments first at the level of municipalities and then at the level of alliances of provincial cities. It progressed to centralized procurement guided by government at the level of provinces and then cross-regional alliances, and finally it is moving in the direction of centralized bidding procurement organized at the central-government level. In this process, the degree of coordination has constantly improved, scale has increased, and the results have been conducive to gaining quantity in exchange for price.

Second, the process is going from bidding purely on the basis of price to bidding that specifies both price and quantity. It is going from an agreement 'in principle' to procure a certain quantity but with no measures to ensure compliance, to a process that not only defines quantities explicitly but that uses a variety of mechanisms to ensure that promised quantities are actually purchased. This long-discussed topic in the centralized procurement of drugs is finally beginning to be resolved, which realizes the trend of a greater respect for orderly development.

Third, (coverage by insurance) is progressing from just commonly used medicines to more innovative drugs. Centralized procurement of drugs for inclusion in the reimbursement list is gradually moving toward procurement by category of drug. Based on such procurement by category, (the government) is gradually pushing forward reform of mechanisms that allow for procuring innovative drugs. Negotiating at the national level is enabling such drug procurement mechanisms to develop in a more comprehensive way.

Fourth, centralized procurement is moving from a focus on drugs to the inclusion of medical equipment and materials. In the actual process of centralized bidding and procurement of medicine, tenders have gradually begun to cover the procurement of medical equipment as well. In 2004, the Ministry of Health launched a pilot program to conduct centralized procurement of high-value medical materials in eight provinces and cities directly administered by the central government. The pilot programs included Beijing, Shanghai, and Guangdong. The scope of procurement included such commonly used products as cardiac pacemakers, cardiac intervention devices, and artificial joints. In 2006, the National Development and Reform Commission carried out an investigation of the high prices of medical equipment and solicited public input in the process. It did not in the end release a report, however. In 2007, the Ministry of Health issued a *Notice on further strengthening the management of the centralized procurement of medical devices*. This ruled that

> The Ministry of Health is responsible for managing centralized arrangements in cases where hospitals have few cardiac pacemakers, cardiac intervention devices, and other high-value medical devices and clinical applications, and for managing problems in cases where different places have radically different procurement prices and in cases where prices are unreasonably high.

This presented the opportunity for centralized procurement of medical equipment and materials on a nationwide basis, even though actual unified nationwide bidding happened only once in 2008. In 2013, the Ministry of Health and five other departments issued trial regulations on 'Standardizing the procurement work of high-value medical materials.' This explicitly stated that all high-value medical materials must be bought through centralized procurement, including such things as vascular intervention devices, orthopedic implants, and cardiac pacemakers.

2 The history of deepening reforms that deal with drug procurement mechanisms under the 'new pattern'

There is an inevitable quality to the way China's centralized drug procurement has moved step by step in the direction of national quantity-linked procurement. This has met the needs of the way in which medicine (medicine, drugs, and healthcare) is developing in the country. It is in line with the need to push forward reform. It also echoes the requirements of the new institutional structures that administer China.

2.1 Meeting the needs of development laws

First, reform of the drug procurement mechanisms in China is in line with the inherent requirements of the laws of the country's medical reform. The medical reform is systemic reform. It requires comprehensive reform of six spheres – the so-called six-in-one – including medical services, public health, medical security (insurance), supply of medicines, compensation for medical personnel, and supervisory management by government – in order to achieve the goals of the reform in an effective way. Procurement of drugs is a key aspect of reforming drug supply. Critical considerations include what entity is doing the procuring, what it is buying, and how it is determining price and quantity, as well as related issues such as payment, quality control, and evaluation of results. At the very least, procurement of drugs has to meet two goals: first, lowering the economic burden on the public in an effective way, which means both spending less money and using fewer unnecessary drugs, and second, encouraging R&D on more effective drugs and encouraging their production and use.

Second, reform of drug procurement is in line with the inherent requirements of price-formation mechanisms for drugs. As seen from the conventional laws of economics, a buyer can expect to receive a price reduction by increasing the amount purchased. This 'group purchase' condition is the general law of the market, and applies both to private goods and to public goods. As seen from the perspective of 'special products,' such as public goods with a natural monopoly, in general it is impossible to set prices effectively through market competition. One can then adopt administrative public services to set price, which is equivalent to setting up a direct price-control system, or one can use negotiating and bidding by buyers to establish price. The latter is better at using the function of the market in price discovery. In practice, government intervention in the supply of drugs and medical equipment (through either price or procurement) has been the universal law of healthcare and medical systems. Because of this, centralized procurement through bidding is more in line with the economic requirements of a market and also with international trends in drug procurement as part of the ongoing development of medical and healthcare systems.

2.2 Complying with the requirements of reform

First, reform has been carried out in line with the need to reduce the excessive speed at which medical and healthcare costs are growing. On the one hand, China is facing a situation in which both the rate of economic growth and the rate of increase in revenues from public finance slowed down once its economy entered the stage of 'a new normal' (lower growth). On the other hand, China's medical expenses have continued to rise at a fast pace. Between 2009 and 2018, their average compound rate of growth reached 14.2%. Between 2009 and 2018, spending per capita on medical and healthcare costs rose dramatically, increasing at an annual compound rate of 13.6%. Pressures on families, public finance, and the entire economic system have been enormous. According to an article in *The Lancet*, China's medical expenditures already match those of middle- to high-income countries, and they are increasing at an annual rate of more than 10%. Since 2009, China's healthcare expenses have increased at a faster rate than GDP growth, but in some years, they have increased at a rate of more than two times the rate of GDP growth (Figure 2.2).

Second, reform in the drug procurement arena is echoing the way reform proceeds in stages in China, from 'increment reform' (i.e., reform of the increment) to 'reform of the underlying basics.' Since the 21st century but particularly since the New Medical Reform began in 2009, China's medical reforms have mainly been reforms of the increment. This includes the deepening of reforms in the areas of public health, medical services, medical safeguards (insurance), and drug supply. Examples would be increasing the subsidy standard for per capita basic public health service fees, resuming rural cooperative medical service, establishing basic medical insurance for urban residents, and building more public hospitals in counties and health centers in townships. After a decade of reform, however, the available space left for such reform is shrinking. Whatever was easy to resolve has

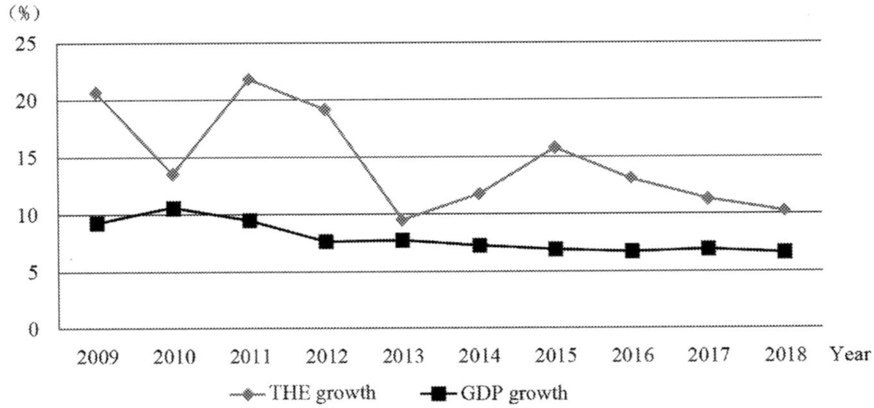

Figure 2.2 Growth Rate of GDP Compared to the Rate at which Total Healthcare Expenditures (THE) are Increasing in China

Data Source: China Health Statistical Yearbook

been resolved. By now, we have reached a point of having to gnaw at very hard bones, which means we must engage in reform of structural mechanisms that have to do with the underlying system itself. This includes procurement mechanisms for drugs, and it includes adjusting the entire pattern of the interests of stakeholders. It means carrying out reform of the underlying basics. Reform is now entering deeper waters.

Third, reforms have reflected the importance that drug costs play in overall reform. The outstanding challenge in China's healthcare sphere remains the fact that medical care is too expensive and too hard to access. In recent years, total costs of drugs have risen at an annual rate of 11.9%. The cost of drugs as a percentage of total healthcare costs is high compared to international levels. Medical reform is not just a matter of drug reform, since drug reform is simply treating the symptoms of the problem. Treating the symptoms must have some effect, however, if the entire body is to get well. We must remain problem-oriented and tackle the drug issue first, resolve the most obvious contradictions – this too is an important principle of reform.

One of the most urgent tasks of China's overall medical reform has been to control the costs of medical treatment and the spending on drugs and medical equipment. That has meant controlling the cost of drugs. For one, it has meant controlling drug prices and, in this regard, going from administrative setting of prices to bidding- and procurement-based pricing became a key priority. Second, however, it has meant controlling the quantity of drugs that are prescribed. Markups and kickbacks have been the most direct and obvious incentives in the practice of over-prescribing drugs. Eliminating markups therefore became a break-through point in achieving reform.

Fourth, reform has responded to the need to address short-term issues first – the so-called dividends required of reform. All six stakeholders with an interest in the subject have different demands for medical reform, including patients, doctors, hospitals, drug companies, health insurance, and the government. Patients want to lower their cost of healthcare; doctors and hospitals want to increase their income or at the very least do not want it to go down; drug companies want to grow and develop and come up with innovative medicines; the medical insurance fund wants to be sustainable; while the government wants public finance to be able to bear up under healthcare costs. In the short term, it is impossible to achieve all these objectives simultaneously, so 'reform' has to be selected from among them. In the short term, trying to lower astronomically high prices and curb unsound use of drugs, and thereby controlling drug costs to a reasonable extent, has been the necessary option (Figure 2.3).

2.3 Echoing the requirements of the new administration system

China's National Healthcare Security Administration (NHSA) was established in 2018, consolidating some of the responsibilities of several other government bodies. The Ministry of Human Resources and Social Security had previously handled the basic medical insurance programs of urban employees and urban residents, as well as maternity insurance. The National Development and Reform Commission had previously handled price management of medical services; the National Health Commission had previously handled functions of the New Rural Cooperative Medical program. The Ministry of Civil Affairs had handled functions relating

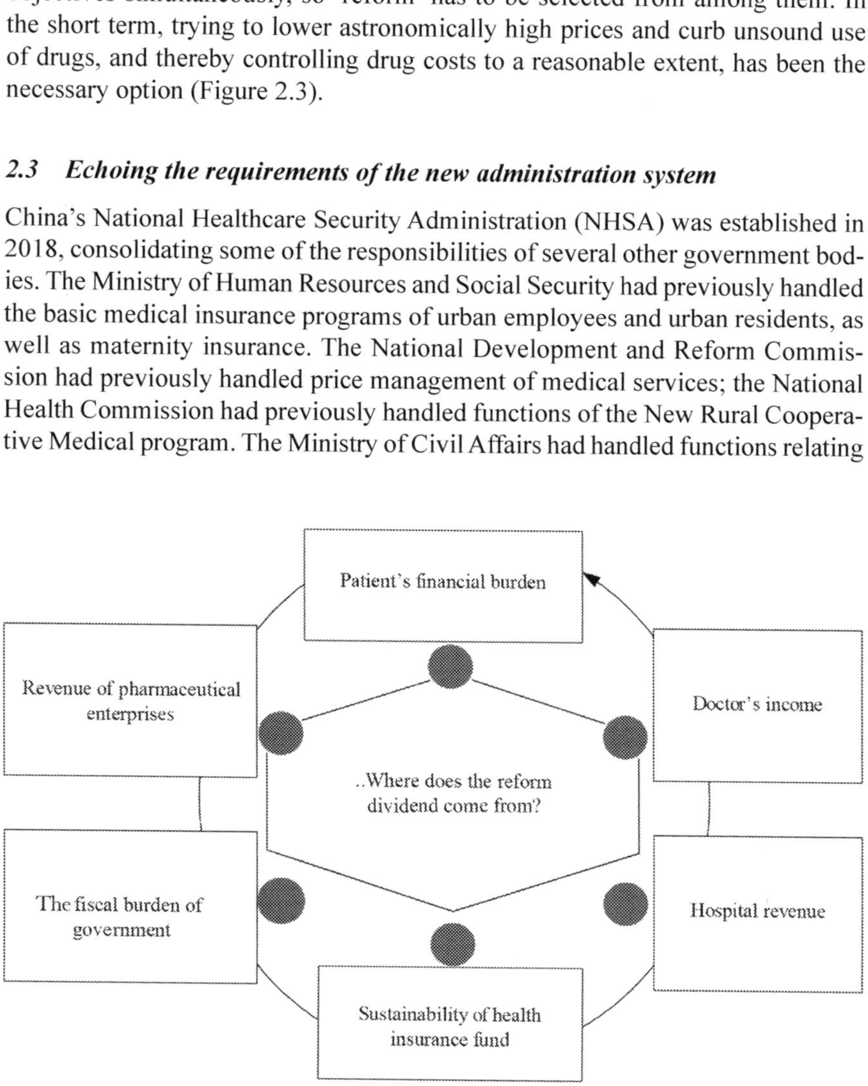

Figure 2.3 Source of China's 'Medical Reform Dividend'

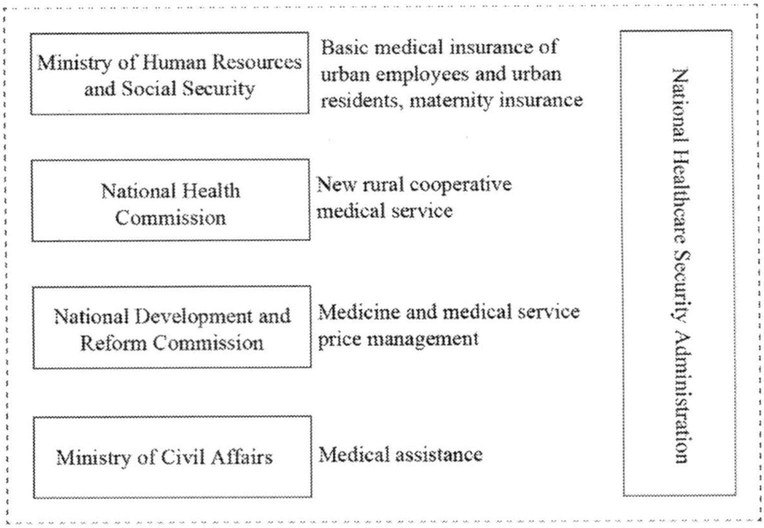

Figure 2.4 Structure of the Functions of the National Healthcare Security Administration

to medical assistance, and the pricing and procurement of drugs. All of these tasks were now assumed by the NHSA.

All functions relating to social medical insurance programs were now brought under the aegis of the NHSA (Figure 2.4). This has not yet involved a complete institutional reorganization of social medical insurance programs, but it has realized unified management of the basic medical insurance of the country. To a certain degree, this has created the nature and the capabilities of a 'single payer' system. The ultimate financial burden of the country's medical insurance fund falls on those who are insured, which means patients, but medical insurance departments are directly responsible for handling the finances. As the 'payer,' therefore, the medical insurance fund must improve the efficiency with which funds are utilized. It must achieve reasonable control of spending out of the fund. The old adage says it best: 'spending other people's money on yourself leads to waste; spending your own money on yourself is most efficient.' This economic principle means that having a 'Single Payer' to a certain degree became quite important. Directly handling procurement now became an important reform orientation for drug procurement mechanisms. It signified that drug procurement will be taking on much greater responsibility in controlling costs.

3 Reform of drug procurement under the 'new pattern:' achievements and challenges

As noted, the NHSA was set up in 2018, and in November of the same year, the CPC Central Committee held its 5th session on Comprehensively Deepening Reform. At this meeting, a pilot program was passed, called the *Pilot program on nationally organized centralized drug procurement and use*. The formal initiation of the first group of pilot locations to carry out centralized procurement and use of drugs followed. Four cities directly under the administration of the central government (Beijing, Tianjin, Shanghai, and Chongqing) and seven provincial-level cities (Shenyang, Dalian, Xiamen, Guangzhou, Shenzhen, Chengdu, and Xi'an) were selected as pilot cities. A total of 31 types of medicine (with designated specifications) were chosen for the pilot program.

Given positive results of the initial pilot program, in September of 2019 the program was expanded. The 'nationally organized centralized drug procurement program that specified quantities' was launched in a cross-regional alliance that was based on the experience not only of the 11 initial cities but also the provincial bodies that had followed on in executing their own centralized drug procurement programs. Twenty-five types of drugs were included in the expanded program.

In 2019, the State Council issued a notice called *Notice of the 'Leading Group on deepening reform of the institutional structures of the medical, pharmaceutical, and healthcare systems' with regard to promoting the experience of institutional reform in Fujian province and Sanming City*. This confirmed in explicit terms that, in 2020, the scope of medicines under the nationally organized centralized drug procurement program that specifies quantities should be expanded, as per unified deployment of the plan by the central government. On December 29, 2019, the 'joint procurement office for nationally organized centralized drug procurement and use' issued a bidding document that marked the formal launch of procuring the second batch of drugs in the process. The main difference between the first batch and the second batch was that the program had gone from being a 'pilot' to nationwide implementation. On January 16, 2020, the NHSA issued a notice called the *Notice on launching the process of procuring and using the second batch of nationally organized centralized-drug-procurement drugs*. This notice did not make any mention of the word 'pilot' in its language, which signified that the program of linking quantity to procurement was already launched on a nationwide basis. Specific cities were no longer chosen as pilot sites. Instead, the procurement alliance was composed of all provinces together with the Xinjiang Production and Construction Corps. The alliance was to carry out bidding and implementation simultaneously throughout the country. All public hospitals and military hospitals were welcome to participate. Non-governmental medical institutions and retail pharmacies that had been designated as approved for medical insurance could participate as they wished on a voluntary basis. On January 17, 2020, the bidding for the second batch of drugs was formally launched. Thirty-three medicines were involved, ranging from drugs for diabetes and high blood pressure to anticancer treatments and treatments for rare diseases. One hundred twenty-two companies were present on-site to submit bids.

3.1 Achievements of the reform

The pilot program achieved notable results.

Performance of the first batch of drugs put up for centralized quantity-linked procurement was excellent. Eleven cities were involved and 31 generic drugs, of which 25 went into planning for the centralized procurement process. In terms of the direct impact on lowering prices, a comparison could be made with the same drugs in the same cities in 2017. Compared with the lowest procurement prices of these drugs in 2017, the average price drop of 22 generic drugs with winning bids was 51.55% (Figure 2.5). The greatest drop in prices came to 96%. With respect to original (patented) drugs, the price cut for Gefitinib tablets came to 76%, for Fosinopril Sodium tablets it came to 68%. The prices of these drugs came in at 25% less than prices in surrounding countries. Entecavir tablets (0.5 mg, RMB 0.62/tablet) manufactured by CHIA TAI TIANQING for the treatment of chronic hepatitis B had the greatest price decrease – up to 95.496% in terms of the planned-for-selection price.

The initial national drug procurement program had a tremendous impact on the prices of drugs in pilot cities. Xiamen City is an example: the manufacturers of the 25 types of drugs that were selected for procurement are all located outside of Xiamen. Some of their drugs had never been sold before in Xiamen. The maker of one drug, namely Atorvastatin Calcium tablets, is based in Beijing. Not only had it never sold this drug in Xiamen before, but the drug had never been used in all of Fujian province. Prior to this time, some 85% to 90% of hyperlipidemia used for hypertension came from overseas drug companies. The price for this drug as listed on the Fujian website was around RMB 53. The price of the drug that won the bidding in this round, of exactly the same specifications, was RMB 6.6. In short, the new procurement process enabled the public to have access to low-price high-quality medicines. In Guangzhou, before the 'procurement program with specified quantities in 4+7 cities' began, centralized procurement took place with the provincial-level procurement platform as the unit in charge. This resulted in procurement of drugs that were produced within the province. After the

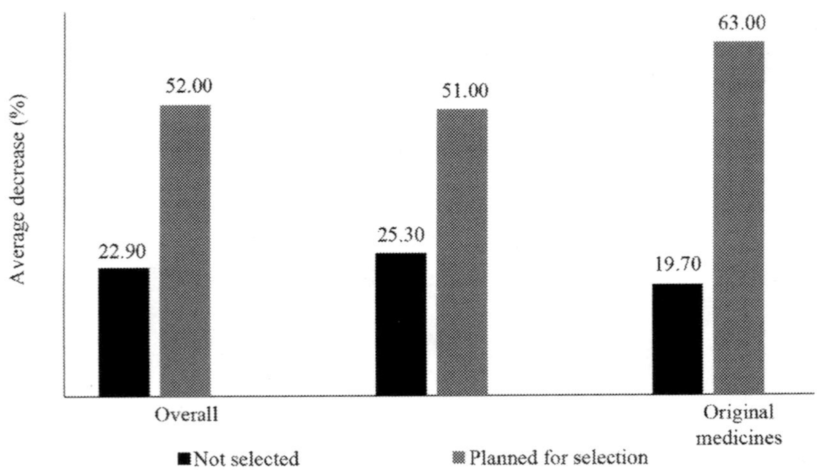

Figure 2.5 Average Price Reductions of Medicines Planned for Selection in '4+7' Pilot Cities and Eligible Medicines that were not Selected

following program started up, procurement by a cross-regional alliance, prices of bid-winning drugs within the city were significantly lowered. Although some of the bid-winning drugs were imported original medicines, most were generics that had passed the consistent-quality evaluation. The program effectively reduced the enormous financial burden on people who had been paying the higher prices for a long time.

With respect to grassroots medical institutions, the policy of drug procurement with specified quantities was a success – it provided low-priced medicines and an abundance of different types of medicine. At the same time, the policy greatly improved the operating environment of these institutions. It saved them money on medications, it reduced the fees they were charged by medical insurance and, under the medical insurance cap system, it reduced their financial pressures.

3.2 Characteristics of reform

Centralized drug procurement mechanisms were practiced for more than a decade, but never achieved the results that had been hoped for, whereas procurement that was 'nationally organized and that specified quantities' went very quickly from being a pilot program in certain cities with only certain drugs to being used in most cities with more drugs, and then nationwide with even more drugs. In this process, it was able to lower prices of drugs very substantially. This success can be attributed to the following several factors.

First, it enjoyed the close attention of high-level leadership. Reform of drug-procurement mechanisms was closely watched by the CPC Central Committee and the government's top leaders. Under such powerful determination, a program that was complex and affected the interests of a broad range of stakeholders nevertheless managed to start off well.

Second, it enjoyed collaboration among departments. The key to the success of 'government-organized centralized procurement which specified quantities' was not merely that prices and quantities were linked, but that (more) quantity was traded for (lower) prices. At least three other core factors contributed. One, drug quality was monitored and had to pass a test. In order for the public to have faith in the drug, generics had to be evaluated for consistency. Two, drug companies were reimbursed on time. Their accounts receivable period was shortened, which reduced their cost of capital – and this required the coordination of health insurance payments. Three, procurement and use of the drugs were integrated, which required not only the guarantee of reasonable procurement prices but the guarantee that doctors would use the medicines in their prescriptions. This required coordinating the administration of medical institutions. Once the National Health Security Administration was set up and then initiated the drug procurement reform, therefore, the actual success of the reform was carried out by a number of departments working together, including the National Health Commission, National Medical Products Administration, Ministry of Finance, and China Securities Regulatory Commission.

Third, reform was promoted in a strategic fashion. The national centralized bidding and procurement process required quality guarantees, cooperation with drug companies, and even more important, the very real use by doctors and hospitals. Pushing forward the policy was very much like playing chess, in that it proceeded step by step. The first step was to eliminate the markup on drugs completely, so that hospitals would no longer have an income incentive off (selling) drugs. The second step was to launch a 'consistency evaluation,' to guarantee the quality of drugs. The third step was to organize the actual bidding and procurement in a centralized way that specified quantities, so that prices truly came down. At the same time, medical insurance payments had to follow on immediately and funds had to be in place to make that happen – this allowed drug manufacturers to have the confidence to lower their prices. The fourth step was to readjust the incentives by which hospitals were funded, to ensure that hospitals were willing to use the centrally procured drugs. In overall terms, steps two and three could basically be accomplished by departments working on their own. Steps one and four had to be the result of the 'three medicines' working in concert with one another. They even required the cooperation of the ministry of finance and the securities regulatory commission in 'rectifying' the performance of drug companies with respect to financial statements and taxes, and listing requirements for listing on the market. Taking these actions was a strategic way to push forward reform.

Fourth, reform was improved upon as it went along. During the 'first batch' pilot program of the 4+7 cities, the rule that just one company could win the bid was broadly criticized. What if the production capacity of this company turned out to be insufficient? If it ran into problems, and there was no fallback, then what? This rule was not, in fact, set in stone. During the first procurement, only 16 companies won bids, but as the number of drugs being procured increased, it was decided that 'no more than three' per type of drug could win. That meant that 45 companies were selected. By the time of the second batch, 'no more than six' became the rule, and a total of 77 companies were selected. Allowing more companies to be selected meant that more producers who invested in consistency evaluations had the opportunity to join the circle.

Fifth, reform was supported by companies. There are still companies who take a wait-and-see attitude and who still have doubts about the whole procurement process. Nevertheless, many companies are enthusiastically embracing this opportunity. Some, for example, are using their winning bids to take their drugs onto a national market, or at the very least to certain provinces. This particularly applies to companies that previously had a very small market.

Finally, reform has enjoyed the support of the public at large. During the pilot program, many voices were raised in opposition – some called for the end of the program or at least a delay. After the 'first batch' pilot ended, some continued to express opposition and tried to delay or prevent further expansion of the plan. That the reform was consistently pushed forward was due not only to tremendous support at the highest levels, but it was due to the fact that the benefits of reform were apparent and patients themselves truly benefited. The great mass of people therefore was reassured by the idea of deepening the reform. After the completion of the 'first batch,' many areas that had not been in the pilot program quickly volunteered to join the experiment and then implemented the same standards as the national procurement effort. This too was a major factor behind the ability to expand the pilot program.

3.3 Challenges to the reform

There are still doubts about this reform, and there are indeed areas in which the design of the system needs improvement.

Some of the questions include the thought that the drop in drug prices may not be sustainable. Once enterprises that win bids lower prices to a substantial degree, will they have to operate at a loss? Will they still be able to guarantee quality medicines? The non-exclusive model of selecting bids may help curb inherent problems in a monopoly-bid system, but on the other hand will it lead to unfairness in the system, since neighboring provinces might supply the same products for different prices? Once bid-winning enterprises lower their prices substantially, despite the guarantee of greater quantities, they will still be reducing their margins. Will this affect the ability of the industry as a whole to be more innovative? Once companies win bids, it may well be that they have to cut their number of employees – will that lead to unemployment problems? And so on.

In point of fact, it has actually happened that medicines could not be adequately supplied under the quantity-linked procurement program. Yunnan province is one example. In June 2020, the provincial Healthcare Security Administration issued a notice saying that there would be inadequate supply of eight of the types of medicine selected for inclusion in the 4+7 program. Due to the impact of COVID-19 in 2020, supply disturbances could be due to suspended production or they could be just because supply could not catch up with demand. Analysis has been done on information reported by some provinces on their implementation of the expanded 4+7 program – according to this analysis, the highest completion rate of single products during three months of execution of the program came to 400%. What this means is that the drug-usage figure that had been used prior to procurement, for reporting to authorities (which is also the base figure used for calculating procurement amounts), was far lower than the actual use figure of the drugs. As reform is pushed forward, the older the procurement quantity is, the more it approaches the usage quantity – procurement amounts may exceed the production capacity of drug companies as time goes along.

Attention should be focused on two key aspects as we seek to improve the existing procurement mechanisms. First, can hospitals actually guarantee use of the drugs that national centralized procurement is buying? The NHSA and the National Health Commission, among other departments, have set forth documents and related policies that promote the use of these drugs and that monitor their required use by hospitals. Nevertheless, over the long term we must resolve the issue of incentive mechanisms that persuade doctors to actually prescribe drugs that have won selection bids. Second, what should the division of labor be between central and local (governments) in the drug procurement process? From the standpoint of drug supply, China has issued 168,000 approvals relating to drugs; 50,000 products are under production, and 4,700 companies supply 7,700 types of drugs. From the standpoint of drug usage, China includes 31 provinces, 332 prefecture-level cities, 28,000 hospitals, 920,000 grassroots medical institutions (basic-level or community), and 450,000 retail pharmacies. It is impossible for the national body involved, the NHSA, to organize procurement on behalf of all of these. A division of labor between the NHSA and local authorities needs to be clarified.

3.4 Analysis of stakeholders with respect to the reform

In the course of policy reform, it is inevitable that some persons will gain more in the way of interests and others will lose what they already had, given the realities of limited resources and how they are distributed. The primary stakeholders with regard to changes in drug procurement systems include government, drug companies, medical institutions, doctors, and patients. Those benefiting from the changes will do their best to help further reform of the system. Those who stand to lose will put up a certain amount of resistance. The results of the reform of mechanisms that apply to drug procurement are in fact the results of a contest, or a battle if you will, between stakeholders. It is necessary, therefore, to analyze these stakeholders as we explore policies that will deepen drug procurement reform.

3.4.1 Government

The government has adopted drug-procurement reform in order to lower drug prices and solve the problems that people have in accessing affordable care. Reforming the mechanisms involved has been a key measure. In the more than 40 years of reform, China's drug procurement system has been through three main stages, from the earliest 'total administrative control' to the later 'relaxed administrative controls,' to the current system of 'centralized procurement.' In this last stage, exploratory measures have come up with such things as 'raising the government level at which centralized procurement takes place,' using a 'two-invoice' system in order to shrink the number of intermediate transactions, gradually eliminating the markup on drugs, and finally using a quantity-specified form of procurement as the primary means of procuring drugs. The system is aimed at ensuring that patients can obtain medicines at a lower price, which also helps build a good image for the government.

In the course of actually implementing reform of drug-procurement mechanisms, however, government still faces certain difficulties and challenges. The 'two-invoice system' has been a shock to small- and medium-sized drug companies. In trying to transform their internal systems, some of these have simply failed and are either closing or being acquired. What this means is a reduction in government tax revenues from pharmaceutical companies. Under the impetus of maintaining their own interests, local governments will tend to be lax about implementing reform policies, or policies will be implemented but in unintended ways.

3.4.2 Drug companies

Drug manufacturers are the suppliers of medicines and their goal is to realize the greatest economic profit for themselves. China has a large number of drug companies and the industry has made significant progress – these companies manufacture the majority of drugs used in the country. Nevertheless, they are still constrained by such factors as operating on too small a scale, being too numerous, and having limited innovative capacity. China's government adopted measures to implement 'centralized bidding and procurement mechanisms' in order to lower exorbitant drug prices and address the problem of people not being able to afford medical care. Drug prices did indeed fall to a degree, and to a degree this spurred the development of drug companies. Nevertheless, given that the drug procurement system still has problems, including that the 'upgrading' to a higher level of government procurement needs improvement, drug companies have been somewhat negatively impacted. It should be said that drug companies are stakeholders that are substantially affected by the drug procurement system.

Positive influences of reform on drug companies include the following:

1 Reforms have corrected (rectified) improper behavior in the course of drug buying and selling. Before the implementation of the centralized drug procurement policy, each and every drug company made its own connections with each medical institution. In order to make sure its own drugs were smoothly and effectively introduced to the medical institution, each company had to carry out PR activities with each step of the drug procurement process in that particular institution. This required an enormous amount of money and human effort. Only by maintaining extremely close relationships with an institution could a company ensure that its drugs would be sold. The central effort of each company was therefore placed on public relations as opposed to R&D. Once the system of centralized drug procurement was implemented, each company now had to compete on the basis of price and occupy market share on the basis of price. This reduced the PR links in the company's selling process and allowed it to put more energy into R&D and production. Not only did this clean up the market environment, but it contributed to greater production.
2 The reform has served as an impetus to consolidate the pharmaceutical industry, and it has helped transform and upgrade the industry's operating modes. The original saying with regard to drug selling was 'sell by adding a commission.' This changed to 'sell by adding quantity,' which meant that price competition became more intense. Once the policy of procurement with specified quantities was implemented, companies that had very little in the way of initial investment were hard put to get results by lowering prices in the midst of intense price competition and attempting economies of scale. (For larger companies), quantity-linked procurement eliminated the 'systemic costs' they previously had to pay, it got rid of activities relating to market promotion and selling, it improved operating and administrative

efficiencies and production results and thereby lowered per unit costs. These companies were able to expand production and thereby achieve economies of scale. Small- and medium-sized companies faced pressures and limitations once the procurement with specified quantities policy began, to the extent that the pharmaceutical industry as a whole saw a re-allocation of resources. Instead of being characterized as 'small, too many, dispersed, and rough and ready,' China's pharmaceutical industry is now gradually transforming itself into being 'large, few, concentrated, and defined by excellence.'
3 Reform contributed to standardizing drug distribution procedures

The 'two-invoice system' both standardized procedures and posed new challenges to drug distribution companies. In seeking to maximize profits, each segment of the drug-distribution process added in a markup to price. Each time a product was transmitted to the next link in the process, the price would go up, to the extent that China's drug prices were overly high. As the 'two-invoice system' gradually began to replace the 'multiple invoice system,' a number of unnecessary channels were eliminated. This reduced unnecessary costs in the course of distributing drugs. It regulated and standardized drug distribution procedures.

The negative impacts of reform on drug manufacturers were mainly as follows:

1 Prices of drugs that won the bidding for 'procurement with specified quantity' accepted prices that were much lower, but the costs of drug manufacturers rose steeply. The situation in China was opposite to that in other countries, where the rule for generic drugs was 'low profitability, low price.' In China, generic drugs generally were distinguished by having 'high profitability and high selling prices.' The procurement mechanism that tied price to quantity signified that if a company wanted to gain relatively high market share, it had to push down its prices. Although low drug prices relieved the problems of patients to a degree, in terms of the high costs of medical care, low prices unavoidably impacted corporate profits. Some companies found it hard to continue operations. Others decided to accept prices below their production costs just to maintain market share – they made up the difference by raising prices on the drugs that were not within the centralized procurement program in order to stay profitable overall. This was, of course, contrary to the whole purpose of the centralized procurement system.
2 Drug manufacturers were overly aggressive in offering low prices, to the extent that quality could not be guaranteed. Some drug manufacturers who were forced into accepting low prices actually camouflaged an increase in prices by lowering quality. They cut corners on production costs, while not vouching for quality. The primary task of the drug procurement system has been to safeguard drug quality, yet China's drug procurement system does not have a regulated industry standard in that regard. It therefore risks having companies reduce active ingredients, among other things, which means that the rights and interests of consumers are not protected.

3.4.3 Medical institutions and doctors

The system of centralized procurement of drugs had the effect of shrinking and limiting the scope of doctors' choices. To a degree, it changed the interest relationships that medical institutions and doctors had enjoyed with income from drugs. It changed the whole situation described as 'subsidizing medicine through (selling) drugs.' However, the attitude of doctors and institutions toward the drug procurement system was influenced by whether or not hospitals could in fact make a reasonable profit and whether or not doctors could in fact earn a reasonable income. This attitude affected the results of the drug procurement system.

Although patients are the ones who take medicines, they cannot decide on how much to take and which kinds to take – doctors and hospitals have enormous autonomy in this regard. The salary levels of doctors in China are, however, quite a bit lower than those in other countries. Moreover, doctors' income has nothing to do with the number of patients they serve. What it has to do with is the number of prescriptions they write out and the price of those prescriptions. This leads to such problems as the willingness of doctors to accept kickbacks from drug companies, their willingness to write out high-priced prescriptions and accept the ongoing high prices of drugs. These problems have long since been hard to tackle.

The two-invoice system made it harder for drug companies to keep channeling benefits to doctors, so many companies found a way around this. They intentionally raised the prices of drugs that were not in the bidding, and channeled the additional benefits to doctors and hospitals. Kickbacks (commissions) that had been part of original sales channels, and fees that had been charged on 'promotion' were now shifted to a new form of channeling interests. Doctors now started writing prescriptions for high-priced drugs that were not in the centralized procurement program. Even though the program lowered prices on some drugs, patients did not really gain actual benefits and the costs of medical care remained exorbitant.

(In addition), in order to maximize their own profit, some medical institutions might under-report the amount of drugs they actually needed during the process of drug procurement with specified quantities. They would then buy the remaining quantity, which they had not reported, directly from the drug manufacturer. They had a much higher incentive to procure drugs in this way, since they could then sell the more costly drugs to patients at a higher profit to themselves. In this way, they realized the same goal of maximizing their own profit.

3.4.4 Consumers and patients

Patients are the ultimate beneficiary of China's drug policy. On the one hand, the drug procurement mechanisms have controlled the phenomenon of exorbitant prices to a degree, since prices of drugs on the reimbursement list procured under the centralized system are quite obviously lower. Most of these are generics that have been evaluated for consistency (quality control), but some are also imported 'original-research' drugs. Such lower-price drugs have moderated the enormous economic cost that patients have borne for a long time.

On the other hand, the psychological aspect of taking low-priced drugs also has an impact on China's drug-procurement mechanisms. In the initial period of reforming the drug-procurement system, our purpose was to enable consumers to purchase affordable drugs and receive affordable medical care. Whether consumers were in fact willing to take 'cheap' drugs became an issue in the actual course of implementing the reform. This directly affected the results of the procurement system. Only if consumers are willing to accept and use low-priced drugs will there be any reason for the existence of the current policy of centralized drug procurement with specified quantity. It cannot be denied that some consumers equate 'expensive drugs' with 'good drugs.' They have the mistaken notion that expensive drugs have better results. One of the key points that China's policy needs to address, therefore, is how to turn around this mistaken concept and get consumers to have confidence in drugs that have been procured at a lower price.

4 International examples of drug procurement mechanisms

In its guiding opinion on how a country formulates pharmaceutical policies, the World Health Organization (WHO) states that policies must explicitly define the decisions and objectives and the responsibilities of each party. In more precise terms, policies should state the goals that a country wishes to achieve, the measures or paths by which it aims to achieve them, and the responsibilities of all relevant parties, including public and private. This includes making clear how the course of reform will affect all stakeholders, a point that is particularly important. The WHO goes further in stating that the basic objectives of pharmaceutical policies should include: the ability of any person to access basic medicines on an equal basis and to be able to pay for them; the assurance that all drugs should have guaranteed quality, safety, and effectiveness; and the idea that both medical professionals and consumers should jointly ensure that the therapeutic value of drugs is reasonable and cost effective.

Going further, the WHO also recommends the following steps that policy makers should take into account: organize the procedures of making policy, clarify the key questions and stakeholders with an interest in those questions, do a detailed analysis of the existing situation, set up objectives and tasks, write policy documents, canvas the opinions of all relevant sides and make revisions, sign a formal policy document, and implement the policy on a nationwide basis.

After confirming the objectives of pharmaceutical policies, the key issue becomes determining the course of executing the policy. That is, the issue becomes determining which strategies and actions will achieve the objectives. On this point, the WHO recommends determining the optimum sequence of execution. In the concrete action plan, each aspect should then be spelled out – what is to be done, who is to do it, what resources are needed, which resources can actually be obtained. In addition, the beginning and ending dates of key activities should be determined.

4.1 The experience of and lessons to be derived from some typical countries and regions

In what follows, we provide a brief introduction to drug procurement practices in seven places, namely England, Germany, Japan, Denmark, the United States, China-Hong Kong, and China-Taiwan.

4.1.1 England (Great Britain)

England follows a model of universal medical services that are paid for out of general tax revenue. Nearly free services are provided to the public by public hospitals. These hospitals carry out centralized procurement through bidding. The Commercial Medicines Unit of the Department of Health and Social Care lists drugs according to prices that each manufacturer has reported, and then carries out quality inspections starting at the low-price end of the list. Manufacturers win the final bid by having drugs that are both low-priced and of good quality. In contrast, patented medicines and branded drugs are subject to planned price controls. Prices are fixed, and medical institutions are welcome to purchase them at their own discretion. At the same time, the National Health Service (NHS) is the largest 'payer.' By collaborating with the government and the pharmaceuticals industry association, it controls the pricing of medicines and the profit made on drug sales, particularly patented drugs, and thereby controls the total amount of spending on drugs.

4.1.2 Germany

Germany follows a model of universal medical insurance. It provides the entire public with medical safeguards by having mandatory social insurance that then can be used to compensate where needed. Hospitals have autonomy in procuring medicines, but are also gradually moving in the direction of group procurement through group purchasing organizations (GPO) that purchase drugs from pharmaceutical companies. The specifics of the procurement process are as follows: a medical institution signs a drug procurement agreement with a GPO, the GPO negotiates with drug manufacturers and reaches agreement on centralized purchasing, the hospital then signs a contract with those pharmaceutical companies that have acceptable prices. Meanwhile, the medical insurance fund adopts a 'reference price system' that is organized by the government and associations. It indirectly influences the market price through medical insurance payments. This mainly has the effect of lowering the price of generic drugs.

4.1.3 Japan

The Ministry of Health, Labor, and Welfare is the main department handling medicine, healthcare, and social security in Japan. At the present time, Japan has not developed a unified single model for drug procurement by hospitals. Some medical institutions choose to purchase through a joint group method, while others choose to do their own procurement. These different procurement methods share the same goal, however: obtaining the lowest price possible from drug manufacturers. What's more, Japan has a fairly well-developed system for distributing drugs – drug quality is ensured in the process, which means that drugs can get to hospitals to meet their needs in a timely manner.

4.1.4 Denmark

Denmark also follows a universal medical insurance model. The supply of all drugs for all public hospitals is done by AMGROS (which is a procurement organization used by the five large regions in the country). Depending on their own needs, hospitals decide on the types of medicine they want and they purchase though the e-platform of AMGROS. Hospitals publicly issue bidding announcements, drug companies voluntarily participate in bidding as they wish, and hospitals then evaluate the drugs that have initially been chosen. The results of that evaluation determine which company wins the bid. The European Union guidelines in this respect require that any purchase totaling over 67,000 euros must be put out for public bid. Before issuing bidding announcements, hospitals must draft the price standards at which they estimate major drugs will be purchased. AMGROS puts out public announcements for the bidding process in advance.

4.1.5 United States

The United States has a highly market-oriented medical system. Drug procurement and the pricing of drugs primarily make use of the market, but Group Purchasing Organizations are gradually becoming specialized intermediaries in the process. Their participation improves the efficiency of the medical market. Once Group Purchasing Organizations are authorized to do so by medical institutions, they consolidate orders from all institutions and sign agreements with suppliers. Large-sum orders give the GPOs the ability to request price discounts from drug manufacturers. Having lowered the price at which drugs are procured, they then are able to take a certain management fee from hospitals.

4.1.6 China-Hong Kong

China's Hong Kong region also follows the model of universal medical services. The ultimate payer in this case is the Hospital Authority, which is in charge of guiding the bidding and pricing system of drugs for public hospitals. Hong Kong adopts various ways of procurement that is done by categories for drugs that are incorporated in a 'use' list of medicines. These ways include direct procurement by hospitals, competitive negotiations, and centralized bidding and procurement. First, the method of centralized bidding and procurement is adopted for any drug for which annual total use value exceeds HKD 1 million. Any patented drugs in this category are subject to a separate bidding process. Non-patented drugs go through a public bidding process. Generally the contracts that result from these processes are valid for two years. Second, the Hospital Authority centrally coordinates the procurement of drugs that range in annual cost from HKD 50,000 to HKD 1 million. The Authority chooses a supplier and the transaction price through negotiations, and the quantity used throughout Hong Kong serves as the base quantity figure. This is a form of procurement based on 'centrally' coordinated quotations. Third, hospitals may directly purchase drugs that come to an annual value of less than HKD 50,000. The *Materials Supply and Management Manual* is used as reference in this case.

4.1.7 China-Taiwan

The Taiwan region uses a universal medical insurance model. Medical institutions have the authority to procure drugs themselves, depending on their own needs. The price is determined by direct negotiations between the supply-and-demand parties, but at the same time, the Taiwan Health Insurance Bureau exercises controls over the prices of drugs that are covered by medical insurance. New drugs are priced through comparison with international prices.

The important ways in which these countries and regions handle drug procurement provide us with a number of ideas about how to deepen drug-procurement reform in China.

1 Speed up the market-oriented aspects of centralized drug procurement

Drug procurement is highly market-based in the United States, Germany, Denmark, and Japan. Market intermediary organizations, such as GPOs, play a major role in the process. Medical institutions do not need to disperse their energies by handling the purchase of medicines as a kind of 'food' that feeds their system. At the same time, government is not overly involved in the process of procurement. In the early period of Reform in China, this country also adopted the use of intermediary organizations to purchase drugs from drug companies for medical institutions. Later, however, government began to play a larger and larger role, and went from being the regulatory supervisor overseeing drug procurement, to the body that actually executes procurement. This led to a situation in which it was very hard for government to be fair and just. One of the biggest problems facing China's reform is how to use the decisive role of the market in allocating resources and how to apply that to the process of procuring drugs. China must hold fast to the functions and responsibilities that have to do with regulatory supervision. It should pass related laws and policies as fast as possible and it should construct a drug procurement platform that is transparent and fair. We must emphasize that there is no contradiction between wielding the 'third-party' force of the market and having the government guide and organize procurement of drugs.

2 Focus on the economic practicality of drug procurement models

The main purpose of most drug procurement activities is to lower price. In China, many people believe that the efficacy of generic drugs is far below that of original-research drugs. In fact, the efficacy of these two is quite similar, while the price of original drugs is five times that of generics. Medical institutions in China would indeed prefer to buy original-research drugs and patented drugs, in order to gain a higher profit for themselves, which has led to high drug prices in the country. Greater use of low-priced generics, which have results that are essentially the same, could greatly lower what patients have to pay for drugs.

3 Focus on conducting evaluations both during and after drug bidding and procurement

Quality testing should cover the entire process of drug procurement. Merely carrying out evaluations at the time of bidding is insufficient – they should also be done after drugs have been procured. Advanced countries have developed a unified standardized set of testing criteria that measures the quality of drugs that have been procured. In China, the quality of drugs can vary greatly due to irregular and improper behavior of drug manufacturers. A company may lower prices during the procurement process, but then actually increase its profit by using deceptive ways to improve margins. These include adopting using inferior ingredients, substituting second-rate products for good ones, and so on. In some parts of the country, there is fundamentally no quality testing at all in the process of procuring drugs. Companies that are selected in the bidding process are determined solely on the basis of whether price is high or low. Even if quality testing is done in the course of procurement, demands on quality are different in each part of the country and testing criteria are also not the same. This leaves room for a great deal of latitude in making decisions. At the same time, patients should be able to voice their complaints or make the results of their use of a drug known – that is, once a drug starts being used, there still is a need for testing and evaluation of quality. This is to avoid having the poor behavior of some drug companies, who may lower quality after winning a bid, affecting the recovery of patients.

4 Put in place a form of management that handles drugs by category, and implement different procurement strategies depending on specific drug characteristics

Different procurement measures should be adopted that are targeted at different categories of medicines. Centralized procurement systems should be used in the case of medical institutions who use large quantities of drugs and whose expenditures on drugs are substantial. The model here is Hong Kong, where the Hospital Authority mainly purchases common medicines used by public hospitals in a centralized way. The larger quantity improves its bargaining power and lowers price. For patented drugs, or original-research drugs, such centralized procurement is unnecessary due to the smaller quantities involved. The medical institution may be allowed to make its own decisions in this regard, depending on its own needs.

4.2 Summing up the situation in other countries

4.2.1 Main problems with drug procurement

In looking at other countries, the main problems that exist in drug procurement that need to be overcome include the following: inadequate and imperfect rules and organizations pertaining to the process, and inadequate government regulation; lack of experience in personnel at procurement departments in dealing with a market environment; lack of complete and detailed policies on procurement, and an insufficient systemic approach, leading to lack of standardized action in the most basic operations; inadequate government funding or the problem of irregular timing of funding; different procurement systems among different parts of a single country, leading to inconsistencies; lack of accurate market information; lack of procurement personnel who have been trained for the specific purpose. In overall terms, the problems that are coming up in the process of drug procurement in other countries are not only related to the unique nature of pharmaceuticals but are also the result of poor management.

4.2.2 Basic principles behind drug procurement

In other countries, basic principles mainly include the following:

1 Different functions and responsibilities should be undertaken by different departments, committees, or individuals. Such functions include selection, quantifying, product needs, advance selection of suppliers, bid opening, and so on. Each of the relevant parties should also have a sufficient amount of technical know-how and enough resources to fulfill the corresponding functions.
2 Drug procurement must be transparent and the entire process must be carried out according to formally established procedures.
3 Procurement must follow a reasonable plan, and performance evaluations of people involved in procurement must be carried out on a regular basis, which includes an annual internal audit.
4 The procurement carried out by government departments must be confined to drugs in basic medicine catalogues or national/regional prescription catalogues.
5 The names of drugs on documents calling for procurement bids must ensure that the names of common drugs do not appear in a different guise – that is, labeling must avoid the problem of new wine being poured into old bottles.
6 The quantity of drugs to be procured must be based on real need and a reasonable estimation of quantity. Only when drug suppliers feel that the purchase amounts are accurate and reasonable will they be willing to offer a lower price.

7 Mechanisms to ensure that the funds are available for procurement must be well in place, as well as mechanisms to ensure the timely use of the funds.
8 Medicines should be procured in the maximum possible quantities, in order to ensure economies of scale.
9 Procurement done by the public sector should adopt a variety of competitive methods, except when quantities are small or procurement is done for some kind of crisis.
10 The commitment made to a single source must be respected, that is, it is necessary to buy all contracted items from a supplier who holds a contract.
11 Advance investigations of potential suppliers should be carried out. Suppliers who have been selected should agree to go through a process that evaluates their product quality, reliability of service, timely delivery of product, and financial soundness.
12 Procurement procedures and systems must ensure that all drugs being procured meet national quality standards.

4.2.3 The division of labor between the central government and local governments in drug procurement

First, centralized drug procurement and decentralized procurement both have their pros and cons. From an international perspective, there are five main types of supply systems, including centralized pharmacy systems, voluntary supply by intermediaries, dispersed procurement, private distribution systems, and fully private supply systems.

In various systems, central and local responsibilities differ in the main links they handle in the drug procurement process. Such links include holding bidding procedures and then signing contracts with suppliers, handling storage and distribution of drugs, monitoring and regulating quality, and so on. In the centralized model, for example, the advantages are that the government keeps control over the entire system, which is beneficial in making sure policies are thoroughly implemented; also government can achieve its goal of lowering fees by increasing procurement quantities. The disadvantages are that it calls on greater manpower for support, it demands relatively more in the way of materials, communications, and management, since government has to manage the entire process, and it lacks incentives to improve efficiency. Given the insufficient nature of healthcare resources, this often ends up with low availability of (affordable) drugs.

Second, in the course of centralized bidding and procurement, the division between central and local governments is influenced by the degree to which medical insurance is centrally coordinated. In international examples, the government level at which medical insurance is centrally coordinated is generally high, which enables more strategic procurement of drugs (Table 2.1).

Table 2.1 The Characteristics of and Division of Responsibilities in Various Types of Drug Management Systems

System Type	*Characteristics*	*Responsibility Division*		
		Contract Signing with Suppliers	*Storage and Distribution*	*Medicine Quality Control*
Central pharmacy	Traditional supply system Medicine procurement and distribution in the charge of unified government institutions	Central pharmacy	Central pharmacy	Central pharmacy, medicine regulator
Intermediary agency for autonomous supply	Large-quantity procurement, storage and distribution in the charge of autonomous or semi-autonomous agencies	Autonomous agency	Autonomous agency	Medicine procurement office, autonomous agency, medicine regulator
Decentralized procurement	Decentralized ways for bidding and procurement Suppliers directly distributing medicines to various areas and main medical institutions	Medicine procurement office	Supplier	Medicine procurement office, medicine regulator
Private distribution	Medicine procurement office signing contract respectively with suppliers and a distribution system The contracted distribution system storing medicines and distributing them to various areas or main medical institutions	Medicine procurement office	Distribution system	Medicine procurement office, distribution system, medicine regulator
Fully private supply	Private wholesalers and pharmacies in charge of medicine supply	Private enterprises in charge of procurement and distribution		Medicine regulator

5 Policy recommendations

In China, resolving the problem of unaffordable and inaccessible medical care is the starting point and end point of the country's overall medical reforms. The pharmaceutical industry is also carrying out reform that revolves around this goal, since the industry is an important component of medical reform. In specific terms, this means achieving a drop in the prices of drugs and medical equipment through reform of procurement methods. Such reform is meant to resolve the issue of 'unaffordable' medicine. It is meant to enable the public to enjoy access to high-quality low-cost drugs by formulating industrial development goals that allow for independent R&D and greater manufacturing capacity in the pharmaceuticals industry. Such reform also involves safeguarding the quality of drugs and medical equipment by strengthening regulatory controls over quality. Again, the aim is to ensure that all people have the right to obtain high-quality but reasonably priced medicines.

Given that the realities of various countries are different, the goals for drug policy are necessarily also different. In China, enabling each person to enjoy the right to health is the most important and the most basic consideration. This takes into consideration the country's current economic, medical, and healthcare situation. For the short term, therefore, the goal is to lower drug prices as much as possible by using such methods as centralized procurement. The idea is to enable the people of the country to obtain more effective and more affordable drugs. At the same time, this means encouraging the production of generic medicines, by concentrating forces on producing drugs that the country urgently needs for common diseases and for frequent diseases. For the longer term, we need to establish production of low-cost, high-results generic medicines as well as medical equipment and materials, and we need to set up systems to deliver them. We should be able to form an independent and complete pharmaceuticals and medical equipment industry on this basis. Not only will this become a key force in independent innovation, but (the pharmaceutical industry) should be an important force for economic growth. For these reasons, the important reform measure that the government is currently organizing, namely the centralized procurement of drugs with specified quantities, is a way to start a policy rooted in immediate circumstances that will have very long-range importance.

5.1 Focus on the importance of setting goals

Although different medical and healthcare systems may face different problems, their goals are the same – that is, to provide high-quality, low-cost, timely, reasonable health services to patients. In the course of reforming drug procurement systems, it is imperative that we be clear about the goals of reform, and also that we make sure all relevant parties are familiar with these goals. Reasonable and clear reform goals are a prerequisite for making sure that the entire society is behind the reforms.

We first should therefore firmly define the parts of reform on which we intend to put most effort. This means specifying the direction of reform for both the market and local government in order to increase their level of support and coordination. In this regard, we must be determined to carry through with supply-side structural reform. We must adhere to the plan to 'vacate the cage in order to change the bird in the cage,' which means vacating medicines in favor of services (as a way for hospitals to bring in income) and vacating common medicines in favor of innovative new medicines. This leverages the procurement value of medical insurance, and forms a stable pattern of 'collective procurement of common drugs and negotiated procurement of new drugs.'

Right now, the emphasis should be on exchanging medicines for services. This refers to saving on the cost of drugs in order to create more usable capital, particularly insurance funds, and then using those to pay for hospital services – both by raising the prices of those services and allowing greater reimbursement by insurance. This helps optimize the way in which medical and drug resources are allocated. On this basis, from now on we should use the funds saved from procurement to purchase innovative drugs. We should realize a situation in which the medical fund purchases drugs according to a 20/80 principle: 20% of the funds are used to purchase 80% of common medicines, while 80% of the funds are used to purchase innovative medicines. Not only does this satisfy the demand for basic medicines, but it tries to maximize the quality of medical care.

5.2 Focus on the importance of making more systemic decisions

In the medical and healthcare system, any new policy in one department will affect overall behavior in other departments. Actually achieving the goals of reform depends on whether or not adequate attention has been paid to the behavior of the system in general. Drug procurement is a procedure that involves systems. It touches on various aspects, including quality control, management of bidding and procurement, delivery of drugs, and so on. At the same time, drug procurement is one of the key aspects in the entire system of managing drug supply. It involves such issues as drug selection and the reasonable prescribing of drugs. Furthermore, the management of pharmaceuticals is just one part of the entire medical and healthcare system. Reforming this part must be accompanied by corresponding (changes) in the funding and incentive mechanisms of medicine and healthcare, reform of the medical and healthcare services system, and the medical insurance system.

5.3 The importance of stakeholder involvement and cooperation

Clear goals are, of course, a prerequisite, but even more importantly there must be a clear plan and effective implementation of that plan. Many reforms have failed due to weak implementation. Because of this, all parties involved in the medical system must be proactive in participating in the reform. At the same time, reform of the drug procurement system affects the interests of related systems – coordinating those interests and the interests of individuals is the most important guarantee that reform will be successful.

Right now it is particularly important to increase the degree to which doctors and hospitals cooperate with reform. This means speeding up reform of the way doctors are compensated, rationalizing the current incentive system so that doctors' incentives are no longer tied to drugs. In practicality, this involves using a portion of the money saved through centralized procurement and giving it to hospitals. This will benefit the extent to which hospitals are happy to cooperate (with reform), but it will not provide a direct incentive to doctors. For that reason, one possible solution may be to use a portion of the saved insurance costs and put that toward rewarding doctors. This concept has been thought of as a kind of special way of purchasing doctors' services.

As for encouraging drug companies (to cooperate with reform), we should lean in the direction of generic drug companies whose drugs have passed consistency evaluations. We want to encourage drug companies to participate in evaluations and lift the overall quality level of China's generics. At the same time, with respect to the procurement of innovative drugs, we should integrate that with the process of 'bidding for drugs with specified quantities' and lean in the direction of the innovative drugs that companies who have won the bidding are producing. This is to encourage innovation in such companies. Meanwhile, we should take real advantage of the role of associations. We need to strengthen their role in such key processes as drug selection, price negotiation, and medical and healthcare technology and evaluations, in addition to strengthening the role of the government and the market in drug procurement. Associations are the spokespeople for the industry but they also self-regulate the industry through industry standards and regulations. They seek to create better space into which the industry can grow.

As for patients, it is inevitable that some will want to exchange bid-winning medicines for some other medicine, whether for objective or subjective reasons. In addition to guiding their behavior through payment incentives and scientific education, the emphasis here should be on strengthening evaluations of treatment effectiveness and, through the resulting evidence, try to change patients' behavior.

5.4 The importance of discriminating among different environments

Looking at how other countries handle their drug procurement, no one unified model is suitable for all. The systems operating in 'successful' market-economy countries may be incapable of solving the problems that developing countries are facing. In most countries, reforms of drug procurement systems are tied in to the local situation in terms of the economic, political, and medical and healthcare systems of the country. This is necessary in order to implement creative measures. For example, in some countries the system of centralized negotiated procurement is suited to a medical services system that is dominated by public institutions. Some countries use electronically based bidding in their procurement systems, because it is aligned with reforms of their overall government procurement systems.

Every country has its own situation. The foundation on which medical insurance and medical treatment can develop in a given place – the managerial capacity, communications systems, level of informatization, and so on – are all different. It is necessary to proceed according to actual circumstances in both coordinating from an overall perspective and adjusting at the local level. Right now, the situation in China is that the country must adhere to the principle of procuring drugs by category, and it must use different procurement methods depending on the nature of the drug. Supply must also take into consideration differences among different parts of the country.

5.5 The importance of the proper balance between centralized procurement and improving efficiency

Centralized procurement is an important way to improve the efficiency with which drugs are ultimately supplied to patients. However, it requires large amounts of organizational capital which in turn lowers the efficiency of the process – the key is to focus on raising overall efficiency.

China should, therefore, research how to make the process of centralized procurement by state organizations more professional; it should gradually transition from procurement methods that rely on direct administrative forces to procurement that is conducted by professional platforms.

5.6 The importance of regulating medicines

Drug procurement is procurement of a special nature – it requires a control system that regulates medicines. This is particularly true in developing countries, where the information asymmetry between those supplying and those using drugs is severe. For this reason, it is even more important to strengthen the role of government when it comes to implementing control systems that apply to medicines. It is important to strengthen regulatory supervision of drug quality.

China should adhere to the principle of 'guaranteed quality and reasonable price.' It should establish comprehensive and unified standards on quality and price, using procurement data from each province, and it should set up an evaluation platform that evaluates drugs in a unified and standardized way. In the course of bidding and procurement, drugs should be ranked from lowest to highest in price, and then evaluated in combination with quality, as a systematic way to determine whether or not a company's product will be selected. Evaluation experts can carry out a rating of drugs by comparing such factors as the production capacity of companies and their record on sample tests. Based on the score of such a rating, the experts then can go in the order from top to bottom in deciding which drugs to select.

5.7 The importance of evaluation and adjustments

It is critical to keep firmly in mind the original objectives of reform. As reform proceeds, it is also important to confirm the practicality of reform steps and make sure they are doable. After carrying out a sequence of reforms, it is always necessary to look back on them and ensure that they conform to the goals that were originally established. It is also necessary to ensure they are corrected in reasonable ways when evaluations show that there are new circumstances. The success of reform depends on the support of a very broad spectrum of stakeholders. The process of looking back over what has been done and making adjustments must be done in ways that are helpful to garnering the support of these stakeholders. Many successful reforms in the sphere of drug procurement came about in just such a gradual and incremental way. In Thailand, for example, centralized negotiated procurement systems began to appear in 1990, but only after 1997 were they applied nationwide. In Chile, the electronic procurement system basically was only set up in 1998, after seven years of constant evaluation and adjustment.

5.8 *The importance of transparency*

Fairness is the key to attracting outstanding suppliers and obtaining optimal prices. The possibility of corruption lurks in non-transparent procurement processes. Whether or not corruption actually exists, the possibility that it does is detrimental since suppliers, medical institutions, and the public at large will have no trust in such a system. Complete disclosure of price information is of ultimate importance. This includes not only prices of competitors but also prices of similar types of drugs in other markets. Many countries therefore require that manufacturers disclose not only the prices within a country but also their international prices.

In the implementation of its reform, China must firmly adhere to the principle of open and transparent information. Using transparency and openness, the country should be able to remold the behavior of stakeholders.

5.9 *The importance of information technologies*

One disadvantage of centralized bidding by government lies in the fact that such a system often cannot get drugs to patients in a timely and effective manner. This is especially true when the procurement institution has very loose control over delivery channels, and when its ability to coordinate the whole system is limited. For these reasons, it is important to focus on the importance of information technologies and to improve China's level of information technologies.

In an era in which information technologies are constantly advancing, we should listen to the emphasis of President Xi Jinping at a meeting of the CPC Central Committee on the Deepening of Reforms:

> We must focus on applying the new generation of information technologies to China's medical, healthcare, and pharmaceutical sphere. [New information technologies] can remold how this sphere is managed, as well as its modes of service. They can optimize the allocation of resources and upgrade the efficiency of medical services.

By relying on 'informatization' and full use of the Internet+, China can realize a closed-loop system in its drug supply. Profits can be achieved in the supply chain through pooling end-user demand. Win-win solutions can be achieved through using innovative business models as well as direct compromise in negotiations at the upper end of the process. Not only does this reduce the ultimate cost of drugs to society, but it improves the efficiency with which drugs are supplied.

Bibliography

BianJie. (2020). Shuffling in the second batch of drug procurement with target quantity. *Medicine Economic Reporter*, March 5.

Centralized drug procurement in the new situation: Past, now and future. *Official WeChat account "Chinese Medical Insurance"*, 2018. https://mp.weixin.qq.com/s/HZUHc2PnLP-bYvol9OLt1A

Centralized drug supply promoted in Zhenjiang. *Soft Science of Health*, 1998 (06): 13.

Chen Guangtai & Hao Yuantao. (2009). Deficiency and suggestion on medicine purchasing system. *Modern Hospital*, 9 (01): 9–11.

Chen Hao & Rao Yuanhong. (2019). Practice and thinking on the pharmaceutical procurement with target quantity in the new era. *China Journal of Pharmaceutical Economics*, 14 (07): 19–26.

Chen Qiulin. (2010). *Influence of the Medical Health System on Health Performance*. Peking University.

Fu Hongpeng. (2015). Suggestions of the improvement of public hospitals drug procurement mechanisms. *Chinese Hospital Management*, 35 (02): 13–15.

Fu Hongpeng, Su Jianting, Shan Nan & Wang Xuetao. (2010). Introduction of drug centralized purchase of Bureau of Hospital Management in Hong Kong. *Health Economics Research*, 9: 38–40.

Gao Herong. (2018). Achievements and challenges of the drug procurement system over the 40 years since the reform and opening up. *Frontiers*, 21: 81–87.

Generic drugs will be shuffled and original drugs embrace development opportunities. *China Powder Industry*, 2020 (01): 55–57.

Hu Shanlian. (2019). Analysis on economics theoretical basis and impact in drug bulk purchasing with quantity. *Soft Science of Health*, 33 (01): 3–5.

Huang Yushu & Tao Libo. (2020). Influence of centralized drug procurement with target quantity on Chinese pharmaceutical industrial concentration: A perspective of industrial economics. *China Health Insurance*, 2: 64–67.

Li Cuicui & Fu Hongpeng. (2018). A study on the evaluation of the "two-bill system" in drug procurement. *Health Economics Research*, 5: 49–51.

Li Dongsheng. (2019). Impact of quantity-based procurement in "4+7" cities on community-level medical institutions. *Physician Online*, 26: 9–10.

Li Nan. (2018). Impact of drug bidding on the marketing modes of pharmaceutical enterprises. *Technology and Market*, 25 (06): 192–193.

Luo Sainan & Ma Aixia. (2008). The mode of pharmaceutical purchasing management in USA and Japan and the inspiration to our country. *Shanghai Medical & Pharmaceutical Journal*, 6: 258–260.

Peng Jing. (2011). *Evaluation Studies on the National Essential Medicine System Based on the Stakeholder Theory*. Anhui Medical University.

Sara Bennett, Jonathan D. Quick & Germán Velásquez. (1997). *Public-Private Roles in the Pharmaceutical Sector: Implications for Equitable Access and Rational Drug Use*. WHO/DAP. www.who.int/medicines/library/dap/who-dap-97-12/who-dap-97-12.pdf

Song Daolan. (2013). *The Defect of the Current Centralized Pharmaceuticals Purchase System and Improvement*. Southwest University of Political Science and Law.

Sun Jie. (2020). The second batch of drugs procured with target quantity to land in Jiangyin. *Jiangyin Daily*, April 25.

Tan Qingli, Yang Siyuan, Li Wenjing & Zhang Wanping. (2020). Effect, key problems and countermeasures of drug procurement with target quantity in "4+7" cities: A case study of Guangzhou. *Health Economics Research*, 37 (04): 46–50.

Tan Zaixiang & Fan Shun. (2019). Challenges and countermeasures of pharmaceutical enterprises under the background of centralized purchasing of drugs "4+7". *Health Economics Research*, 36 (08): 13–15, 19.

Wang Lijie, Jin Chunlin, Duan Guangfeng, Tian Wenhua & Wang Linan. (2013). Inspiration of the international practices on improving bidding and procurement mechanism of essential medicine in China. *Chinese Health Economics*, 32(09): 78–79.

Wang Lixian & Yang. (2020). Problems in the practice of the "two-invoice system" and countermeasures. *China Collective Economy*, 11: 11–12.

Wang Yiran. (2019). Xiamen: What else did the quantity-based procurement bring besides quantity. *China Health*, 5: 85–86.

Wang Yun. (2014). Current status, experience and inspirations of the drug manufacturing and circulation system in UK. *Review of Economic Research*, 32: 86–112.

WHO/EDM/PAR. (1999). *Operational Principle for Good Pharmaceutical Procurement*. www.who.int/medicines/library/par/who-edm-par-99-5/who-edm-par-99-5.pdf

World Bank. (2001). *Technical Note: Procurement of Health Sector Goods*. www.worldbank.org/html/opr/biddocs/health/health-tn-ev2.doc

World Health Organization. (2002). *Practical Guidelines on Pharmaceutical Procurement for Countries with Small Procurement Agencies*. www.wpro.who.int/pdf/PHA/Practical_guidelines.pdf

Yu Changyong. (2020). Practical effect of the pharmaceutical procurement with target quantity in "4+7" cities and institutional concerns. *Journal of Southwest Minzu University (Humanities and Social Science)*, 41 (04): 34–39.

Zhang Yubo, Chen Yang, Sun Kexin & Huang Li. (2018). Discussion on the development direction of drug circulation enterprises under the "two invoice system". *China Pharmacy*, 29 (05): 577–579.

Zhao Chenhao, Liao Tongquan, Zhang Chun, Wei Xiaoyan, Huang Jingbin, Tang Ziyun & Qi Deguang. (2020). Operation effect of pilot hospitals for drug procurement with target quantity. *Hospital Administration Journal of Chinese People's Liberation Army*, 27 (04): 385–388.

Zou Wujie, Zhang Jingyuan, Guan Xiaodong & Shi Luwen. (2016). The development and thinking of drug centralized procurement policy in China. *Drug Evaluation*, 13 (10): 18–20, 61.

3 Research on drug price-formation mechanisms

Wang Zhen

1 Executive summary

1.1 The root cause of price distortion in China's drug prices: 'the problem lies in medicine, not in drugs'

Distorted drug prices are a concentrated expression of the many problems in China's sphere of medicine. Exorbitantly high drug prices, the over-prescribing of drugs, and inflated costs relating to drugs have plagued the country since the start of Reform and Opening Up. The composition of the price of a given drug in China goes beyond the normal costs of production, distribution, and profit and includes such things as fees for hospitals and doctors' services. These are the fees that lead to the phrase 'subsidizing medicine through the sale of medicines.' In addition to such fees are the other fees to get around all kinds of controls. This last kind of fee (or cost) is a pure waste of social resources, and it is the most unreasonable part of drug prices. From an economic standpoint, normal production and distribution costs, plus profit, come to around one-third of the total price of a given drug, while fees paid to hospitals and doctors come to another 40%.

This kind of distortion in drug prices is fundamentally rooted in the supply side of China's healthcare and medical services. It could be said that China's drug price problems stem from 'medicine' as a system and not from 'drugs.' The system for pricing drugs in China has been through several changes since the start of Reform and Opening Up. During the planned-economy period, prices were set entirely through administrative fiat. By the 1980s and 1990s, a two-track system of pricing involved both administratively determined prices and prices determined by the market, and that further evolved to a two-track system of pricing which involved a ceiling on the administratively determined price and a market-determined price. In 2015, the administrative fixing of prices was completely eliminated. A singular price-formation mechanism that was determined primarily by the market came into effect.

Such changes in price-formation mechanisms, as well as changes in corresponding policies and regulatory systems, did not, however, resolve the problem of exorbitant drug prices and distorted drug price mechanisms. Instead, such changes constantly generated new distortions.

DOI: 10.4324/9781003325345-3

Between 1997 and 2013, the government adjusted drug prices 32 times. The consequence of trying to adjust them downward, however, was that they continued to go up. In addition to reforming price-formation mechanisms, the government also initiated other related measures to try to control the situation. These included, for example, controls on the practice of adding markups, setting rules on the percentage of drug-price differentials, the 'two-invoice system,' a zero-markup system, government-led centralized drug procurement, and so on. Without a single exception, all of these policies have, up to now, failed to get at the root of the problem. They have not been able to mitigate the distortion in drug prices.

(As noted previously), the deep-seated cause of this situation lies on the supply side of China's medical services. China's public hospitals are 'administratively' managed. This leads to the simultaneous co-existence of excessive incentives and inadequate incentives. Under the completely planned-economy system, medical institutions lacked any incentive to improve performance and therefore were inefficient. In the 1980s, the greatest problem in the medical sphere in China – which includes drugs, medical services, and healthcare – was that supply was insufficient due to this extreme inefficiency. In order to provide incentives to get hospitals to deliver more services, an initial reform was carried out that increased their operating autonomy. The reform encouraged hospitals to be inventive in generating income. However, even as this encouragement was going forward, the administrative control system that applied to hospital institutions continued to exist. No appropriate system was set up to pay doctors for their services or hospitals for their services. Given this situation, the sole means by which hospitals and doctors could get paid lay in manipulating the prices of drugs. A pattern gradually developed that is known as 'paying for medicine through drugs.'

The second part of this situation includes the monopoly position that hospitals enjoy under the protection of the administrative system, and the way public units are staffed by doctors who rely on the hospital's *bianzhi* system. This system appoints hospital personnel, including doctors, as staff in a hierarchical structure and graduated pay system. It is similar to a civil service system, but with Chinese characteristics. China's public hospital institutions are not only the recipients of administrative protection, but they also enjoy all kinds of financial subsidies, some overt, some hidden, and the right to use public funds. The administrative monopoly leads to a situation described as 'those who excel cannot rise to the top, and those who are inferior cannot be gotten rid of.' Neither incentives nor constraint mechanisms are effective in such a situation. If administrative controls over hospitals are relaxed, then the phenomenon of 'seeking self-interest' takes hold – taking advantage of both the administrative monopoly and public resources. Medical institutions become profit-driven and profits are gained mainly by distorting the price of drugs. Herein lies the primary cause of China's drug price distortion.

1.2 The international model for pricing drugs: market-based pricing guided by reimbursement standards

In the United States and the main countries of Europe, the market mainly determines the pricing of drugs, but there is generally also government intervention through public policies at various stages. When drug expenses are borne by the public (including via social security and government payments), a country's reimbursement standards are key in determining the price of drugs. To sum up, the price-formation mechanisms for drugs in major countries are: market-determined prices as guided by medical insurance reimbursement standards.

Market-based drug pricing guided by the reimbursement standards of medical insurance has two benefits. It controls drug prices within a specific range and keeps them from rising too much. But second, it also provides medical providers and drug companies with plenty of margin. This creates the incentive for both to keep their prices within a reasonable range. The core part of this incentive mechanism is that medical providers carry out procurement themselves – they thereby keep the price differential between the payment standard and the actual procurement price of the drugs.

However, in order for the pricing mechanisms as described earlier to be workable and to have good results, certain conditions must apply to medical services providers. First, medical services providers must be independent entities operating on their own initiative, taking responsibility for both profits and losses so that there are inherent constraints on internal incentives as well as external competition. This is the case whether or not the institutions are public or private and whether they are for-profit or non-profit entities. Second, medical services providers have to be part of a sufficiently competitive pattern. If they cannot decide on their own operations and are not responsible for their own profits and losses, then they fundamentally have no incentive to lower the actual procurement prices of drugs. The reason is that profits and losses have no effect on them. If they cannot be part of a competitive situation, they lack the external constraints that competition brings into play. A medical services provider that enjoys a monopoly will use its monopoly position to the utmost – it will adopt highly opportunistic behavior, such as the over-prescribing of drugs.

1.3 Centralized drug procurement, reimbursement standards of drugs covered by medical insurance, and price-formation of drugs

In contrast with countries that have fairly mature price-formation mechanisms for drugs, in China, the problem of exorbitant prices has not been resolved. Price distortions still exist, despite the fact that China eliminated the setting of prices by administrative fiat some time ago and moved in the direction of price-determination done primarily by the market. In 2015, the reform of drug price-formation mechanisms in China required that any drug included in the reimbursement list for insurance purposes had to be adjusted to conform to insurance reimbursement standards. Over the past few years, various regions have carried out experiments and explorations into how to do this and have come up with two main measures. The first is to use the price at which a drug won the bidding in centralized procurement as the insurance reimbursement standard. The second is to use a linkage mechanism of lowest prices as the insurance reimbursement standard. In this case, the lowest bid-winning price in a nationwide or region-wide area becomes the reimbursement standard. Both of these methods are different from the way prices are set in other countries, where either prevailing reference prices or reimbursement standards are used.

The operating philosophy, basic principles, and the underlying incentive mechanisms of 'centralized drug procurement' are different from those of 'reimbursement standards.' Centralized drug procurement uses the monopoly buying power of the payer to carry out strategic purchasing, and it uses the principle of gaining a lower price in return for buying a larger quantity. The basic philosophy behind the use of reference prices and reimbursement standards is that they provide incentives to both buyers and sellers of drugs, including hospitals, clinics, and retail pharmacies. These voluntarily keep prices low in order to gain more margin between the 'reimbursement standard' and the actual buying and selling prices. In other countries, the primary entities carrying out centralized purchasing are such medical services providers as hospitals, clinics, and retail pharmacies as well as drug supply companies. GPOs, group purchasing organizations, provide group purchasing services to these buying and selling entities. What a 'reference price' or a 'reimbursement standard' provides is simply the price at which insurance reimburses. It does not in fact imply any responsibility for actual purchasing. In fact, in England, which has a National Health Service system, even the NHS[1] has no specific responsibility for purchasing. It simply pays retail pharmacies according to the mandated reimbursement schedule (reimbursement standards).

In China, once the National Health Security Administration was established (in 2018), it took on the function of centralized drug procurement. It undertook two measures in order to force down excessively high prices: first, it introduced negotiated drug prices into the process of determining the insurance reimbursement list. For example, through negotiations, it lowered the price of 17 kinds of anticancer drugs. Second, it implemented the key focus of centralized procurement, which is 'procurement with specified quantities.'

Both of these steps followed the line of thinking of centralized procurement, in that they did strategic purchasing by making use of the status of medical insurance as the largest payer. In the short term, these methods may be able to force drug prices lower, but they will have no fundamental reforming effect on the price-formation of drugs.

In the 1980s and 1990s, medical institutions were the main entities buying and selling drugs in China. Starting in 2000, centralized procurement in fact deprived these entities of their drug-buying and drug-selling authority. Such procurement was done first at the prefecture level (of government), and then shifted toward government-guided centralized procurement at the provincial level. Meanwhile, the 'zero markup in drug sales policy' that was initiated as part of the reform of public hospitals also deprived hospitals of their ability to make economic-management decisions about drugs. Nevertheless, several decades of experience now shows

1 National Health Service, as represented by the United Kingdom and the Nordic countries.

that, despite having deprived hospitals of these authorities, exorbitantly high drug prices continue to be a problem.

1.4 Objectives of the reform of price-formation mechanisms with respect to drugs in China

Medical insurance is the largest 'payer' for drugs in China. The practice of centralized procurement can be used in the short term in pricing those drugs and can even be used in negotiations for insurance reimbursement standards. In the long run, however, further reform is necessary. Given the reality that China has already established a universal health insurance system, China may learn from drug-pricing practices of other countries and regions, and its objectives for reform should be the following:

First, prices for drugs should be able to reflect the realities of supply and demand for drugs. Any payments for hospital services and doctors' services should be removed from the pricing of drugs, so that the distortions of 'institutional costs' are completely eliminated.

Second, reform should help encourage innovation. At the same time, it should ensure access to affordable drugs and the sustainability of health insurance funds.

Third, price-formation mechanisms should be based on the market. Health insurance drug reimbursement standards should mainly be used only as a way to make adjustments.

1.5 Separating payment for 'medical treatment' from payments for 'medicines'

In order to realize these functions, we have to carve away the burden of paying for hospitals and doctors' services from the price of drugs. Paying for these things should fundamentally not be the function of insurance reimbursements for drugs. Instead, to realize separate payment for medical treatment and drugs, we should set up a payment system for hospitals and doctors that is solely tailored to that purpose.

Since Reform and Opening Up began, China has never set up a payment system that functions solely for hospitals and doctors. In setting one up, the general direction must be to carry out 'de-administering' reform. Instead, reform should set up a pattern of supplying medical services that is commercially managed, based on competitive practices, and that offers the ability to compare one service to another. From the perspective of what is actually feasible, we first must reform the *bianzhi* system of public institutions, that is, their system of appointed staffing (with its hierarchy of appointed positions). We must 'liberate' doctors from a system that forces them to rely on public medical institutions, and form a pattern whereby doctors are free professionals and can work in different places. When doctors have mobility, we can then form price structures that are aimed just at doctors' services.

The first step in 'liberating doctors' is to reform the *bianzhi* system of public institutions. This means gradually carving away the policy protections and hidden benefits that lie behind the system. It means turning the staffing of public institutions into an instrument of management, a method by which doctors themselves select where they want to work and how they work. Doctors will then rely on their own levels of expertise, as well as their risk and income preferences, in deciding where to work. They will not rely on the institutional policies that apply to the staff-appointments system of public institutions.

Before we can realize this ideal situation, however, we can consider pegging the pay scales of doctors to average wages in non-governmental jobs – that is, we first set up a payment schedule for doctors' services. As for medical insurance, we can gradually set up a system whereby doctors and health insurance sign agreements directly with one another as part of the establishment of a medical insurance/doctors system. Reimbursements from insurance would then be made directly to doctors who have signed up under the medical insurance program.

Second, we should separate out doctors' services from the services of hospitals. With respect to hospitals, reform of pay schedules should be done in line with the reform that is currently under way that will pay hospitals according to category of illness via diagnosis related groups. The particular focus should be on shifting the direct subsidies that public finance pays to hospitals (the supply side) to subsidizing the demand side, and incorporating such subsidies into payments for specific types of illness. This would mean going from a direct annual subsidy-payment system toward a system whereby (the government) purchases services.

1.6 Establish and optimize the payment standards by which medical insurance reimburses for drugs

While separating out payment for medical services and reimbursement for drugs, we also need to focus on a shift in how we handle the pricing of reimbursement for drugs. The current method is primarily centralized procurement, but this should gradually shift toward using medical insurance reimbursement standards. In constructing these standards, we should conduct reform according to the saying 'move forward in the proper sequence and in incremental fashion, and first separate the issue into categories.' The reform should be integrated with our reform of the method of paying medical insurance, reform of public hospitals, and reform of the centralized procurement of drugs. We should focus first on hospitals and later on clinics.

First, synchronize reform of reimbursement standards with reform of the methods of paying insurance. Set up a system of inpatient fees according to type of illness, and incorporate the cost of drugs into the package, together with type of illness costs. Have hospitals conduct drug procurement themselves and manage inpatient medicines. Medical insurance pays in one unified package, according to predetermined payment standards.

Second, gradually carve away the system that requires people to buy drugs from the hospital's own pharmacy – loosen controls and allow prescriptions to be fulfilled on the outside. Before this, however, strengthen supervision over commercial pharmacies. Set up mandatory systems for disclosure of pharmacies' drug price data to authorities, as well as open information to the public at large. Coordinate this with the cultivation of a professional cadre of pharmacists. Have these pharmacists sign agreements with the medical insurance system.

Third, gradually set up medical insurance drug reimbursement standards that are based on price surveys and commercial negotiations. With respect to innovative drugs and high-value drugs, establish payment standards through negotiations as well as the 'price for quantity' program of centralized procurement. Accelerate economic evaluations of innovative drugs, so as to have a basis on which negotiations for reimbursement standards can proceed.

Fourth, with respect to generic drugs, the priority is to push forward consistency evaluations and upgrade quality. Given higher quality, the next step is to speed up the substitution of generics for patented drugs. Strengthen regulatory monitoring of such aspects of generics as quality, safety, and efficacy. Increase regulatory controls, even if a drug has passed consistency evaluations, in order to prevent the kind of opportunistic behavior that some companies may adopt in trying to lower production costs. Having consistency evaluations is a prerequisite for setting up reimbursement standards for generic drugs.

The reimbursement standard for generic drugs will be based on the average market price, but can be adjusted depending on the ability of medical insurance funds to pay. In the beginning stage, we recommend using drug prices of countries that are at the same level of economic and social development as China as reference points in determining China's own drug reimbursement standards.

2 Reform of China's drug-pricing mechanisms and policy options[2]

Issues surrounding drug prices are a concentrated expression of all the various problems in China's medical sphere. Making order out of China's drug prices has been the emphasis and focus of all the medical reforms that have taken place since the start of Reform and Opening Up. Price-formation mechanisms have undergone several changes since planned-economy controls were gradually loosened in the 1980s. In the 1980s and 1990s, prices set by administrative fiat co-existed with prices determined by the market. After 2000, the employees and workers' drug reimbursement list for medical insurance had an administrative limit on the highest price of a given drug. By 2015, all administrative controls were taken off drug prices altogether. A number of other policies came out that were related to drug price-formation. However, in looking at the results of all of these reforms, the way

2 This 'study of drug-pricing mechanism' is the third research in the project 'Implementation of Drug list of Medical Insurance in China' organized by China Development Research Foundation. This report is written by Wang Zhen, a professor of the Institute of Economics, Chinese Academy of Social Sciences. The views expressed in this report are those of the author's and do not reflect the views of the author's employer or other institutions.

drugs are priced has not yet in fact been ironed out. The 'exorbitant' problem still has not been resolved. In some cases, the more we play this game, the worse it gets.

The international experience indicates that the market serves as the basis of price-formation, but even here, administrative controls and monopoly-type buying by medical insurance can also be the prevailing practice. Many commonly used policy implements are key factors in the pricing of drugs – including controls over markup rates, use of reference-price systems, reimbursement standards used by medical insurance, and so on.

Nevertheless, China's price-formation has its own unique characteristics and logic. Specifically, the prices of drugs have never been purely a 'price' issue. Behind prices lie such issues as compensation of doctors, operating mechanisms of public hospitals, and administrative controls over health insurance. Although medical institutions have been through several rounds of reform since Reform and Opening Up, to this day no reasonable systems have been set up by which doctors and hospitals can get paid. As a result, there is no reasonable system for pricing doctors' services. Given this situation, drug prices have taken on the function of paying for the costs of doctors and hospitals in China – that is, they have assumed the function of 'paying for medicine through drugs,' which essentially means funding hospital operations with profits from overpriced drugs. To address the problem of China's drug price-formation mechanisms, therefore, we first must resolve the issue of how to pay hospitals and how to price doctors. Only on that basis can we straighten out drug prices. To a large degree, China's current policy measures with respect to reforming the drug-pricing structures in the country are a matter of resolving this issue of paying for medicine through drugs. When it comes to drug pricing, this is the greatest difference between China and western countries.

With this as the general context for the discussion, the following attempts to answer several questions. First, what in fact are China's drug price-formation mechanisms? What is the process by which prices are formed? What key problems are there? What are the systemic causes of these problems? What should China's price-formation mechanisms look like in the future? How can this reform objective be realized? Before entering into an analysis of all of the specifics, we still need to straighten out the theoretical framework for the subject. At the same time, we review international practices in drug pricing.

3 Drug-pricing policy and theoretical framework

3.1 Theoretical framework

3.1.1 Definition of the equilibrium price

To determine if drug prices are exorbitantly high or unreasonably low, the 'real price' of drugs must be defined. According to general economic theory, a 'real' price is defined as the point when there is an equilibrium between supply and demand. In a completely competitive market, the equilibrium price is the price at which the supply of drugs is equal to the demand for drugs. Naturally, in reality, an equilibrium price is hard to observe given the many intervention policies that exist and also given an imperfect market. Only by using this theoretical 'equilibrium price,' however, can we define how much prices in the real world deviate from equilibrium prices. When drug prices in China are actually higher than a theoretical equilibrium price, they are 'exorbitant' or unreasonably high. When they are lower than the equilibrium price, they can be called 'unreasonably low.'

The market for drugs in the real world is imperfect. As compared to manufacturing in general, it does not satisfy the requirements of a completely competitive market for quite obvious reasons: first, patent protections insert a monopoly element into production processes; second, in procuring drugs, both medical insurance and group purchasing (a buyer's monopoly) affect prices; third, in prescribing drugs, the asymmetry of information between doctors and patients and the behavior of hospitals and doctors influence the price of drugs.

3.1.2 Patent production of innovative drugs and prices of new drugs

The prevailing practice in modern economies is to grant producers of innovative products a period of patent protection, a monopoly, in order to encourage innovation. This is true with respect to drugs in many countries. During the period of patent protection, monopoly producers of such drugs will generally set a fairly high price on them in order to maximize profit. Naturally, behind the high price is the high cost of developing the drug – this goes for both patented drugs and 'original-research' drugs (what are sometimes referred to as reference listed drugs. The Chinese term is original-research drugs). The United States is the largest producer of new drugs. The R&D costs of each new drug that the FDA approves in that country average USD 2.558 billion (see Figure 3.1). In 2016, the investment that the largest ten pharmaceutical companies put into research and development was equivalent to 17% of their gross income. In the aeronautics and space industries, the percentage was just 3%. In the computer and electronics industries, it was just 9%.[3]

Patent protection of new drugs helps drug companies recover R&D costs by allowing them to charge high prices. On the one hand, this encourages innovation, but on the other it leads to rising medical costs. Between these two considerations, there has to be an appropriate balance. The use of generics is the primary policy tool that can help strike that balance – once a patent has expired, governments encourage the use of generics to substitute for innovative drugs and thereby lower drug prices.

3.1.3 Medical insurance and drug procurement

The chain of drug price-formation involves three pricing stages. The first is the *ex factory* price, namely the price at which the manufacturer supplies drugs to the wholesaler. The second is the price at which the wholesaler supplies to the retailer,

3 Scott Fry. *US Pharmaceutical Pricing: An Overview*, 2019, URL: https://axenehp.com/us-pharmaceuticalpricing-overview/.

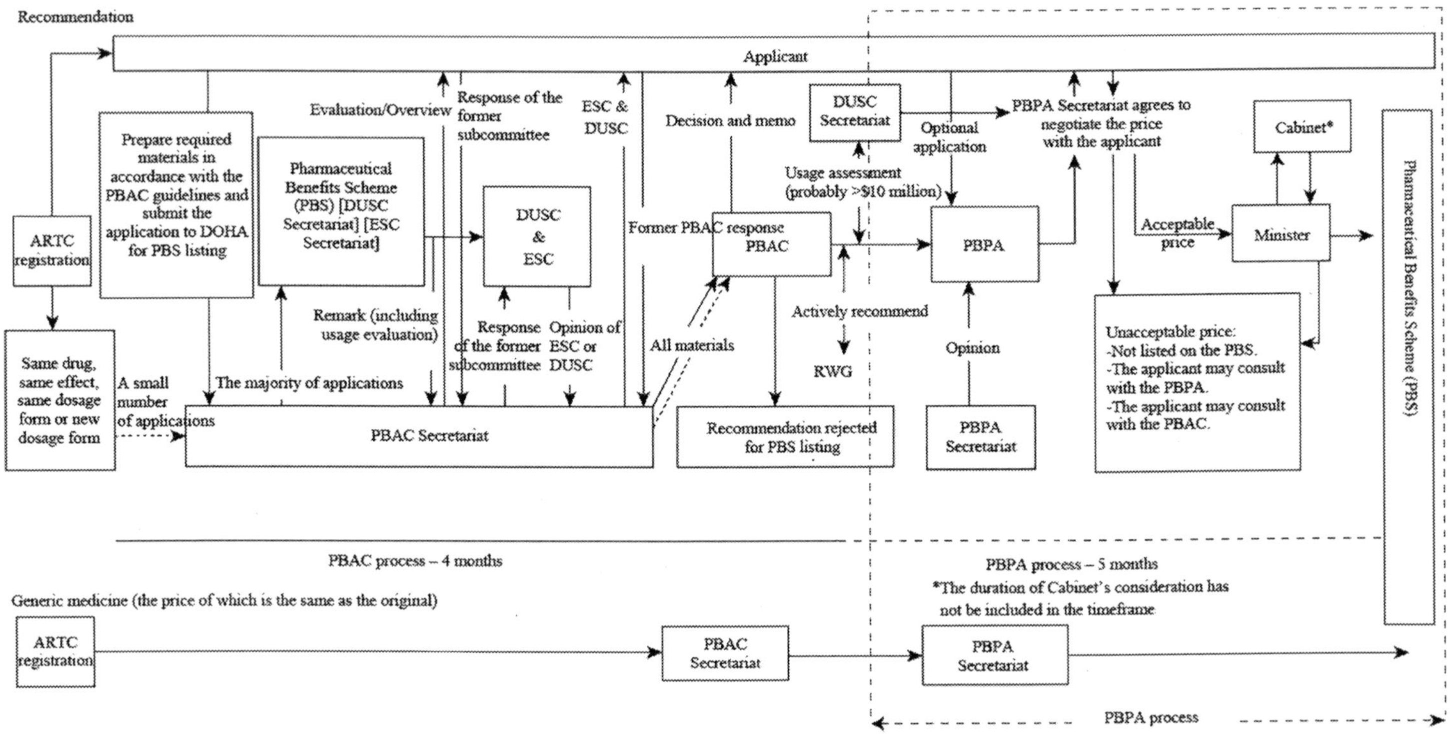

Figure 3.1 Average Development Costs of Different Types of New Drugs Approved by the U.S. FDA (Unit: U.S. 100 Million)

Source: Avik S. A. Roy, The competition prescription: a market-based plan for making innovative medicines affordable, The Foundation for Research on Equal Opportunity, URL: https://freopp.org/a-market-based-plan-foraffordable-prescription-drugs-931e31024e08, 2019

Note: Inflation not taken into account. USD of 2013 is used.

that is, the wholesale price. The third is the price at which the retailer sells to the customer, that is, the final retail price or the consumer price.

Price-formation in the case of drugs is different from other products in that medical insurance, as the largest payer for drugs, is inserted into the process. Modern medical insurance not only provides safeguards against the risk of illness to those who are insured, but it also uses its advantages as a monopoly to affect the price of drugs. This is particularly true in the case of universal medical insurance as well as countries that have a national healthcare system, such as the U.K.'s NHS.[4] In these cases, the drug payment terms (reimbursement) by insurance companies play a key role in the price-formation of drugs. Different companies and regions influence drug prices in various ways, but the logic behind their actions is the same, namely to use the group buying power of medical insurance and their buyer's monopoly to affect prices. Specific models by which they do this include directly mandating prices, and using a 'reference price' system.

3.1.4 The influence of drug use on drug prices

The 'use' of medicines is different from that of other products, in that patients must go through the process of getting a prescription from a doctor before they can purchase and use the drug. In this process, doctors hold an information advantage. In theory, doctors can potentially use this advantage to seek their own maximum benefit. Drug prices may therefore be affected by the prescribing behavior of doctors. The following two factors serve to constrain the impact that prescribing behavior has on drugs.

The first is the extent to which the market for medical services is competitive. A competitive market can help dissolve the information advantage of doctors and thereby constrain opportunistic behavior. In the long term, the possibility that doctors will use their information advantage to their own ends diminishes if a market maintains competitiveness. If a market exhibits the long-term existence of self-serving behavior on the part of doctors, such behavior indicates that the degree of competitiveness in a market is low.

The second factor is whether or not medical services are separate and distinct from the selling of drugs. That is, are pharmaceuticals operated as a separate industry or are the operations of the two combined. In systems in which they are separate, the income of doctors and income from selling drugs are two separate things, which reduces the possibility that doctors will use their information advantage to seek profit. In situations where the two are combined, however, when doctors' incomes and the income from drug sales are mixed in together, it is more likely that doctors will exhibit opportunistic behavior.

4 The NHS (typical countries are the U.K. and northern European countries) is different from social medical insurance in terms of funding (it is funded by government) and operations. But both of them serve as buyer in monopoly.

3.2 Policy framework for drug pricing

In a perfectly competitive market, the real price of drugs is equal to the equilibrium price, at which supply equals demand. The actual price of drugs is subject to different influences, however, in the course of price-formation. Policy interventions can address each of the three stages of drug prices, and can be divided into the two main categories of supply-side policies and demand-side policies.

Supply-side policies are focused on the R&D, production, and distribution links in the supply process. At the R&D stage, most countries extend patent protection to companies in order to encourage drug innovation. This policy has to be balanced with policies that try to control overly fast growth in pharmaceutical costs. While setting up patent protections, therefore, some countries also formulate policies that encourage the substitution of generics. At the production stage, the strictest controls involve prices set by administrative fiat, that is, the government mandates fixed prices of drugs and the manufacturer has no alternative but to price drugs accordingly. A slightly more lenient approach is to set a limit on the price of drugs – in this case, the government sets a ceiling price. The manufacturer can set prices at anything below that but cannot exceed the limit. At the delivery stage, the customary market procedure in most countries is to add a markup to the wholesale and retail prices. Some countries put controls on these markups and mandate a fixed markup rate, or a highest markup rate. In addition, some countries put limits on a manufacturer's profitability (rate) at the production stage and require that the manufacturer set prices that allow for only a certain degree of profitability. In addition, policy interventions can also occur at the tax-revenue stage of drug production. Such interventions can include, for example, value-added tax.

Demand-side policies focus on the users of drugs and the payer of drug costs. These policies are not directly aimed at prices but they influence the way drugs actually get priced. First, policies can seek to control the prescribing behavior of doctors and hospitals. For example, they can draw up the lists of drugs that will or will not be covered by medical insurance, or by the national health system of the country. They can require doctors to prescribe according to specific guidelines, and they can set limits on the total value of prescriptions made by a doctor or hospital. By constraining the prescribing behavior of doctors and hospitals, such policies influence the sale of drugs and their price.

Second, policies can address the patient side of demand. In countries in which medical insurance or a national health system covers costs, drug 'consumption' is actually paid for by a third party, not the end consumer, so it is necessary to put restraints on the consumer. The most commonly used policy in this case is to have the patient pay some of the cost, or a 'co-pay.' The threat of having to pay a high co-pay helps constrain the end-users' behavior. Another policy on the patient side is the use of generic drugs. If a generic drug can be substituted for a patent drug, then medical insurance pays the price of the generic – if the patient wants to use a non-generic, he or she pays the difference.

A third type of policy intervention relates to insurance payment, and this mainly involves the 'reference price' system. The system of using reference prices can be divided into two parts, one that uses external reference prices and one that uses internal reference prices. 'External' refers to using reference prices for drugs that are outside the boundaries of the country or region. These are taken as reference to help determine the prices of drugs inside the country or to determine the reimbursement standards of medical insurance. 'Internal' refers to the prices that are determined by group negotiations or through drug price surveys within an area. These then are used to determine the country's drug prices or insurance reimbursement standards.

Table 3.1 summarizes the drug-pricing policies generally used by the European Union and some OECD countries. Naturally, these policies are not adopted by every country or region, since different countries adopt policies that apply to their

Table 3.1 Drug-Pricing Policies of the EU and Some OECD Countries

Supply Side		
Innovation and R&D	Patent protection	Grant patent protection to innovation medicines. Allow monopoly and high prices of innovative drugs.
	Generic substitution	Encourage generic substitution.
Price regulation	Fixing price	Fix prices of all drugs or drugs covered by medical insurance (government pricing)
	Price cap	Set a price cap for all drugs or drugs covered by medical insurance. Enterprise's price shall not exceed the price cap.
	Markup regulation	Regulate markup rate in distribution.
Profit regulation	Profit control	Control the maximum profit (rate) of pharmaceutical companies, requiring pharmaceutical companies to set drug prices in accordance with the mandated maximum profit rate.
	Tax benefit	Regulate VAT or other taxes concerning drugs.
Demand side		
Doctors/ Hospitals	Positive list	Medical security or NHS only pays for drugs in the list.
	Negative list	Medical security or NHS pays for drugs not covered in the list.
	Guidelines	Doctors must prescribe in accordance with the guidelines. Drugs not covered in the guidelines are not reimbursed.
	Spending cap	Set a spending cap of prescription drug fees for doctors and hospitals.
Patients	Co-pay	Patients pay part of the drug fees.
	Generic substitution	Medical security reimburses according to prices of generic drugs, and patients pay for the remaining part.
Payment of medical insurance	External pricing reference	Determine drug prices according to drug prices in one or several countries or regions.
	Internal pricing reference	Determine drug payment price through negotiations or mean price surveys.

Source: T. Stargardt & S. Vandoros, Pharmaceutical pricing and reimbursement regulation in Europe, *Encyclopedia of Health Economics*, 2014(3): 29–36.

Sabine Vogler & Katharina Habimana, Pharmaceutical pricing policies in European countries, 2014, Vienna: Gesundheit Osterreich, URL: https://pdfs.semanticscholar.org/32a8/48962eb48cd5045a2752a91ecce475424f77.pdf.

Monique F. Mrazek, Comparative approaches to pharmaceutical price regulation in the European Union, *Croatian Medical Journal*, 2002, 43(4): 453–461.

Paula Tele & Wim Groot, Cost containment measures for pharmaceuticals expenditure in the EU countries: a comparative analysis, *The Open Health and Policy Journal*, 2009, 2: 71–83.

own situations. Some countries are inclined in the direction of using government interventions in price-formation, while others are more inclined to let the market determine prices. Still other countries are in between, and emphasize the role of commercial negotiation. In what follows, this report (Table 3.1) gives an overview of the specific policies of four typical countries and regions with respect to drug-pricing policies.

4 Review of the drug-pricing policies of four typical countries and regions

The following describes the drug-pricing policies of four countries and regions: the United States, Germany, the U.K., and Taiwan, China. These four have been chosen because each is a prime example of different ways to fund medical and healthcare systems. The United States has a system that combines public medical insurance with private medical insurance. Germany has a typical social medical insurance system. The U.K. has a National Health Service system that is based on funding from public finance, while Taiwan, China, has a universal health insurance system. The second reason for choosing these four is that each has its own way of coming up with drug pricing. The United States is the largest manufacturer of innovative drugs in the world, and it also has the highest medical costs and drug expenses in the world. Its patent protection system has a strong impact on the price of drugs. As a social medical insurance country, Germany uses a well-seasoned reference-price system for determining drug prices. In the U.K., the National Health Service adopts a value-based payment system. The system that Taiwan, China, still implements is similar to that of mainland China in that it mixes together medical treatment and the prescribing of drugs.

4.1 The drug-pricing system in the United States

One distinctive feature of the U.S. drug-pricing system is its high degree of market competition. R&D, production, sales, procurement, and usage – all stages in the process are based on market competition. On top of this market competition, however, the country also uses a considerable amount of public intervention policies in coming up with its drug-pricing system.

4.1.1 Patent protection for innovative drugs, and generic substitution

The United States is the largest producer of innovative drugs in the world and is indeed the center of global innovation in this sphere. This is intimately related to the country's patent protections for innovative drugs. Back in 1938, the United States passed the *Food, Drugs, and Cosmetic Act*, which set up the Food and Drug Administration (FDA). This required a permitting process for drugs that were new to the market. In 1962, the *Kefauver Harris Amendment* required that all drugs undergo clinical trials to test for safety and effectiveness before going on the market, a provision that included both innovative drugs and generic drugs.

However, one aspect of this Amendment was that it set a fairly short period for patent protection of innovative drugs. Meanwhile, generics had to go through the same clinical-trial process as innovative drugs, which meant that it took a long time for them to reach the market. Not only was this was detrimental to the development of innovative drugs, but it also held generics back from reaching the market once patents on innovative drugs had expired.

In 1984, Congress passed the Hatch-Waxman Act, also known as the *Drug Price Competition and Patent Term Restoration Act*. This attempted to strike a balance between patent protection and the substitution of generics. It extended protections of innovative drugs to 14 years.[5] Meanwhile, not only could generic drug manufacturers carry out trials during the time when patents were still valid, but their drugs could be allowed on the market by just producing evidence that the effective ingredients of these generics, and their bio-equivalent results, were similar to those of innovative drugs.

The substitution of generics has an extremely obvious effect on lowering drug prices. Comparative research undertaken in 12 countries shows that prices decline by as much as 66% from the price of the original drug within one to five years after the expiration of that drug's patent.[6] Countries in the research included the United States, Canada, Australia, the U.K., Germany, and France. The speed at which generics force prices to decline once a patent expires has been called the 'Patent Cliff.'

Despite the impact that generic substitution has on lowering prices, however, the great majority of total payments for drugs in these countries continues to be spent on innovative drugs. In the United States, the largest producer of innovative drugs, more than 80% of prescriptions prescribe generics, but the majority of actual expenditures on drugs is for innovative drugs. In 2016, the country prescribed USD 333.9 billion worth of innovative drugs and USD 50.1 billion worth of branded generic drugs. It prescribed only USD 36.1 billion worth of non-branded generic drugs (Figure 3.2).

4.1.2 Public medical insurance reimbursements for drugs

The United States uses a classic 'mixed system' of coverage for medical safeguards. In 2016, Medicare, Medicaid, CHIP, and other publicly funded programs covered 37.3% of the total population. Private health insurance (both for-profit and not-for-profit) covered 67.5%. Within the publicly funded component, Medicaid provided coverage to 19.4% of the population and Medicare provided coverage to 16.7%. Within private health insurance, employers provided medical insurance

5 Before the Hatch-Waxman Act was enacted, the average patent term was nine years. After the Hatch-Waxman Act was enacted, the average patent term was extended to 11.5 years. Jinxi Din. A preliminary analysis of patent term extension in the U.S.: Lessons from Hatch-Waxman Act to promote the pharmaceutical industry in China. *Chinese Journal of Pharmaceuticals*, 2006 (09).

6 Gerard T. Vondeling, Qi Cao, Maarten J. Postma, et al. The impact of patent expiry on drug price: A systematic literature review. *Applied Health Economics and Health Policy*, 2018 (16): 653–660.

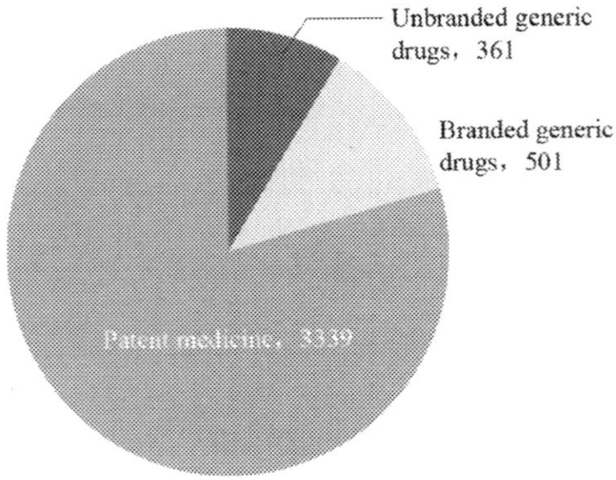

Figure 3.2 Spending on Prescription and Generic Drugs in the U.S. (2016; Unit: USD 100 Million)

Source: Avik S. A. Roy, *The competition prescription: a market-based plan for making innovative medicines affordable*, The Foundation for Research on Equal Opportunity, URL: https://freopp.org/a-market-based-plan-foraffordable-prescription-drugs-931e31024e08, 2019.

coverage for 55.7% of the total population, while individuals who purchase coverage directly constituted 16.2% of the population.[7] Although public health insurance does not cover the majority of people, and constitutes only 40% of total insurance costs, policies relating to insurance reimbursement for this kind of insurance have a very large impact on drug prices.

Medicare reimbursement of drugs comes in three categories, Part A for drugs used by inpatients in hospitals, Part B for such drugs as injections that must be used either in a clinic or the outpatient clinic of a hospital, and Part D for some prescription drugs (self-managed drugs).[8]

The *Centers for Medicare and Medicaid Services* (CMS)[9] authorizes private insurance companies to handle the reimbursements of drugs under Part D. Companies design various Part D plans – the rates and also services of these Part D plans are different and the insured person may select an option that suits their needs. Medicare is responsible only for the subsidized portion of the cost, as well as for supervising the overall operation, but it does not handle the specifics of individual plans.

7 Jessica C. Barentt and Edward R. Berchick. *Health Insurance Coverage in the United States: 2016, U.S. Department of Commerce, Economics and Statistics Administration*. U.S. Census Bureau. Population covered by different insurance plans overlap, so, the sum is over 100%. In fact, in 2016, about 10% of people in the U.S. were not covered by any medical insurance.

8 Patients can take self-administered drugs, such as most oral medications, on their own, though such drugs are prescription drugs.

9 CMS is a division under the U.S. Department of Health and Human Services. It is in charge of public medical insurance and medical aid.

Medicare has formulated payment standards for drugs used in clinics under Part B. It makes payments to the hospital or the physicians' clinic according to these standards, irrespective of the price at which the hospital or clinic has bought in the drugs. The hospital or clinic is responsible for any profit or loss due to the price differential. The CMS payment standards use the Average Sales Price (ASP), a market average, and add on 6% markup (ASP + 6%).[10] For single-source drugs, the ASP is determined by taking the average in different markets. For multiple-source drugs, the ASP is determined by taking the average of the generic name of the drug. Drug suppliers must provide the CMS with semi-annual reports of drug prices, which are used by CMS to determine payment standards.

In the 1980s, Medicare began using a system of advance payment to hospitals according to Diagnosis Related Groups.[11] Drugs under Part A of Medicare were then tied to the hospital's services – that is, the payment for drugs was a specific and fixed amount, depending on the type of illness. Given this change, hospitals now had to exercise control of all costs it incurred for a given illness group, including the cost of drugs. Hospitals still purchased drugs from CMS according to the CMS payment standards by illness group. The principle behind this payment model was similar to the principle behind payment standards, namely that hospitals, as medical service suppliers, would negotiate harder with drug suppliers on the pricing and quantity of drugs.

4.1.3 Group purchasing of drugs and drug pricing

Given drug payment standards by which hospitals were reimbursed, and given the way in which payments were bundled with services, hospitals were now motivated to negotiate with drug suppliers for the most beneficial price to themselves. The ability of a single hospital, or clinic, or pharmacy to negotiate with drug suppliers is limited however. The transaction costs are also high. For this reason, such buyers turned to Group Purchasing Organizations. These had already begun in the 1960s, when Medicare and Medicaid were set up, but they now grew rapidly. By today, more than 97% of medical services providers have joined either one or more Group Purchasing Organizations. Roughly 72% of the drugs used in hospitals are purchased through such groups. This kind of collective buying of drugs actually began in 1910 in the United States, but developed only slowly until the appearance of Medicare and Medicaid. In the 1960s, the appearance of public medical insurance and its method of reimbursing for drugs gave hospitals the incentive to negotiate with drug suppliers in order to receive kickbacks. This lowered their actual purchase price. GPOs developed rapidly in this environment. Their services

10 MEDPAC (Medicare Payment Advisory Commission). Medicare and the health care delivery system. *Report to the Congress*, 2017, URL: http://medpac.gov/docs/default-source/reports/jun18_medpacreporttocongress_sec.pdf.

11 NORC at the University of Chicago. *Trends in Hospital Inpatient Drug Costs: Issues and Challenges*, 2016, URL: www.aha.org/system/files/2018-01/aha-fah-rx-report.pdf.

to medical service providers include, first, lowering the transaction cost by going through a professional pharmaceutical buyer, and second, negotiating with drug suppliers from a monopoly-buyer position.

GPOs in fact receive 'kickbacks' on drug prices by using their monopoly buyer status. This, however, is illegal under the U.S. legal system. Because of this, as GPOs developed, the United States began passing legislation that exempted GPOs from legal liability when they took such kickbacks on drug prices. In 1986, Congress revised relevant laws to say that the price kickbacks between GPOs and drug suppliers did not contravene U.S. laws.[12] In 1991, the Department of Health and Human Services signed a 'safe harbor' provision that implemented specific rules in this regard, and that set 3% of the purchase price of drugs as the fee that drug suppliers could pay to GPOs.

In theory, GPOs that carry out group purchasing of drugs should help lower the actual buying price of drugs and thereby the total costs of medical care. However, there is no empirical evidence[13] to show that this is so. Some research on the subject believes that GPOs actually are motivated to increase the price of drugs, since they are allowed to earn 3% of the purchasing price. At the very least, they wish to keep drug prices at a fairly high level, which makes it hard to reach the goal of lowering overall costs. Other research believes, however, that GPOs have plenty of reason to try to lower drug prices given the intense competition in the business. The U.S. Government Accountability Office has done an investigative survey which has not yet produced any definitive evidence.[14] Whatever the case, GPOs are an indispensable and major part of the price-formation of drugs in the United States.

4.2 Drug-pricing policies in Germany

Germany comprises the largest market for pharmaceuticals in Europe. In 2016, the country's total drug sales volume came to EU 40.98 billion (USD 44.2 billion). Germany's pricing system is based on market-determined prices. Any drugs entering Germany, whether patented or generic, need only receive a permit from the European Medicines Agency (EMA) and they can then be sold on the German market and the *ex factory* price of the drug can be set as the manufacturer wishes. However, Germany is also a classic case of social medicine insurance. Over 90% of residents are covered by statutory health insurance. The remaining 10% must, as per legal requirements, participate in private health insurance plans. In 2015, within the total healthcare costs of EU 344 billion, statutory insurance paid out EU 200 billion, or 58%. Government and individuals paid out EU 113.5 billion,

12 Safe harbor provisions.

13 Marilyn M. Singleton. Group purchasing organizations: Gaming the system. *Journal of American Physicians and Surgeons*, 2018, 23(2): 38–42.

14 GAO (US Government Accountability Office). Group purchasing organizations: Funding structure has potential implications for Medicare costs. *Report to Congressional Requesters*, 2014, URL: www.gao.gov/assets/670/666644.pdf.

or 33%.[15] Given this, it is clear that Germany's medical insurance has a decisive impact on drugs and payment systems in the country.

Three price concepts should be clarified in order to understand Germany's drug-pricing system. The first is the *ex factory* price, which the manufacturer determines. The second is the reference price, which is provided by the health insurance company. The third is the actual selling price that hospitals or clinics charge for drugs. The key to Germany's drug-pricing system, however, is the 'drug reference price' which medical insurance puts forth.

4.2.1 Reference prices for drugs

Germany's medical insurance reimburses for drugs according to a reference price. This price is divided into two parts, one 'external' and one 'internal.' The external reference price is linked to prices in other countries or regions, whereas the internal reference price is self-determined according to relevant rules and regulations. Once the reference price is formulated, each critical illness fund pays hospitals or pharmacies according to that standard.

In Germany's medical insurance system, however, greater use is made of the internal reference system. In formulating this internal price, distinctions are made between innovative drugs and generic drugs.

Reference prices of generic drugs are calculated on the basis of the average sales price of all drugs in a relevant cluster. Clusters are made up of common-name generic drugs that have the same ingredients (chemical components, etc.).

The procedures for determining reference prices of innovative drugs are more complex. After a law was passed in 2008 called the *Health Insurance Competition Enhancing Act*, Germany's medical insurance went from being a 'passive recipient' to playing a more active role in formulating prices. First, a cost-benefit evaluation is done of the marginal therapeutic value of a given innovative drug in establishing a reference price. An innovative drug first must pass review by the European Pharmaceuticals Management Administration (EMA) in order to be sold on the German market, after which companies are free to set their own prices. If they want to be reimbursed by medical insurance, however, then they must apply to the Federal Joint Committee (G-BA).[16] This body authorizes the Institute for Quality and Efficiency in Health Care (IQWiG) to evaluate the 'marginal therapeutic value' of the drug in doing a cost-benefit assessment. Each assessment takes one

15 IGES Institute. *Reimbursement of Pharmaceuticals in Germany*, 2018, URL: www.iges.com/e15094/e15095/e15096/e17469/IGES_Reimbursement_Pharmaceuticals_2018_WEB_ger.pdf.

16 Germany's statutory health insurance is operated by independent sickness funds. In 2012, there were 136 sickness funds in Germany. Sickness funds across the country form the National Association of Statutory Health Insurance Funds (GKV-S). The GKV-S, the National Associations of Statutory Health Insurance Physicians and Dentists, and the German Hospital Federation join together and form the Federal Joint Committee (GBA). The GBA is a public legal entity in Germany. It develops policies concerning services of hospitals and physicians, payment policies of health insurance, reference prices of drugs, etc.

year, during which time the drug goes through numerous hearings and external critiques. After one year, the G-BA issues an assessment report on the marginal therapeutic-added of the drug. If this indicates there is *inadequate* additional value, then the drug is put directly into the group of generic-drug reference prices. If there is *sufficient* value-added, then the National Association of Statutory Health Insurance Funds (GKV-S) determines a reference price that is based on both the value added and the negotiations that it holds with the supplier of the drug.[17]

The previously mentioned reference prices are for prescription drugs sold in clinics and drugs used in the outpatient clinics of hospitals. For drugs used by patients staying in hospitals, Germany's medical insurance uses a DRGs–PPS payment system (Diagnosis Related Group – Prospective Payment System). The cost of drugs is incorporated into the illness category and insurance pays the sum together as a package. The medical-services provider determines the purchasing and price of drugs, which is arrived at by negotiations with the drug supplier. Germany's medical-services providers therefore also make tremendous use of Group Purchasing Organizations in order to lower prices.

4.2.2 Policies relating to the distribution and prescribing of drugs

In addition to systems that regulate reference prices of drugs, Germany has formulated policies that apply to the distribution and prescribing of drugs. The first type of such policies relates to distribution markups. Generally speaking, a specific markup rate applies to different stages of the process. A markup of 6% to 12% is added to the base *ex factory* price, for example, to come up with the wholesale price. Retail prices add 3% to the wholesale price.[18] Second, there is a mandatory discount at the retail level with respect to 'critical illness funds.' If a certain drug has not been entered into the reference-price system, then the seller of the drug must grant the fund a specific discount: for drugs that are still under a patent, that discount is 7%; for non-patented drugs, it is 6%. In 2016, 81% of all drugs had been placed in reference-price groups. The rest were all required to grant the corresponding discount to funds. Third, Germany places regulatory controls on the prescribing of drugs by doctors. These include a total annual budget for drug prescriptions that each doctor must stay within, a maximum limit on large prescriptions, guidelines for prescribing by doctors, and so on. Fourth, constraining mechanisms apply to how patients themselves use drugs. Each time a patient purchases drugs, a fixed sum of 5 to 10 euros must be paid as a fee. If the drug being purchased is within a reference-price group, and the actual price exceeds

17 Martin Wenzl and Valerie Paris. Pharmaceutical reimbursement and pricing in Germany. *OECD County Profiles*, 2018, URL: www.oecd.org/health/health-systems/Pharmaceutical-Reimbursement-and-Pricing-in-Germany.pdf.

18 T. Stargardt and S. Vandoros. Pharmaceutical pricing and reimbursement regulation in Europe. *Encyclopedia of Health Economics*, 2014 (3): 9–36.

the reference price, then the patient has to pay this fee. In 2016, 84% of all drug costs were paid for by insurance. The remaining 16% was paid for by individuals.

4.3 The drug-pricing system of the U.K.

The NHS (National Health Services) is the healthcare funding and services system of the U.K.[19] Unlike the funding of the social insurance system in Germany, funds for the NHS come entirely from general tax revenues. They do not come from premiums paid by individuals. The Department of Health in the U.K. and the NHS Management Committee, which is under the Department's jurisdiction, manage all affairs that have to do with the NHS. Among these are drug-pricing policies and drug reimbursement policies. One notable feature of the supply of medical and healthcare services in the country is its highly developed network of general practitioners (GPs) as well as its community hospitals and community pharmacies. General practitioners provide more than 90% of medical services and are the primary suppliers of NHS medical services. Publicly funded hospitals are primary in supplying medical services of hospitals in general, but they still only provide around 10% of all medical services. Although the NHS system is directly operated by government, in terms of its management model the NHS is based on market-oriented practices. For example, the general practitioners who constitute the bulk of medical service providers in the country are all in private practice. Meanwhile, the pricing system of drugs in the country is also market-based. The U.K. does not institute administrative controls over the *ex factory* price or the actual price of drugs, but it does in fact influence drug prices through a number of policy measures. This is done to coordinate two objectives, namely affordability (and therefore accessibility) of drugs, and control over total medical costs. These policies apply to three main areas: first, allowing drugs access to reimbursement depending on their value; second, pricing policies relating to innovative drugs; and third, pricing policies relating to generic drugs.

4.3.1 Access to reimbursement that is based on assessing value

In order to be reimbursed by the NHS, innovative drugs or new drugs that seek to enter the U.K. market must go through a pharmaco-economics evaluation, which looks at the therapeutic value of the drug. The National Institute for Health and Care Excellence (NICE) is the entity that carries out this process. It was set up in 1999, and its mandate is to determine whether or not drugs that have already passed the European Management Administration (EMA) requirements can be sold on the U.K. market. To do this, NICE mainly uses a cost-benefit analysis that is based on Quality-Adjusted Life Years (QALYs). If the cost of a new drug is below a certain

19 The NHS in U.K. consists of NHS England, NHS Scotland, NHS Wales, and NHS North Ireland. They have the same structure and follow the same principle, but each part is individually funded and managed. In this section, we are talking about NHS England.

threshold of QALY, that is, if using this drug leads to benefits that exceed QALY costs, then NICE recommends that the drug be entered into the NHS system. The threshold of drugs for general diseases is between 25,000–30,000 pounds per QALY. In other words, if a drug can result in savings of one QALY, then its cost must be less than 30,000 pounds. For drugs that are used at the end of life, the threshold can be raised to 50,000 pounds. For rare diseases that affect fewer than 1,000 people, the threshold can be raised to 100,000 to 300,000 pounds.[20]

4.3.2 Pricing of innovative drugs

NICE determines whether or not a new drug in the U.K. market will be covered by the NHA, but it does not intervene in drug pricing. The prices of innovative or branded drugs are mainly subject to intervention by the Pharmaceutical Price Regulatory Scheme (PPRS).

First, it must be clarified that drug manufacturers have the freedom to set their own prices if they wish. They participate in the PPRS on a voluntary basis. The Ministry of Health in the U.K., as representative of the 'payer,' and drug suppliers jointly hold negotiations on how to execute the plan. A new round of negotiations is held every five years. Naturally, if a given drug supplier does not participate in PPRS, the supplier must still abide by price regulations that are similar to those set forth by PPRS.

The main objective of the PPRS is to formulate price ceilings on innovative drugs for which the NHS will reimburse costs. This does not mean direct determination of a specific price as the ceiling. Instead, it involves setting a limit on the profit rate of the manufacturer of the drug. The manufacturer can set any price that allows the profit rate to come in below the limit set by the PPRS. Between 2013 and 2018, the return on sales to manufacturers was 6%, as determined by the selling price of drugs. The return on investment was 21%. If the actual profit of a given manufacturer does in fact exceed the limit as prescribed, then the surplus amount must be returned to the NHS in the following period, either through a reduction in price or through a discount.[21]

4.3.3 Pricing of generic drugs

Prices of generic drugs in the U.K. are established mainly by the market. The payment standards for generic drugs that are reimbursed by the NHS are determined

20 Leo Ewbank, David Omojomolo, Kane Sullivan and Helen McKenna. The rising cost of medicines to the NHS: What's the story? *The King's Fund*, 2018, URL: www.kingsfund.org.uk/sites/default/files/2018-04/Rising-cost-of-medicines.pdf.

21 Steven Morgan. Summaries of national drug coverage and pharmaceutical pricing policies in 10 countries. *Working Papers for the 2016 Meeting of the Vancouver Group in New York*, 2016, URL: www.commonwealthfund.org/sites/default/files/2018-09/Steven%20Morgan%2C%20PhD_Ten%20Country%20Pharma%20Policy%20Summaries_2016%20Vancouver%20Group%20Meeting.

by the Drug Price List of the U.K., which is revised once a month.[22] Once prices on this list are confirmed, the NHS makes reimbursements to pharmacies with which it has signed agreements. These pharmacies carry out their own negotiations with drug wholesalers or manufacturers. If the negotiated price is lower than the Drug Price List, then the pharmacy keeps the margin. The principle behind this way of operating is similar to that used by Germany in its own reimbursement standards for drugs.

In 2005, the U.K. government passed an act which makes it mandatory for NHS pharmacy contractors to provide relevant data about drug manufacturing and distribution. This was done in order to control the differential between prices on the Drug Tariff and actual prices at which drugs were being sold. Based on such information from pharmacies, the Department of Health may adjust prices on the List as a control over pharmacy profits. At the same time, in order to keep pharmacies from operating at a loss, the Department of Health adopted two additional measures. First, the Drug Tariff now included a service fee that NHS paid pharmacies for the various services that pharmacies provide. Second, if actual drug prices that pharmacies have to pay for drugs begin to surge past the prices established by the Tariff, then pharmacies may petition to the NHS for additional payment.

Generic drugs are used mainly in community healthcare settings in the U.K.[23] In 2016–2017, 81% of the total cost of prescription drugs in the U.K. came from doctors in such community healthcare locations.[24] This enormous use of generics in the U.K. has helped the country keep drug costs at a relatively low level.

4.4 *Drug pricing under the universal health insurance system of Taiwan, China*

Funding for medical safeguards in Taiwan, China, covers the entire population under a universal health insurance system. Similar to that of Germany, the system provides 'social medical insurance,' but it is not tied to employment and does not mainly serve those who are employed. Residents of Taiwan participate in health insurance at six specific levels or categories. Each has a different method of paying premiums and also a different rate. People employed by companies share the cost of premiums with their employer. Those who are unemployed share the cost with the government. Low-income groups are fully paid for by government. The Central Health Insurance Bureau is under the jurisdiction of the Department of

22 Emil Aho, Pontus Johansson and Gunilla Ronnholm. International price comparison of pharmaceuticals 2017. *Dental and Pharmaceutical Benefits Agency*, 2018, URL: www.tlv.se/download/18.60fc571b1618606ac975dd4d/1533558140914/internationell_prisjamforelse_av_lakemedel_2017_rapport_engelska180213.pdf.

23 Extensive use of generic drugs in primary care is closely related to GPs' record of generic names alone in prescriptions in the U.K.

24 House of Commons Committee of Public Accounts. Price increases for generic medications. *Sixty-second Report of Session 2017–19*, 2018, URL: https://publications.parliament.uk/pa/cm201719/cmselect/cmpubacc/1184/1184.pdf.

Health and Welfare, but in terms of operations, it is an independent organization that is responsible for its own profits and losses. It is responsible for managing the servicing the entire health insurance system of Taiwan. In terms of medical services providers, more than 70% of such entities are private (this includes pharmacies, clinics, and hospitals).

A person who is insured in Taiwan pays only a fixed fee when buying drugs from a pharmacy or clinic. If the total amount to be paid by health insurance comes to less than NT$ 100 (Taiwan currency), then the individual pays nothing. If it is between NT$ 101 and 200, the individual pays NT$ 20, and if it exceeds NT$ 1000, then the individual's cost is capped at NT$ 200. As for the drug costs during a hospital stay, the individual pays between 5% and 30% of total costs, and drug costs are not calculated as a separate amount.

Taiwan's drug payment policies consist of two types. One is for insurance coverage of drugs during hospitalization and the other for either outpatient or clinic purchases of drugs.[25] For hospitalization, payment standards are figured according to type of illness and illness group (Diagnosis Related Groups). Drug costs are included as a package in the illness group and are not charged separately. Taiwan's universal insurance system is the single largest payer for healthcare services and drugs. As such, its drug reimbursement standards are decisive in influencing the pricing of drugs.

4.4.1 Payment standards for new drugs

Health insurance in Taiwan classifies 'new drugs' into two categories for purposes of payment. It rates these two in terms of new ingredients, new dosage form, new way to administer the drug, new therapeutic efficacy, and whether or not the drug has new clinical value. Type 1 includes ground-breaking innovative drugs while Type 2 refers to new drugs. The Type 2 category is again divided into those drugs (such as 2A, Me-better) that show a notable improvement over the therapeutic value of existing commonly used drugs, and those drugs where the therapeutic value is nearly the same as that of existing new drugs (2B, Me-too). Payment standards for Type 2 new drugs make use of external references – that is, they adopt the median figure of a given drug price in ten countries (the United States, Japan, the U.K., Canada, Germany, France, Belgium, Switzerland, Sweden, and Italy). The payment standard for the Type 1 category generally is set according to the median price of the drug in ten countries; for Type 2, it is set according to the lowest price in ten countries. In actual implementation, the health insurance authorities and drug suppliers may also negotiate on the basis of the therapeutic value of the drug and its actual volume of use.[26]

25 Zhang Jie, Xiong Xianjun and Li Jinghu. Medicine prices and payment management in health insurance system of Taiwan. *China Health Insurance*, 2015 (4).

26 Wang Yanan, Guan Haijing, Liu Guo'en and Sun Lihua. Pharmaceutical procurement and reimbursement schedule in Taiwan. *Chinese Journal of Health Policy*, 2015 (8).

4.4.2 *Payment standards for generic drugs*

Compared to other countries, the Taiwan region does not in fact use a large quantity of generic drugs. In 2014, generics occupied just 47% of the total volume of drug usage. From the perspective of the demand side of the equation, the self-pay requirement of insurance is not high (a fixed payment amount). Given people's doubts about the quality of generics, this means that demand for generics can stay low. Second, the low use of generics is also related to how the drug payment standard is formulated in Taiwan, since this is based on a determination of the active ingredients and is not concerned about whether or not the drug is a generic.[27]

Generic drugs are classified into Ranks A–D, depending on whether or not bio-equivalent tests are conducted, whether the dosage form complies with the quality management system for medicine manufacturing of PIC/S, whether the drug is approved for marketing by the FDA in the United States or the EMA in Europe, and so on. The payment standard for Rank A drugs is the same as drugs in the same group covered by the health insurance. It goes down in descending order for Ranks B–D. The payment standard of Rank D drugs is no more than 80% of other drugs in the same group.

4.4.3 *Adjustments of drug reimbursement standards, and surveys of drug prices*

The payment standard by which health insurance makes reimbursements is not equivalent to the actual price of the drug. Instead, it is the amount that health insurance pays hospitals and pharmacies. The actual price of procuring a drug is a price that hospitals and pharmacies determine themselves together with drug suppliers. This kind of payment mechanism provides hospitals and pharmacies with the incentive to push down the actual price of procurement as low as possible in order to derive the differential between the actual price and the price at which they are reimbursed by insurance (the 'payment standard').

Pharmaceuticals and medicine are a 'mixed' or combined industry in Taiwan, which leads some hospitals and doctors to use their authority in prescribing drugs to over-prescribe in order to gain more price differential and a higher income. In the Taiwan region this is known as 'the black hole of drug prices.'[28] To resolve this problem, Taiwan's health insurance authorities have created mechanisms for adjusting drug payment standards – by adjusting the standards, they can reduce the margin between payment standards and the 'actual price' at which drugs are procured. They thereby try to control the 'black hole of drug prices' and reduce the amount that health insurance has to pay out. In addition to such adjusting, Taiwan

27 Wu Jiuhong and Li Hong. Probability of production and use of generic drugs in Asia. *China Journal of Pharmaceutical Economics*, 2018 (11).

28 Chen Jing, Zhao Xizi, Zhao Liang and Shi Luwen. Experience and enlightenment of drug price regulation in Germany, Japan and Taiwan area of China. *China Pharmacy*, 2017 (25).

conducts a price survey every two years. The payment standard of patented drugs is adjusted based on the 'weighted average market trading price' (WAP), while the payment standard of generic drugs is adjusted based on the 'group weighted average market trading price' (GWAP).[29]

4.5 Summary of drug-pricing practices in other countries

Price-formation of drugs in the major OECD countries and regions is mainly determined by market forces. However, policy interventions at different stages of the process are also common. When public funds reimburse for drugs (including social insurance and direct government payments) the 'payment standard' can be said to play a decisive role in price-formation. Because of this, price-formation mechanisms in major countries can be summed up as market competition that is guided by the payment standards of health insurance.

This system, that is, market-based drug pricing that is guided by the payment standards of health insurance, does two things: it helps to control drug prices within a specific range and prevents excessive increases in price, and it provides a sufficient price margin between the demand side (medical services providers) and the supply side (drug suppliers). It thereby provides incentives for both sides to keep the actual price of drug procurement low. The core element of the incentive mechanism is that medical services providers carry out their own procurement and take in the differential between the payment standard and the actual procurement price.

To make the system as described work and have good results, medical services providers must conform to certain requirements. First, they must be independent entities handling their own operations, able to make their own decisions, and responsible for their own profits and losses. Second, they must be situated in a sufficiently competitive pattern. If they are not independent, responsible for their profits and losses and so on, they fundamentally will have no reason to try to lower the actual price of drugs. If they are not part of a competitive pattern, then a monopoly medical services provider will make use of its monopoly status to engage in tremendously opportunistic behavior. For example, it will over-prescribe drugs, prescribe inappropriate drugs, and so on.

A proper drug-pricing mechanism maintains a good balance between drug innovation and generic substitution, and also a good balance behind the professional autonomy of doctors and a degree of control over medical expenses. Doctors stand in a critical position, between medical services and drug usage. A proper system not only must respect their professional autonomy, but it must design all kinds of regulations that serve to constrain doctors' behavior.

29 Lai Xinquan, Xue Song, Li Hai, Wang Guohua, Zheng Chaohui and Huang Zhangxin, et al. Survey of healthcare system, health insurance and healthcare and medicine price management in Taiwan. *Market Economy and Price 6*, 2014 (6).

5 The evolution of China's price-formation mechanisms for drugs, and pricing policies

5.1 Drug pricing in the planned-economy period

China's price-formation mechanisms for drugs were born out of a planned economy. After Reform and Opening Up, they continued to transition through a number of changes. To understand the current situation and its problems, it is necessary to understand the changes in the systemic structures behind drug pricing and changes in policy since Reform and Opening Up.

During the planned-economy period, China's healthcare safeguards consisted of three different parts. First, employees of public institutions and government organs were under a publicly funded medical system. Medical expenses were paid for through direct appropriations from public finance. Second, employees of State-Owned Enterprises and collective enterprises were under a medical system of 'labor insurance.' A labor insurance fund was formed out of fees paid by enterprises (or out of the non-operating cost of enterprises).[30] Part of this fund was used for paying medical expenses of employees and their families. Third, 'rural cooperative medicine' applied to rural areas, and was funded by the business organizations of rural collectives. On the supply side, medical services were mainly provided by public medical institutions. The finances of these institutions were operated on the basis of 'centralized inputs and centralized expenditures,' that is, they lay within the planned-economy management system.[31]

Drug manufacturing, distribution, and sales were all handled under the aegis of the planned management system. They were operated under centralized government commands, according to planned production, planned purchasing, and planned allocations. With respect to the distribution of drugs, drugs were collectively purchased and exclusively sold to designated buyers in a system that had three tiers or government levels of wholesalers and one tier at the retail level. At the retail end, a system was practiced that had begun in the 1950s. In order to incentivize medical institutions and also provide subsidies due to their losses, the system allowed public medical institutions to add a markup on drug sales that was calculated on the basis of the price at which the drugs entered the institution. The rule was that the markup could not exceed 15% of the drug price.[32]

30 According to the *Opinions on Several Rules in Financial Operations of State-run Enterprises (draft)* issued by the Ministry of Finance in 1969, enterprises shall no longer draw from labor insurance security, and employee's pension and medical expense, etc. shall be recorded as non-operating costs.

31 Various measures were taken in different periods. For more information, please refer to Zhu Heng-peng, Zan Xin and Xiang Hui. Evolution of financial compensation mode and de-administration in reform of public hospitals. *Economic Perspectives*, 2014 (12).

32 Wu Jiexiong. Recognition on the presupposition of cancelling hospital drug price addition. *China Pharmacy*, 2005 (20).

5.2 The loosening of controls on drug prices and ensuing chaos

In the early part of Reform and Opening Up, the biggest problem confronting the medical and healthcare sphere was inadequate supply of medical services and drugs. Supply was inefficient – it was hard to get medical care at all, let alone get into a hospital. This was the state of affairs in general, not only in rural areas that lacked medicine and doctors, but also in large cities with concentrations of industry and population. Even here, the lack of sufficient hospital beds and services was common.[33, 34, 35] Due to this, the overall tendency in the early part of Reform and Opening Up was to relax controls in the areas of medicine and healthcare. On the one hand, this meant loosening the planned management system that governed the institutions providing medical and healthcare services. It meant increasing the operating autonomy of such institutions, emphasizing economic incentives for both the institutions and their medical personnel, and allowing medical institutions to 'pool any leftover (funds) and keep them back for your own use.'[36, 37] On the other hand, this meant loosening planned management controls over drug production and distribution. It meant encouraging local drug manufacturing companies to carry out reform, expand production, and increase supply.[38]

The administrative control system that applied to drug prices was also gradually relaxed. Drug pricing went from being completely determined by the planning system to a 'two-track' price system in which prices set by administrative fiat co-existed with negotiated prices in the market. In 1986, the State Administration of Medicine released a notice on 'the price management list for the pricing of medicines and medical products.' This summed up the existing price-formation mechanisms as being 'the co-existence of government-set prices, government-guided prices, and market-adjusted prices.' Drug prices were divided into three categories: first, drug prices that were centrally controlled (by the State Administration of Medicine); second, drug prices over which control was delegated down to the provincial level of government; and third, other drugs not on the list, which were to be priced through market adjustments. Enterprises were allowed to set prices on this last category according to their own operating circumstances.

This kind of two-track system played a considerable role in encouraging drug production. Drugs had been in short supply for years, and this effectively changed

33 The Ministry of Health. Wuhan municipality takes measures to address difficulties in getting medical treatment. *Hospital Management*, 1983 (11).

34 Qingdao Municipal Bureau of Finance and Qingdao Municipal Bureau of Health. Promote development of healthcare through economic methods. *Finance*, 1980 (01).

35 Ouyang Jing and Yu Zhiping. An important method to address difficulties in getting medical treatment: Survey of hospitals for employees in Heilongjiang and Liaoning on services to the public. *Hospital Management*, 1982 (01).

36 The Ministry of Health, The Ministry of Finance and The National Bureau of Labor. *Opinions on the Experimental Work of Strengthening Economic Management in Hospitals*, 1979.

37 The Ministry of Health. *Report on Several Policies in Medical Reform*, 1985.

38 Wang Xiangting. Remarks of Wang Xiangting at the national biochemical and pharmaceutical conference in 1986. *Chinese Journal of Biochemical and Pharmaceutics*, 1986 (01).

that and also spurred the development of a drug manufacturing industry. However, the two-track drug-pricing system also brought on intensely negative side effects. The chaos in drug pricing reached a peak in the early 1990s. Drug prices were effectively divorced from prices set by government; high prices, high rebates, and high kickbacks became the norm.

First, there was the problem of an enormous proliferation of drug manufacturing companies. In the early 1980s, China had only around 500 pharmaceutical companies, but by the mid-1990s, it had more than 6,000.[39] These could mainly be characterized as 'small, dispersed, and second-rate.' Over 90% were small-scale companies with no ability to reach economies of scale or to manufacture according to GMP standards.[40] Second, there were rampant irregularities in the distribution process. Once reforms did away with the planned system of a three-tiered wholesale and one-tiered retail distribution process, all kinds of companies came in to fill the distribution space and carry on the purchasing and selling of drugs.

Given local protectionism, these small, dispersed, and second-rate companies were able to carry on business by various means. They expanded market share mainly through price competition. Given the two-track pricing system that was still in effect, however, this kind of price competition did not have the effect of washing out the dregs and letting the best companies win. Instead, it bred a large number of improper ways and means. First, large quantities of drugs escaped the scope of administrative pricing – by camouflaging drugs as 'new drugs' through various disguises, prices became market-based. Up until 1996, the catalogue of prices that had been put out in 1986 still had just 100 types of drugs. Of these, the central government set prices on 67 types. The prices of the rest were determined at the provincial level. For example, Hebei Province set the prices of 90 types of drugs, Shandong set prices of 42 types, Liaoning of 41 types. Among the 67 types for which prices were (supposedly) set by the central government, however, only a very small number actually used a unified set price – penicillin would be one example. Most of the others either had to stop production or had to be disguised in various ways and come out under a different name.[41] In 1991, sales of new drugs accounted for 38.4% of the total. This rose to 42.98% in 1992. Less than 30% of the drugs that were supposed to be priced by the central government were actually priced this way.[42]

As noted, once drug pricing broke loose from administrative controls, the situation entered a morass of 'high prices, high kickbacks, and high rebates.' By the time a drug reached the hands of a patient, the actual production cost as a component of the price was less than 30%. The other 70% was made up of rebates and kickbacks in the course of distribution. Wholesalers took a discount of 5% to 10%;

39 Ma Kai. Deepen drug pricing reform and rectify drug pricing orders. *Price: Theory & Practice*, 1997 (2).

40 Yin Li. An exploration of the causes of rising drug prices. *Price: Theory & Practice*, 1997 (11).

41 Shang Yingcai. Status quo of drug prices and measures to strengthen regulation. *China Price*, 1997 (7).

42 Xin. On drug pricing reform. *Soft Science of Health*, 1994 (7).

medical units took a discount and also a rebate that added up to around 30%; on top of these came the kickbacks to doctors and drug salespeople.[43, 44]

In 1994, the State Council issued a Notice that was meant to resolve problems in the sphere of drug pricing and to straighten out the mechanisms by which drugs were priced. This was called *Urgent notice on further strengthening the work of administering medicines*. This called for a rectification of problems that existed among certain regions and departments with respect to drug production and distribution. The emphasis was on the fact that numerous areas were contravening laws and regulations on how to administer drug procedures. Not only were they launching drug manufacturing companies and operating enterprises that wreaked havoc with proper procedures, but in the buying and selling of drugs, they were engaging in such improper behavior as giving and taking bribes and kickbacks.

In 1996, the State Planning Commission issued *Interim procedures for administering drug prices*. This carried forward extensive reform of the way drug prices were administered, but its overall objective was still to find a way to combine administrative prices with market-determined prices. It divided drugs into three categories for purposes of management. First came drugs for which government set the price, with the central government and provincial government units dividing up administrative responsibilities. Such central control covered the manufacture and business dealings of monopoly-type drugs, those which had broad clinical applications, some basic therapeutic drugs which were produced in quantity, and certain special drugs such as Type 1 psychotropic drugs, narcotics, contraceptives, medical devices, and so on. Second came drugs for which enterprises had autonomy in setting their own prices. Third came drugs that were priced according to relevant regulations: drugs were priced according to a fixed markup rate and sold according to the price differential from the actual buying and selling price. Hospitals could sell drugs at a markup rate that generally was not to break through 15%. As for imported drugs and new drugs, the *ex factory* price was to be determined by the manufacturer itself, and the retail price was to be set according to the prescribed markup rate, together with the allowed profit rate when selling the drug.

In 1998, the National Planning Commission issued another notice called *Notice on improving drug pricing policies in order to advance the way drug prices are administered*. First, this re-set the profit rate on sales of new drugs. Second, it introduced the principle of 'higher price for higher quality' on common drugs over which the government exercised price controls. If a manufacturer could prove that their product was clearly higher in quality, safety, clinical effectiveness, and so on, the manufacturer could apply for a one-off special price. Third, it placed limits on the percentage of a selling price that could be added as a 'sales fee.' The fee could not exceed 25% for original-research drugs, and 10% for generics.

43 Research Group of Xiamen Municipality Price Regulation Bureau. Why medical expenses remain high: Survey and analysis of medical expense and drug prices in Xiamen. *Great Tide*, 1999 (3).

44 Research Group of the Institute of Market and Price and Cao Jianjun. Study of pricing for drugs and medical treatment. *China Price*, 2001 (05).

The trend during this period was to strengthen administrative controls over drug prices as part of the overall reform of the institutional structures that handle drug pricing. Administrative controls were placed on everything from *ex factory* prices to selling prices, and interventions even extended to markup rates and profit rates on sales. These measures, however, did not in fact resolve the problems of exorbitant prices or the practice of using kickbacks and rebates. To evade the administrative controls, some companies simply continued the practice of giving kickbacks to medical institutions by such hidden subsidies as sponsorships to conferences, payments for promotion campaigns, and so on.[45, 46]

5.3 Setting up medical insurance for employees, and reform of drug-pricing mechanisms

One of the major events that occurred in the late 1990s was the establishment of 'basic' medical insurance for employees of enterprises in urban areas. This inserted a new element into the sphere of medicine since medical insurance funds were now the unified 'payer' of drug costs and medical services. In order to ensure the safety of those insurance funds, it became necessary to carry forward reform of the chaotic drug-pricing structures.

In 2000, the Economic Restructuring Office of the State Council and other departments issued a joint opinion called *Guiding opinion (directive) on reform of the institutional structures of medicine, drugs, and healthcare in cities and towns*. This called for adjustments to drug prices as follows:

> Drugs on the reimbursable list of basic medical insurance, preventive medicines, essential pediatric drugs, and special drugs operated under monopolies, are to have prices either set by government or guided by government. Where conditions allow, a unified national retail selling price may be formulated. Prices of other drugs may be determined on an independent basis by manufacturers according to pricing methods as prescribed by the government.

That same year (2000), the State Planning Commission issued a notice called *Notice on the opinion on reforming the administration of drug pricing*. This confirmed the situation with respect to administering drug pricing – that is, it approved a method that combined government-set prices with market adjustments. It also specified the scope of drugs for which government set prices, specifically, that the government put a ceiling price on drugs that were incorporated in the reimbursement list of the Basic Medical Insurance. Among these, Type A drugs in the list were priced by the central government, and Type B were priced by the administrative departments in charge of pricing at the provincial level.

45 Liu Gang. Problems in drug pricing and advice on countermeasures. *China Price*, 1998 (10).

46 Wang Yang. Introduce competition to deepen pricing reform for medicine and medical treatment. *Price: Theory & Practice*, 2000 (10).

This round of reform also made the regulations more explicit with regard to one-off special pricing. A manufacturer could apply for such pricing if its drug was clearly more effective and safer than the same kind of drug being produced by other manufacturers, or if the drug was able to treat problems in a shorter time and at lower cost. This regulation was aimed at the fact that numerous manufacturers at the time were applying for such special pricing for their 'new' drugs, which were nothing but old drugs in a new guise – different dosage forms, specifications, or packaging. Prices simply continued to rise, however, and drug-price inflation became a highly controversial topic in medicine at the time.[47]

In order to combat this kind of behavior on the part of drug manufacturers, in 2005 the National Development and Reform Commission issued a ruling called *Regulations on price differentials of drugs (for trial implementation)*. This mandated specific price differentials or comparative ratios for drugs that were the same as drugs on which the government either set prices or guided prices but that had different packaging materials, specifications, dosage forms, and so on. In 2006, the National Development and Reform Commission, the Ministry of Finance, and other departments again issued an opinion called *Opinion on going a step further in rectifying the disorder in market pricing of drugs and medical services*. This required companies to abide strictly by the rules on price differentials and ratios. Furthermore, it ruled that a markup of no more than 15% could be added to a price, with the buy-in price used as the basis. This increased controls over the way the market was allowed to 'adjust' drug prices. It meant that prescription drug prices previously subject to market adjustment were gradually being brought under the purview of government price-setting.

5.4 Two-track drug pricing

Since the start of Reform and Opening Up, reform of China's drug-pricing mechanisms has been carried on within the overall framework of reform of the country's institutional structures that deal with medicine, drugs, and healthcare. To a large extent, drug prices have been a concentrated expression of the many problems in the sphere of medicine, as well as a flashpoint in the course of reform. Exorbitant prices, the way prices are divorced from the true value of drugs, and the way corruption has marked the buying and selling of drugs have all become driving forces behind many attempts to reform the institutional structures of medicine in China. After nearly two decades of reform, by the time of the 2009 New Medical Reform, price-formation mechanisms of drugs in China had gradually settled into a pattern. This was characterized by a two-track system that included government-set prices and market-negotiated prices.

First, the two-track price-formation mechanism involved the co-existence of prices set by administrative means (government) and prices adjusted by the

47 Chen Wenling. Why drug prices remain high: investigation of drug pricing problems and thinking. *Price: Theory & Practice*, 2005 (01).

market. Drugs on the list covered by Basic Medical Insurance were set by government, as well as such things as psychotropic drugs, narcotics, and so on. All others were set by the market.

Second, the basic principle behind the way government set prices was 'cost plus a markup.' In distribution, it was 'add specific markup rates in succession.' The purpose was to repay the manufacturer and distributor for costs and add in a specific amount of profit. The theoretical premise behind this way of doing things was that drugs that cost the same on the supply side would have the same value on the demand side, no matter what kind of thing the drug might treat. If the cost of producing a drug was high, its price should be high, and the quantity that a buyer might want to purchase should not have any real influence on price.

Third, drugs were categorized according to quality. The corresponding impact on price-formation was known as 'superior quality, superior price.' Ever since this concept was put forth in the 1990s, it has been preserved as a principle to follow with respect to how to handle price controls on drugs. Therefore, if a given drug is proven to be superior to another drug in terms of quality, safety, and clinical results, the maker of that drug can apply for one-off special pricing status. As a result, the drug breaks out of the government's price-control system.

5.5 The New Medical Reform and a unified (one-track) system of price-formation mechanisms for drugs that is primarily market-based

In the early days of the New Medical Reform, policies accepted the two-track system as a price-formation mechanism for drug pricing. After the Reform began in 2009, the National Development Reform Commission and the Ministry of Human Resources and Social Security issued an opinion called *Opinion on reforming the price-formation mechanisms of drugs and medical services*. This proposed measures to deal with the situation, and it upheld the 'two-track' feature of the drug-pricing system that had been in place since the start of Reform and Opening Up. At the same time, in coordination with New Medical Reform policies to do with adjusting prices of medical services, it made an attempt to 'straighten out' (rationalize) price levels of drugs and medical services.

The purpose of the two-track drug price-formation mechanism was, of course, well intended. On the one hand, it aimed to ensure access to affordable drugs through the use of administrative controls on drug prices. On the other hand, it aimed to ensure that the market played a role in encouraging innovation and rewarding superior companies while washing out inferior ones, through competition.[48] However, in actual practice the two-track system had not yet achieved its intended results. Chaos prevailed in the market for drugs and prices were exorbitant, accompanied by all kinds of corruption and 'gray' behavior. During

48 Chen Wen. Policy options for pharmaceutical price regulation. *Chinese Journal of Health Policy*, 2008 (03).

this period, administrative price-control measures were used repeatedly to try to bring the selling price of drugs down, but the actual selling price of drugs simply remained high. At times, hospitals were adding an actual markup rate that went as high as 42%.[49] Meanwhile, manufacturers were highly inventive in finding ways to break out of the bonds of administratively set prices. The most common way to do this was to apply for a one-off special price for a so-called 'new' drug. In 2004, the National Pharmaceutical Regulatory Bureau received more than 10,000 such applications for new drugs. Among these 10,000 applications, not a single one had any new chemical ingredients. Meanwhile, during the same period, the FDA in the United States received 148 applications, of which 36 had innovative chemical compounds.[50] Given this situation in China, the National Development and Reform Commission yet again revised the *Regulations on drug price differentials and ratios*. These now re-oriented regulations on differentials and ratios in the direction of such things as average costs, results of clinical applications, treatment costs, level of production technology, ease of use, and contribution to development of the industry.

However, no matter how you look at it, the two-track system as a price-formation mechanism has already come to the end of its road. While stimulating drug production, the system has also brought on disastrous problems. On the supply side, prices of medical services have been strictly controlled in public hospitals, so institutions have funded their operations with overpriced drugs. Drug prices have become the focal point for conflicts of interest, while high prices, high kickbacks, and large discounts have simply become the norm. Drug manufacturers have found numerous ways to circumvent controls on government-set prices,[51] but exorbitant prices have become a problem that is very hard to eradicate after more than 30 years.

At the outset, the 2009 New Medical Reform maintained and extended the two-track system of drug-pricing policy. Drug prices did not, however, reflect supply and demand in the market, nor did they in fact encourage innovation, and the actual price at which drugs are sold has not gone down. Given this situation, the way in which China's drugs are priced had to undergo fundamental reform.

In 2015, the National Development and Reform Commission, together with six other departments and commissions, jointly issued an opinion called *Opinion on pushing forward reform of drug pricing*. This completely eliminated administrative pricing of drugs, except for narcotics and Type 1 psychotropic drugs. 'We eliminate pricing of drugs by government . . . such that the actual price at which drug transactions take place is primarily determined by market competition.' This

49 Zhao Zhenji. Game behind price reduction. *China Drugstore*, 2005 (11).

50 Liu Ping, Fu Wenjun, Ying Xiaohua and Chen Wen. Theoretical study of drug price administration in China. *Price: Theory & Practice*, 2008 (01).

51 Zhu Hengpeng. Endogeneity of regulation and its consequences: a case study of medical and pharmaceutical price regulation. *The Journal of World Economy*, 2011(07).

marked the transition of drug pricing from the two-track system to a sole price-formation mechanism that is primarily determined by the market.

The new method of forming prices adopted a 'negative list' as a price-setting principle. Medical insurance departments determine the reimbursement standards for drugs on the reimbursable list; prices of patented drugs and drugs produced by a monopoly producer are determined through multi-party negotiating; drugs outside the health insurance reimbursable list, such as immunological drugs, preventive drugs, nationally supplied free anti-AIDs drugs, and contraceptive devices are priced via bidding and procurement or negotiations. Narcotics and Type 1 psychotropic drugs are subject to maximum *ex factory* prices and maximum retail prices; and except for these things, all other drugs are freely priced by the market.

5.6 *Sales utilizing the two-invoice policy and the zero-markup policy, and centralized drug procurement*

Given the ongoing problem of high drug prices[52] and resulting unreasonably high insurance payments, China has gradually developed three policy approaches that are outside the normal scope of price-mechanism reforms. These are the two-invoice system, eliminating markups on drugs, and centralized procurement of drugs.

5.6.1 Two-invoice system

What this policy means is that only two invoices may be made out in the process of distributing drugs. One invoice is made out by the drug manufacturer when it sells to the drug distributing company, and the second is made when that company sells to a medical institution. One of the reasons for the persistence of exorbitant drug prices is that there have been too many links in the chain of distribution. The reasoning behind the two-invoice system was that if you control the number of invoices as a policy tool, you may be able to reduce the unnecessarily high costs brought on by all the links in the system.[53] This policy measure was first proposed in Guangdong in 2006, in its campaign for Transparent Drug Procurement. Afterwards, Sanming City in Fujian province also adopted it as a part of centralized procurement.[54] In April 2016, a standing committee meeting of the State Council determined that it should be implemented in centralized procurement procedures at all publicly funded hospitals. In 2017, the General Office of the State Council determined that the policy should be implemented on a nationwide basis in 2018,

52 Liu Yang, Guan Xiaodong and Shi Lu Wen. International comparison of drug price level in China. *China Drugstore*, 2012 (48).

53 Hu Shanlian. The theory and practice of 'two-invoice' system in the drug procurement. *Health Economics Research*, 2017 (04).

54 Dai Jin. Fujian implements 'two-invoice' policy. *China Hospital CEO*, 2010 (06).

as stated in *Various opinions on going further in improving reform of the policies relating to drug production, distribution, and usage*.

However, the results of the two-invoice policy indicate that it has had no noticeable effect on drug prices.[55, 56, 57] The reason is that it does not address the fundamental cause of exorbitant prices. In practice, the impact of the two-invoice system has been canceled out by other forms of price manipulation. Behind all of this is the systemic cause of the problem: public hospitals maintain their operations through income that is derived by inflating drug prices.[58]

5.6.2 Zero markup for drugs

Another view on the exorbitant cost of drugs focused on the markup that hospitals charge. This led to a policy that supplemented the policy on distribution links, called zero markup. The practice of earning income off drugs to maintain hospital operations has been going on since the planned-economy period.[59] In the 1980s and 1990s, income from drug markups indeed became the primary source of income for hospitals. Income from drugs constituted more than 50% of total income at one point (see Figure 3.3). In order to limit excessive amounts of such income, in the mid-1990s various policies such as *Interim measures on the administration of drug prices* put a cap on markups of 15%. Under such restrictions, namely the controls on maximum markups, hospitals began to favor the most expensive drugs in order to boost their incomes. Given that hospitals have a monopoly on the sale of drugs to patients, suppliers of drugs were also motivated to increase their own sales by inflating the cost of their wares, so they raised prices of drugs. This led to a phenomenon in drug marketing that was called 'the higher the prices, the greater the sales.' A policy of eliminating markups altogether therefore was seen to be one way to straighten out this situation.

As policies, eliminating drug markups and implementing 'zero-markup drug sales' were first tried at the grassroots level in medical and healthcare institutions, with regard to the 'basic pharmaceuticals system.' In 2009, the Ministry of Health and other departments proposed that all grassroots-level medical institutions use 'basic pharmaceuticals,' and that they use a zero-markup policy when selling these medicines. This proposal came in the opinion called *Opinion on implementing the*

55 Huang Runqing, Duan Wenyue, Wang You, Li Caijing, Zha Weicui and Li Fan. Study on problems and countermeasures in implementing two-invoice system in medical institutions: a cast study of Yunnan province. *China Pharmacy*, 2018 (24).

56 Huang He, Sun Jing and Liu Yuanli. Investigation on "two tax bill" medicines distribution reform. *China Pharmacy*, 2017, 28(18): 2456–2459.

57 Han Lirong and Qiao Lu. Evaluation of two-invoice policy. *China Management Informationization*, 2019 (10).

58 Gu Xing. Far-reaching influences of two-invoice policy for medicine. *21st Century Business Herald*, 2016 (04).

59 Yuan Kejian. Abolishment of markup addresses only the symptoms. *Contemporary Medicine*, 2005 (07).

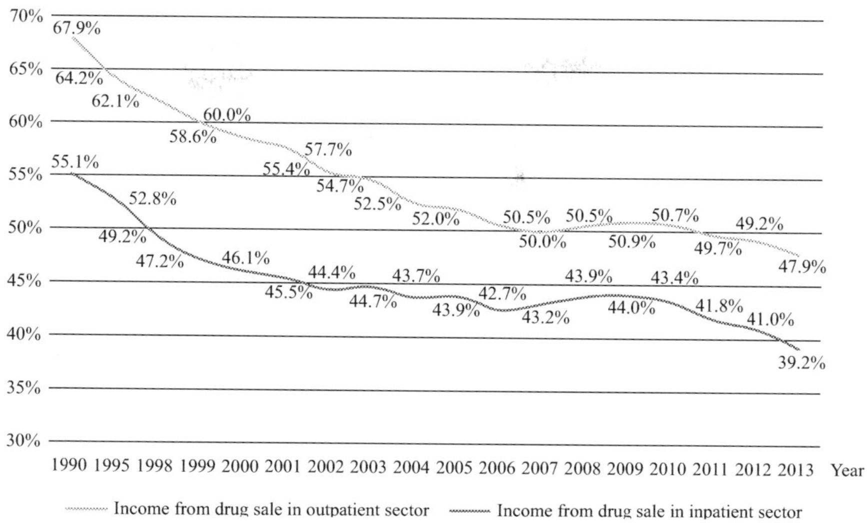

Figure 3.3 Change in Income Derived from the Sale of Drugs in Outpatient and Inpatient Sectors of General Hospitals

Source: China's Healthcare and Family Planning Statistical Yearbook 2016.

Note: The data before 2004 (including 2004) relates to general hospitals under the administration of healthcare authorities; the data after 2005 (including 2005) relates to general hospitals.

national system for basic pharmaceuticals. After this, the reforms of county-level hospitals as well as municipal public hospitals both proposed the same implementation of a zero-markup sale of drugs. In 2017, the National Health and Family Planning Commission and other departments put out a notice on *Launching nationwide comprehensive reform of public hospitals*. This included a provision that called for the zero markup on drug sales, nationwide. Given that such a policy involves a loss of income to hospitals, the policy also called for measures to make up for the loss, including additional support from public finance, increasing the prices of medical services, and improving the efficiency of hospitals.

However, the situation as it stands now does not allow for much optimism, given the way implementation has actually taken place. After eliminating markups on drugs, hospitals found that their total drug costs had not in fact noticeably declined, and drug prices had not been effectively controlled. At the same time, though, examination fees and income from the sale of such things as consumables rose quickly.[60]

60 Hu Dayang, Xu Jinying and Zhang Yan. Analysis of the impact of abolishing the additional cost of drugs on medical insurance funds – based on the practice in Jiangsu province. *China Health Insurance*, 2017 (07).

5.6.3 Centralized drug procurement

During the 1980s and 1990s, medical institutions essentially bought their own drugs. In doing this, however, they were egregious in their self-serving. Drug procurement became a disaster zone of corruption, and prices went ever higher. Starting in the late 1990s, therefore, some parts of China began to experiment with centralized procurement. After 2000, centralized procurement became a nationwide policy, with the first step being purchasing at the prefectural city level. Within the scope of each city, intermediary organizations would carry out market-based procurement. Starting in 2006, China began centralized procurement at the provincial level that was guided by the central government. Such centralized procurement, done through a bidding process at the provincial level, then was extended to a nationwide system as China implemented a Basic Pharmaceuticals System in 2010. The system included such features as bidding by manufacturers and the combination of bidding with procurement, price being linked to quantity, the two-invoice system, and centralized payment. In 2015, the General Office of the State Council issued an opinion called *Guiding opinion (directive) on improving the centralized procurement work of drugs by public hospitals*. This reconfirmed the approach of conducting centralized procurement at the provincial level.

The theoretical basis for adhering to this form of centralized procurement was that the buyer now became a monopoly and therefore could force prices down. Over a decade of experience now shows, however, that centralized procurement procedures have no apparent use when it came to keeping prices down. Prices continue to rise to excessive levels. This has been true whether the centralized procurement is done at the prefectural or the provincial level, and whether it is done through bidding or some other way. What's more, the practice has led to other problems such as inadequate supply, whether or not the winning bid was at a high or a low level.[61, 62, 63]

One theory behind this phenomenon was that medical institutions are not in fact the ones who pay for the drugs. Given China's universal health insurance system, the largest 'payer' is the medical insurance funds, and this has made it hard for centralized procurement to lower drug prices. The funds themselves should therefore take on the responsibility for doing the centralized procurement. Once China's medical insurance administration was set up, therefore, the responsibility for centralized procurement of drugs was shifted from the departments handling the administration of healthcare to the National Health Security Administration. In order to lower the actual procurement price of drugs, the first action this Administration took was to negotiate for including cancer drugs into insurance coverage.

61 Sun Xiao, Fu Shuai and Tan Yingjie. Common problems in centralized bidding and procurement of medicines and countermeasures. *China Health Industry*, 2013 (06).

62 He Changnan and Fu Hongpeng. Analysis on centralized purchasing price of 20 kinds of essential drugs. *Health Economics Research*, 2016 (08), 44–47.

63 Cui Li and Wang Weiming. Discussion on existing problems and strategies of drug centralized bidding. *China Health Industry*, 2017(30).

In return for including 17 types of anticancer medications into the reimbursement list, the manufacturers did lower the prices of these drugs. The second action was to carry out the so-called '4+7 pilot program' by which 11 cities linked quantity to the price of drug procurement. The idea was to lower negotiated prices by guaranteeing the purchase of a certain quantity of drugs. This program has been in operation for too short a time to judge whether or not such linkage has a real influence on price. In the short term, however, it appears that the prices of some drugs have actually gone down even though the 'quantities' involved are fairly small. In the long term, it remains to be seen whether or not this quantity-linked procurement has any effect on lowering prices.

6 The objectives of reform with respect to price-formation mechanisms and the components of drug prices

(As noted at the beginning of this chapter), China's drug prices are a concentrated expression of all the many problems in China's medical sphere. Multiple reforms to do with medicine, pharmaceuticals, and healthcare have been undertaken over the past 30-some years, and the direct reason for every one of these has been excessive drug prices. Despite these, exorbitant drug prices continue to plague the country. Price-formation mechanisms have been through a number of changes – from being determined completely by administrative fiat, to a two-track system of administrative pricing plus market mechanisms, and then to the primary use of market-based pricing. In addition to pricing mechanisms, a number of measures have been adopted in the areas of drug manufacturing, distribution, and sales, as well as the links involved in drug (prescribing and) usage. Despite all of this, the distortion of drug prices has not fundamentally been resolved. Reasons for this lie at deeper levels and do not in fact have to do with drugs themselves. They have to do with the distortion of the supply side of medical services. The root source of drug prices 'lies with medicine, not with drugs.' The distortion of drug prices is simply an indication of the shortcomings in China's medical, pharmaceutical, and healthcare system.

Drug price-formation does not take place in isolation. It is embedded in an underlying web of institutional systems and these systems can even directly determine how drug pricing comes about. In order to understand the peculiarities of China's drug prices, therefore, it is necessary to understand the underlying institutional systems on which drug price-formation depends.

6.1 Institutional background of China's drug-pricing mechanisms

1 The primary suppliers of medical services in China are public hospitals. These medical institutions enjoy a monopoly status that is formed under the protection of administrators. Even though there are quite a few non-public medical entities in the country (see Figure 3.4), public hospitals hold the absolute advantage when it comes to access to resources and supply of services. This includes such things as the number of beds and number of doctors and, on the supply side, to the number of patient visits and hospital discharges. (See Figures 3.4, 3.5, and 3.6.)

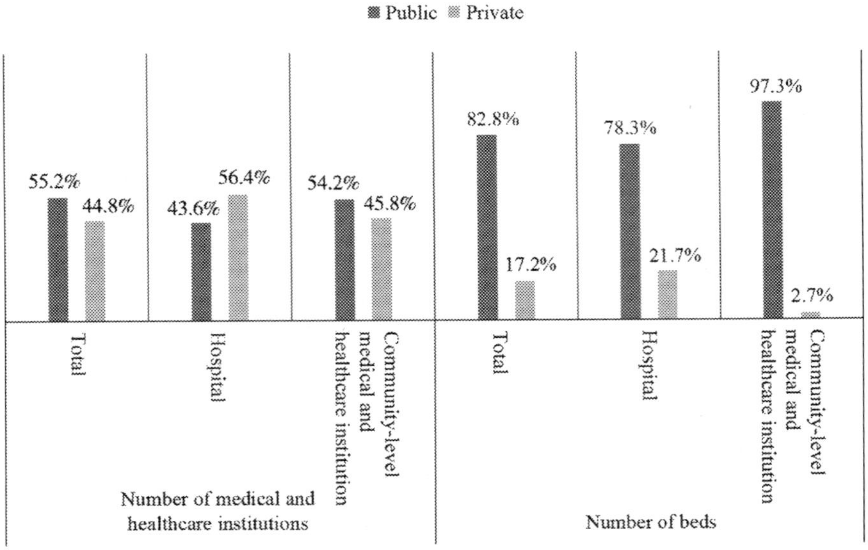

Figure 3.4 Percentages of Public and Private Medical Institutions in China, and their Beds (2016)

Source: China Healthcare and Family Planning Statistical Yearbook 2017

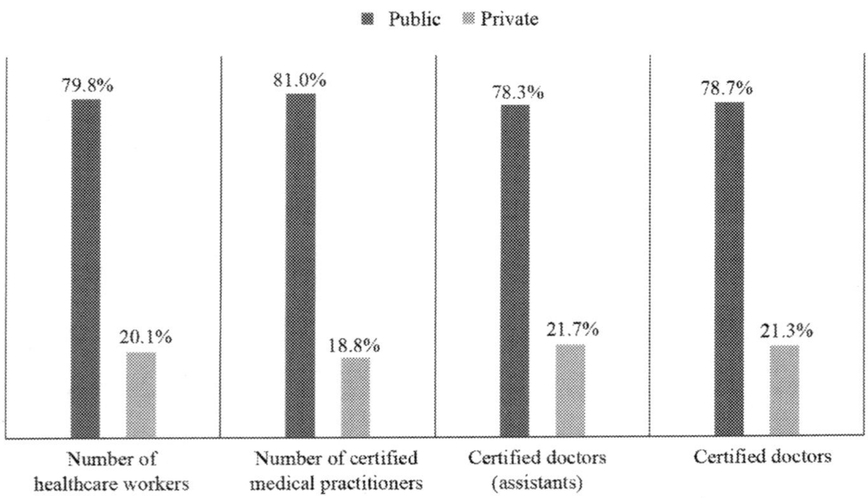

Figure 3.5 Percentages of Public Versus Private Medical Institutions in China, Including Total, Hospitals, and Community Healthcare Institutions, and Percentages of Beds in Each Category (2016)

Source: China Healthcare and Family Planning Statistical Yearbook 2017

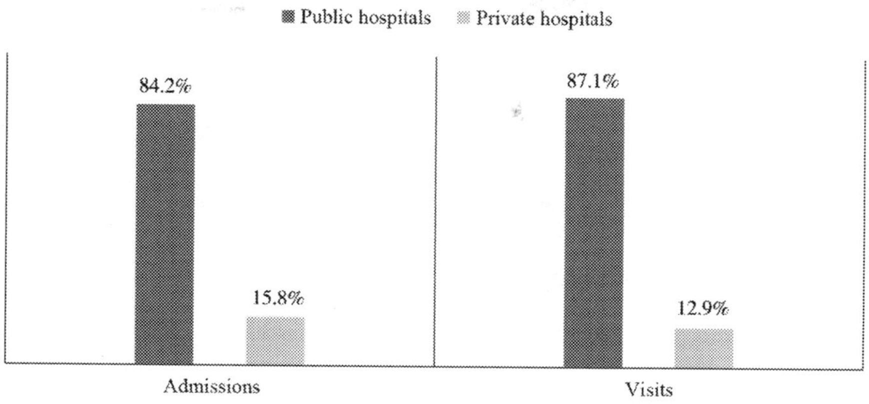

Figure 3.6 Hospital Admissions and Visits to Public and Private Hospitals in China (2016)

Source: China Healthcare and Family Planning Statistical Yearbook 2017

Note: Community-level institutions are excluded.

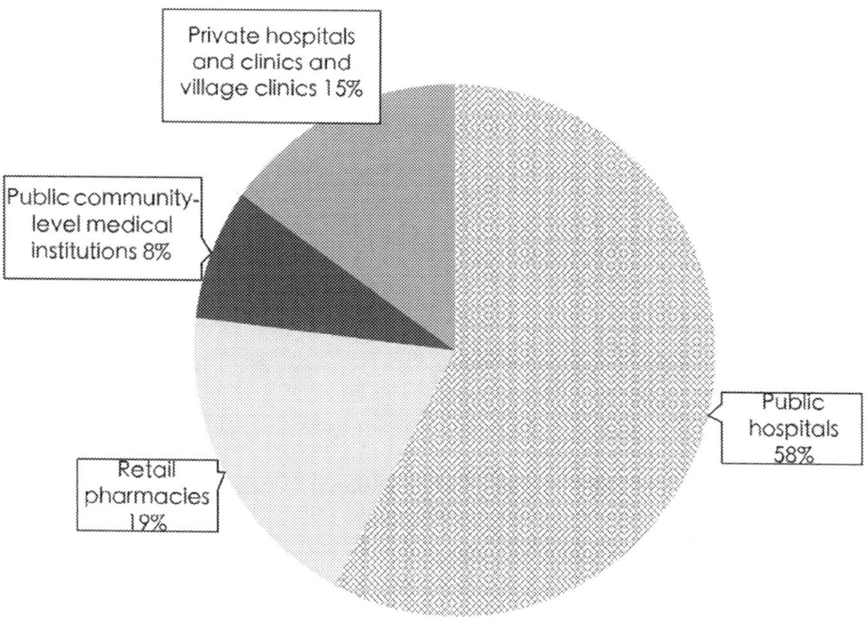

Figure 3.7 Distribution of Drug Retail Channels (2017)

Source: NMPA Southern Medicine Economic Research Institute https://med.sina.com/article_detail_103_1_43310.html

The mode by which China's public medical institutions are governed is distinctive for three reasons. First, they operate under an administrative hierarchy. Resources are allocated according to this hierarchy, from 'grassroots' or community-level healthcare services up to hospitals. Within the hospital hierarchy, Grade 1 hospitals are next in rank to community services, while Grade 3 hospitals are at the top.

Second, governing authority and operating authority are combined, and the 'administration' of a hospital holds a monopoly status. Meanwhile, the administrative departments that govern healthcare services are not only the 'boss' of public hospitals but also the regulatory bodies that oversee the entire industry. This leads to the lack of any competitive pressure from outside public hospitals.

Third, with respect to internal management, hospitals are managed as 'public institutions' that are staffed under the *bianzhi* system (staffing by appointment according to administrative rules). This form of management lacks the incentive and constraint mechanisms that would correspond to a different kind of system. All three of these features lead to a situation in which public hospitals face the dual dilemma of having neither incentives nor constraints. The dilemma comes from the fact that opting for either incentives or constraints would be detrimental. Strengthening controls leads to a lack of motivation to provide medical services; loosening them leads to tremendous amounts of opportunistic behavior.[64] In Chinese, the situation is summarized by the phrases, 'Pulling in (controlling) kills incentive,' while 'letting loose leads to chaos.'

Over 80% of China's doctors (medical practitioners) work in public institutions. The relationship between institutions and doctors is not just one of simple employment, but involves mutual reliance. Doctors and hospitals are tied together due to the linkage created by the country's staffing system of public institutions. Except in special circumstances, public hospitals have no authority to fire doctors. Meanwhile, if doctors want to leave their positions, they face institutional obstacles. This institutional setting is quite different from the situation in most OECD countries.

2 The pharmaceutical and medical industries are intertwined in China's hospitals. Suppliers of medical services are, at the same time, the biggest drug sellers in China. Drugs sold in China, including those sold in the outpatient sector, as well as self-administered prescription and non-prescription drugs, are largely sold from medical institutions. While providing medical services, hospitals are at the same time engaged in the business of selling drugs. In 2017, the total sales volume of drugs in China came to RMB 1.9 trillion, and of this total, RMB 1,247.2 billion or nearly two-thirds (65.6%) was sold by public medical institutions. (These included hospitals at the municipal and county levels, and grassroots medical and healthcare organizations including urban community healthcare service centers and township healthcare clinics.)[65]

64 Wang Zhen. Community-level medical reform and innovation of governance. *Social Governance Review*, 2018 (01).

65 Source of data: *NMPA Southern Medicine Economic Research Institute*. Quoted from https://med.sina.com/article_detail_103_1_43310.html.

3 China has already established a universal medical insurance system. The two main components of the system are the 'basic medical insurance for urban workers,' and the 'medical insurance for urban and rural residents.' Funds collected for these two in 2017 came to RMB 1793.16 billion, while insurance paid out the total sum of RMB 1442.17 billion. This latter amount contributed 39% of the total income of medical institutions in 2017.[66] The National Health Security Administration, established in 2018, consolidated under its jurisdiction the management of three different types of funds – workers' medical insurance, urban and rural residents' medical insurance, and the medical relief and assistance funds. It took on the functions of managing funds, procuring drugs, and adjusting the prices of medical services. The NHSA therefore became the largest 'payer' for medical services and drugs.

From this perspective, China's model of medical insurance is similar to that of Germany and of Taiwan (China). The workers' medical insurance is similar to Germany's social medical insurance, and the residents' medical insurance is even more similar to Taiwan (China's) universal health insurance. Where China's practices differ from those in Germany and Taiwan (China), however, relates to the administrative level of authority handling the business.

In China, medical insurance is localized, so different regions are carved off from one another. Insurance funds are centrally collected, or pooled, mainly at the municipal level of government. Under such localized management, not only is the administrative pooling level of insurance funds in China quite low, but each locality has its own policies and procedures. These policies and procedures include such things as determining the list of reimbursable drugs, premium policies and reimbursement conditions, prices of medical services, prices of drugs, and drug procurement procedures.

6.2 *'Subsidizing medicine through the sale of drugs,' and the various components of drug prices*

In overall terms, drug prices include two components. One is the cost of manufacturing (including the cost of R&D), and including the manufacturer's profit. The other is the cost of distribution, which includes warehousing and storage, shipping and other charges involved in the wholesale and retail processes, as well as profits at the various stages of distribution.

$$P = S + C \quad (1)$$

In this equation, P is the price of the drug, S is production costs together with profit, and C is distribution costs together with profit.

66 Source of data: *China Health Statistical Yearbook 2018*.

In most OECD countries, the medical insurance system reimburses for services and drugs separately, since 'medicine' and 'pharmaceuticals' are operated as different businesses. In addition, medical insurance pays separately for hospital services, doctors' services, and pharmaceutical services. To take the United States as an example: Medicare and Medicaid mainly pay costs to hospitals according to Diagnosis Related Groups; they pay doctors and clinics according to a Physician Fee Schedule. Payments for drugs are divided into inpatient drugs and clinic (outpatient) drugs. Medicare and Medicaid pay according to payment standards, but add a specific markup rate. Hospitals purchase medicines on their own, and their procurement is mainly done through Group Purchasing Organizations (GPOs). In this case, the markup involved, and any price that comes in below the insurance payment standard, is considered to be income to the hospital. In 2016, 38% of the medical expenses of individuals in the United States went to pay for hospital services, 24% went to pay for doctors and clinic services, while just 12% went to pay for prescription drugs. (See Figure 3.8.) In OECD countries, therefore, the components of the price of a given drug include nothing but manufacturing costs, distribution costs, and profit.

In China, however, the situation is far more complicated. Components of a drug price must first include a portion that pays for the services of doctors and hospitals – this is the part that 'subsidizes medicine through drugs.' This part is tied in to, or bundled with, the payment for drugs, but is not solely for doctors' services, for the following reasons. In the planned-economy period, public finance made direct allocations for such fixed capital investments as a hospital's basic infrastructure,

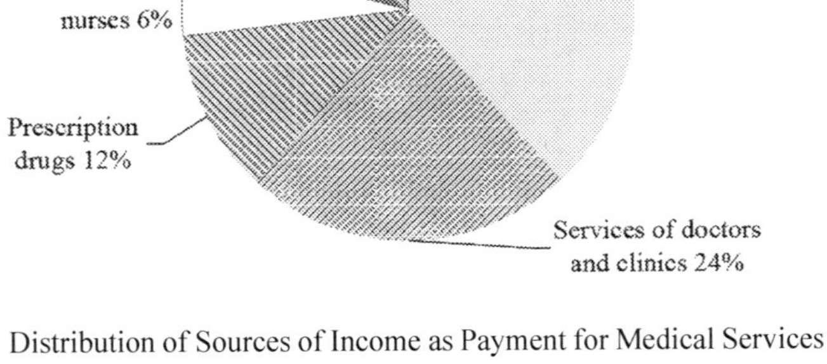

Figure 3.8 Distribution of Sources of Income as Payment for Medical Services in the U.S. (2016)

Source: Cothran, J., 2018, US health care spending: who pays? California Health Care Foundation, www.chcf.org/publication/us-health-care-spending-who-pays/

Note: This figure provides data on individual healthcare services. Public healthcare expenses, etc., are excluded.

its land, its large-scale equipment, and so on. The wages of those who worked in hospitals were also funded directly out of public finance. Theoretically, therefore, under the planned economy, the services of doctors and hospitals should not have required separate payment. However, the way things actually worked is that funds from public finance did not always reach their intended destination. As a result, hospital income was not enough to make up for hospital expenditures. This was the primary reason that, from the 1950s onward, hospitals were allowed to add a markup on drugs that they sold.

Meanwhile, the income from markups that hospitals added to drug prices was, in theory, meant to make up for lost operating income. It was not to be diverted into wage income for doctors. After China began structural reform of its medical and healthcare systems, in the 1980s, institutions were given a degree of autonomy in their operations. This was to increase investment in the medical and healthcare sphere by restructuring incentives in public hospitals. One of the incentives included allowing hospitals to spend any surplus income on the performance-based salary of doctors, after hospitals had covered their operating costs.

However, from the perspective of public finance, government allocations were already covering fixed assets and the salaries of personnel. Hospital fees were therefore allowed to include only things that were not included in 'depreciation of fixed assets and salaries of personnel.' That is, even though hospitals had been granted greater autonomy in operations, it was administratively hard for them to adjust fees from services enough to increase income. All they had left was the window of opportunity that the markups on drugs presented. At the same time, administrative controls were now placed over the extent of this markup, since it was feared that hospitals would use the markup policies to seek personal advantage. Starting in the mid-1990s, therefore, hospitals were obliged to set a fixed markup rate of 15%. Given this predicament, both hospitals and doctors were motivated to elevate the incoming price of medicines, in order to earn a higher income. This has been regarded as one of the root causes of exorbitant drug prices.

In the reform of drug pricing that followed this, markups on drug prices were therefore abolished altogether. Prices of medical services were allowed to increase, which has been one of the main orientations of reform. By 2017, as reform of public hospitals was launched on a nationwide basis, a zero markup became the universal practice among public hospitals. It should be noted, however, that the 15% markup served as an income for hospitals, not for doctors. Abolishing that income has failed to address the problem of doctors making profits off drug sales.

Naturally, the practice of using drugs to help subsidize medicine is not permitted, either in theoretical terms or in the design of policy. In order to combat this practice, and its associated problems of exorbitant drug prices and rampant over-prescribing of drugs, government has passed numerous control measures. The 'two-invoice' policy is a typical example. It is aimed at behavior that 'launders money through the use of multiple invoicing' in the sphere of drug distribution.

These administrative control measures served to add costs to the expenses of hospitals that were in fact attempting to use drug sales to finance operations and pay doctors. That is, the practice of 'using drugs to subsidize medicine' had its own set of costs. This changed the equation noted earlier.

Accordingly, beyond the normal production costs and distribution costs in the composition of drug prices, two additional items have to be taken into account. The 'actual composition' of drug prices now includes H, the payments to hospitals, and Y, the payments to doctors, but in addition, the cost of making these payments also has to be added, call it 'X.' The X part of the equation could be defined as costs incurred as a result of distorting the system. If there were no 'subsidizing of medicine through the use of drugs,' and no kind of administrative controls, then there would be no need for this kind of cost – which is why it is defined as the cost of systemic distortions. From the standpoint of society, this kind of cost is a waste of social resources, pure and simple.

The actual composition of drug prices in China could therefore be expressed as follows:

$$P = (S + C) + (H + Y) + X = P1 + P2 + X \quad (2)$$

To summarize: three components make up actual drug prices in China, the normal costs of manufacturing and distribution plus profit (P1), payments made to doctors and hospitals (P2), and institutional distortions (X).

Selling costs account for the lion's share of the actual composition of drug prices in China. Estimates from multiple sources believe that these take up about 60% of the actual sales price of all drugs.[67] These extremely high costs are paid out to doctors and hospitals under various guises, and are either overt or covert. They appear in such forms as conference fees, business promotion fees, academic promotional fees, market development, market survey fees, and so on.[68]

Going a step further into the composition of prices, normal production and distribution costs (including profits and tax revenue) come to 30% to 35% of the total (P1). Payments to hospitals (H) were, on the surface at least, 15% before the markup was abolished. Kickbacks to doctors vary greatly among different parts of China and at different levels of hospitals, as well as in different medical disciplines. Doctors with different titles also get different levels of kickbacks, and the professional skills and style of the doctors involved play a role. As an overall estimate, the kickbacks to doctors take up between 35% and 40% of the total price of drugs. Costs incurred from inflated invoices, bidding, PR activities of hospitals, and collecting prescription information account for 10–15%, which can roughly be attributed to institutional distortion (X). (See Figure 3.9.)

67 Wang Zhuanghua. Study of drug pricing mechanism from the perspective of cost. *New Wealth Management*, 2017 (09).

68 Gu Huaye, Hu Xinde, Ren Yong and Yang Liu. A preliminary examination of drug prices pushed up by selling costs of pharmaceutical enterprises: a survey of drug pricing mechanism. *Financial Supervision*, 2015 (31).

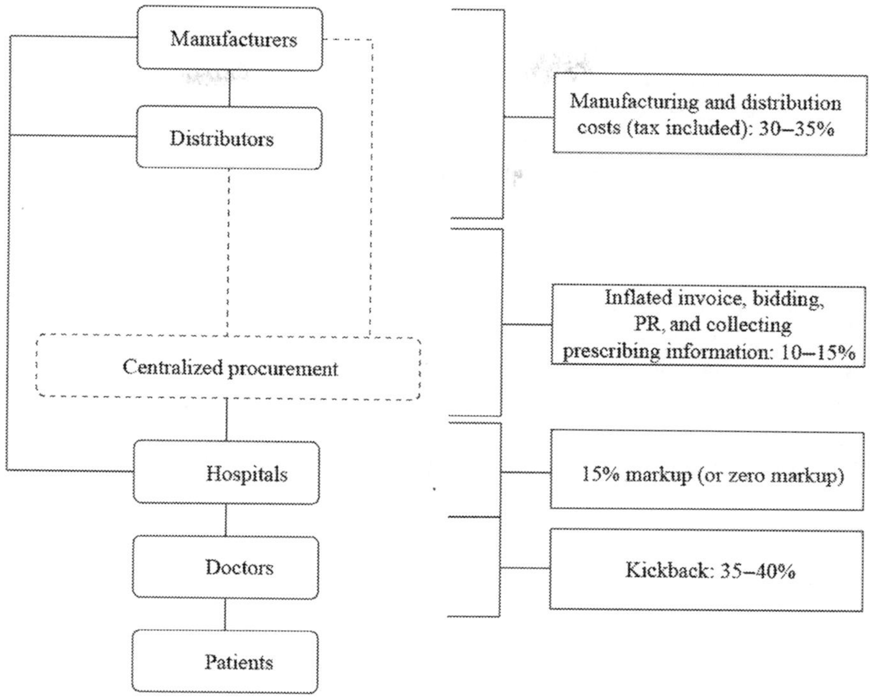

Figure 3.9 Manufacturing and Distribution Components of Drug Pricing

Naturally, these figures are rough estimates. In addition, given the cancellation of the 15% markup, the component of costs paid to hospitals will be changing in volume and share of the total. Looking at the overall trends in drug prices, however, there is nothing to indicate that the exorbitant price situation has been dealt with effectively. Drugs continue to be priced at a very high level, a situation that has not changed.[69] The composition of drug prices as described is pretty much established.

6.3 Objectives of reforming price-formation mechanisms of drugs

'Reasonable' or 'equilibrium' drug prices are those which can reflect both sides of the equation, supply and demand. On the supply side, they reflect the costs of R&D, production, and distribution. On the demand side, they reflect the paying capacity of the payer as well as the therapeutic value of the drug to patients. From this perspective, a 'reasonable' drug price should be equivalent to the sum of

69 Wang Jing, Zhou Wenli, Liu Gang, Zhou Yan'an, Zhou Benhong, Zhang Xianzhou, Zhang Hong and Zou Jun. Study on the situation of price and distribution cost about 63 kinds of drugs and policies of regulation price in Hubei province. *China Pharmacy*, 2018 (08).

production and distributions costs and a corresponding balance of profit, that is, the S + C portion of equation (2).

If the services of doctors and the services of hospitals are completely competitive, in a fully competitive market, then it does not make any difference if payment for these two are stand-alone systems or folded into the price of drugs, since any income that exceeds a situation that is balanced will be washed out in competition.

However, one of the abiding features of the services of doctors and hospitals is that information is not in fact symmetrical, which gives them a 'natural monopoly' status. As a result, they can make use of their information advantage and they are motivated to induce more demand in order to gain 'super-normal' profits. The countries and regions in East Asia have traditionally combined 'medicine' and 'drugs' as a single business, that is, they both prescribe drugs and are the suppliers of drugs at the same time. Among these countries, South Korea, Japan, Malaysia, and Taiwan (China) have been implementing reforms over the past few decades that separate out these two businesses.[70] Case study research indicates that in fact the quantity of prescriptions and cost of drugs declines once drugs and medicine are separated.[71, 72] From this perspective, when doctors and hospitals combine these businesses, it is easier for drugs to subsidize the practice of medicine and for prices to become distorted. The way the pharmaceutical industry should operate in the modern age, therefore, is as a separate industry – the services of hospitals and doctors should be compensated appropriately, but not through the sale of drugs. That is, a 'reasonable price' for drugs should not include the P2 portion of Equation (2). Given that P2 is unreasonable, the X portion of the equation is also unreasonable. A 'reasonable' drug price can therefore only reflect the cost of drugs and the paying capacity of the payer, and the portion of the price that represents the therapeutic value to the patient (P1).

To achieve a reasonable drug price, it is necessary to consider and balance the following three objectives in evaluating drug price-formation mechanisms.[73] First, prices should benefit innovation. This is indispensable for a large country in particular. Second, they should ensure that drugs are affordable and fair, as a social requirement. Third, they should take into consideration the ability of the insurance fund to bear the costs and remain sustainable.

For this reason, the goal of reforming China's drug price-formation mechanisms can be defined as follows: to create a market-based drug-pricing system that uses insurance reimbursement standards as a means of adjustment, in which prices reflect the true supply and demand situation for drugs and serve to stimulate

70 Lou Yi and Wang Shucui. An overview of the context and practice of 'separation of dispensing from prescription' in overseas countries. *Health Research*, 2013 (02).

71 Yj Chou, Winnie C. Yip, Cheng-Hua Lee, et al. Impact of separating drug prescribing and dispensing on provider behavior: Taiwan's experience. *Health Policy and Planning*, 2003, 18(3): 316–329.

72 Masayuki Yokoi and Takao Tashiro. Separating prescription from dispensation medicines: economic effect estimation in Japan. *Global Journal of Health Science*, 2018, 10(5): 88–96.

73 Sabine Vogler and Katharina Habimana. Pharmaceutical pricing policies in European countries. *Gesundheit Österreich Forschungs- und Planungs GmbH*, 2014, Vienna.

innovation while at the same time allowing the public to afford drugs and the insurance fund to be sustainable.

7 Policy options for reform of China's drug-pricing mechanisms

In order to form drug prices that reflect actual supply and demand in the market, the first thing is to strip away the function that prices are currently burdened with, namely the function of paying for the services of hospitals and doctors. That is, the business of 'medicine' (prescribing drugs) must be separated from the business of 'drugs' (selling drugs). To do this, one prerequisite is to set up a payment system for the services of hospitals and doctors. Given that premise, the next step is to take full advantage of the critical role that medical insurance plays in determining prices. That is done by using the payment standards by which insurance reimburses for drugs.

7.1 Separating 'medicine' and 'drugs,' and a payment system for doctors and hospitals

7.1.1 The prerequisite for 'separating medicine from drugs' is a reasonable payment system for hospitals and doctors

As a way to control the excessive rise in drug prices, the policy measure of separating out medicine and drugs began to appear in the minds of policymakers back in the mid-1990s.[74, 75] This way of thinking about reform involved removing pharmacies from hospitals and clinics and setting up a model for selling drugs mainly through commercial (non-hospital) pharmacies. It involved separating the authority to write prescriptions from the authority to fulfill the prescriptions and sell the drugs. Once the idea began, it constantly appeared in various policy documents as a major part of the overall reform of China's medical, pharmaceutical, and healthcare structures. In 2009, when the New Medical Reform brought up the Four Separations with respect to public hospitals, the first on the list was separating out medicine from drugs.

In order to push this forward, a number of concrete measures were passed in the course of implementing the New Medical Reform. The most thoroughly implemented was the 'zero-markup' policy with respect to drug sales, which also involved the greatest readjustment of the interests that were impacted. In 2019, the National Health Security Administration began the 4+7 program of quantity-linked drug procurement, and one of the key goals was to squeeze out the payment fees that drug prices included as payments to doctors and hospitals. The idea was to make drug pricing go back to being a true reflection of supply and demand.

74 Wang Yanbing. On separation of medical care from drug sales. *China Pharmaceuticals*, 1995 (11).
75 Zheng Guochen. On separation of medical care from drug sales. *China Pharmaceuticals*, 1995 (12).

However, these measures have as yet failed to play any fundamental role in preventing the distortion of drug prices. On the contrary, these 'control'-type measures bred a whole new crop of ways to get around the measures that were themselves a new form of distortion. They only served to increase the 'distorted' component of prices. Naturally, in looking at the cases of other countries (Japan and South Korea, for example, as well as Taiwan (China)), substantial obstacles have been erected in order to maintain the status quo. The reason is that separating drugs from medicine impacts deeper levels of entrenched interests, and particularly the professional powers and interests of doctors.[76]

The aim is to go from a situation in which drugs pay for medical services to one in which the services pay for themselves. That is, to transition from having both the fulfilling of prescriptions and selling of drugs serve as income, to a system that depends on medical services for medical income. The first step is to resolve just how to generate such payment for services. Without figuring this out, it will be hard for doctors and hospitals to earn an appropriate income without resorting to even more distorted pricing practices, given information asymmetry and a monopoly on information. Two lines of thought have emerged with respect to how to set up reasonable payment systems.

7.1.2 A payment system based on administrative procedures, and its drawbacks

The first line of thought involves using an administrative solution and paying doctors and hospitals out of public finance budgets. The building of and operating of public hospitals would be paid for by public finance. Payment for doctors would be determined by reference to compensation standards of similar public servants. Underlying this kind of payment system is the principle of compensation according to costs. The total compensation for doctors (total wages) would depend on the ability of public finance (or medical insurance) to pay, with consideration given to how much wages are paid in other government departments. That is, the compensation for doctors would be linked to that of other professions (or similar professions in other countries). For example, the idea has been raised many times in recent years that doctors' salaries are roughly three to five times those of average wages. This is a typical example of compensating according to cost. With respect to how to figure pay scales within the profession of 'doctor,' allocations would be made according to standards set for such things as years of experience, title, academic background, professional rank, and so on. Numerous reform documents have talked about the need to reform the compensation system for doctors and have uniformly said that distribution (allocation) should be made according to performance. 'The more you work, the more you earn,' and 'superior quality, superior pay,' have constantly been proposed, but in actual practice, performance

76 Wang Yaozhong. International experiences of separation of medical services from drug sales. *Health Economic Research*, 2004 (10).

appraisals are a tough subject. Patients cannot provide direct assessments, and the clinical practice of medicine is quite complex. A doctor's 'performance' is evaluated by superiors in the administrative ranking, and there are no objective standards when it comes to 'more work' and 'quality work.' At the end of the day, using administrative means to determine 'distribution' (compensation) still relies fundamentally on title, position, and years of experience. The drawbacks of this method of subsidizing costs are apparent, as follows.

First, it is hard to figure out the accurate positioning of budgetary allocations. This is not because public finance has inadequate resources or because authorities try to keep payment amounts low. Instead, it is due to the difficulty in figuring out costs. Under governance through administrative means, the problem of a 'soft budget constraint' afflicts both hospitals and doctors, that is, the funding source finds it hard to keep the entity being funded within its strict budget. The entity always has an incentive to increase 'costs' in order to get more allocations out of the fiscal authority. Meanwhile, the cost of human labor, namely doctors, is the main cost in medical services. This cost is very hard to estimate, since doctors in China have no job mobility – they cannot easily move from one job to another, so it is hard to measure their value with any accuracy. The core issue that a compensation system carried out by administrative means confronts, therefore, is that 'budget allocations are never enough.'

A second drawback is the co-existence of inadequate incentives and excessive incentives. Under the fully controlled system of the planned economy, the main problem in China's medical sphere was that it was inefficient and insufficient. The first stage of reform therefore focused on expanding the supply of medical services. The main policy in this regard was to loosen controls and allow for more operating autonomy – this was meant to encourage hospitals and doctors to bring in more income through all kinds of ways. In the 1980s and early 1990s, the policy orientation was to encourage hospitals to subsidize their operations through the sale of drugs, to engage in secondary businesses to subsidize the primary business, and to carry on various forms of cooperation with private operators.[77, 78] These measures did indeed stimulate a proactive approach on the part of doctors and hospitals. They swiftly resolved the extreme impoverishment of medical services that had prevailed during the planned-economy period, and indeed the tendency now was an over-supply of services. Starting in the latter part of the 1990s, the problems in China's medical sphere have no longer been a shortage of medical services and drugs, but the opposite – problems now relate to excessive treatments and excessive prescribing of drugs, and consequently the excessive speed with which medical costs have risen.

In order to control this issue of over-incentivizing medical institutions, the New (round of) Medical Reform was begun in 2009. The first step was to launch the

77 Ministry of Health, Ministry of Finance, Ministry of Human Resources, etc. (1989). Opinions on several issues of expanding medical and healthcare services.

78 Ministry of Health. (1992). Opinions on deepening medical reform.

Basic Medicines System on a nationwide basis in grassroots medical and healthcare organizations, as well as a system that created 'two separate lines of administration for revenues and expenses.' The theory underlying these two measures related to the 'over-incentivized' problem in the medical and healthcare industry – and it was felt that the main reason for such excessive incentives was that the income of doctors was linked to the medical services that doctors provided. To resolve the problem, the feeling was that it was necessary to sever the relationship between the quantity of services provided and a doctor's income.[79]

However, after severing the relationship between income and services, medical and healthcare services at grassroots organizations shrank rapidly and their share in total patient visits dropped just as quickly. This happened even though fiscal allocations to these organizations were being increased. (See Figures 3.10, 3.11.) This is also the background to the program re-launched in 2014 that was called 'tiered medical treatment,' that is, medical services tiered by government level. In short, the course of 40 years of medical reform in China indicates that administratively determined payment systems continue to vacillate between 'inadequate incentives and excessive incentives.'

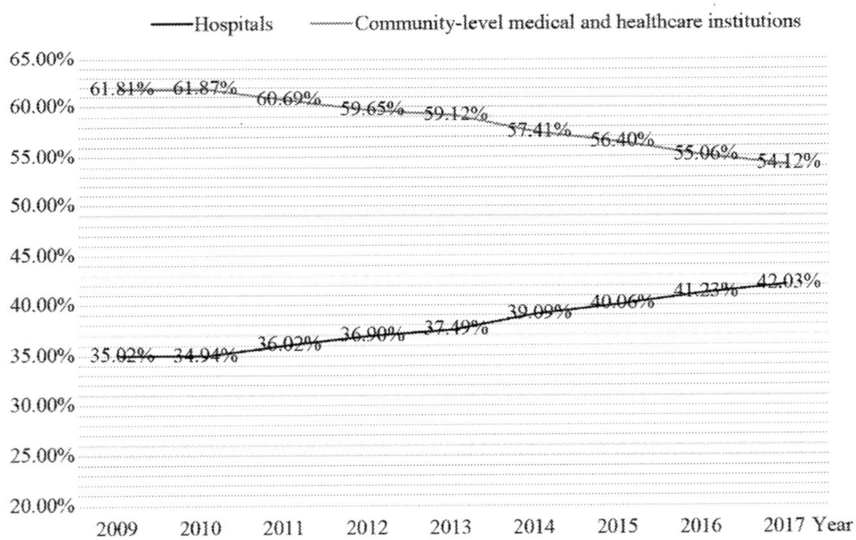

Figure 3.10 Change in the Percentage of Patient Visits to Hospitals and Community-Level Medical and Healthcare Institutions

Source: China's Healthcare and Family Planning Statistical Yearbook

Note: Community-level medical and healthcare institutions include community medical care centers, township clinics, village clinics, clinics, outpatient clinics. Total patient visits of medical and healthcare institutions include those of hospitals, community-level medical and healthcare institutions, specialized medical and healthcare institutions and other medical institutions.

79 Li Ling and Jiang Yu. On issues of public hospital reform. *Journal of Chinese Academy of Governance*, 2010 (04).

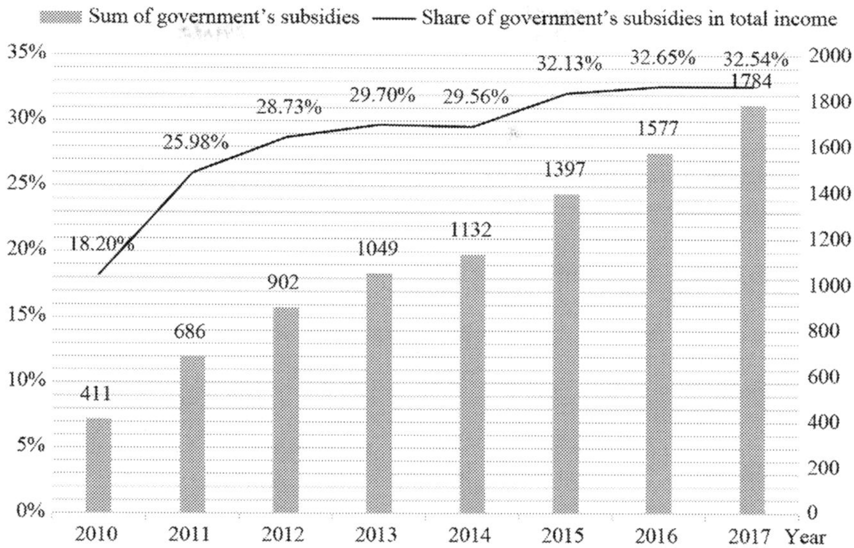

Figure 3.11 Share of Government Subsidies in Total Income of Community-Level Medical and Healthcare Institutions (Unit: CNY 100 Million)

Source: China Health Statistical Yearbook 2018

7.1.3 Building a payment system for doctors and hospitals that is 'socialized'

The second line of thought with respect to payment systems for the services of doctors and hospitals is a system that is 'socialized,' which in this context means that it is operated on a commercial basis by society at large. The basic principle behind such a socialized payment system is that compensation is not made on the basis of costs, but rather on transactions.

The payer, by purchasing services, carries out transactions with the medical services provider. The significance of this kind of transactional relationship is that compensation is not made according to the 'costs' of the medical institution or doctor, but is calculated in a comprehensive way that includes costs, payment capacity, and value to the patient. In such a payment system, based on transactions, if the services that the medical institution and doctor provide are of no value to the payer or the patient, then there will be no compensation. In essence, a socialized payment system based on transactions is a comprehensive payment system based on payment for value.

Such a payment mode is expressed through a competitive system that has a pluralistic supply. In most other countries and regions, the supply of medical services allows public, private, for-profit, and not-for-profit entities to co-exist. Whoever the services provider is, the payer for services deals with them in the same manner, as equal entities conducting transactions in one payment system. Even in the U.K., where reforms are carrying out quasi-market-based reforms, relationships between providers and the government are also shifting from direct administrative control toward the purchasing of services.[80] More than 90% of the supply of medical services in the U.K. is provided by general practitioners, and these are mainly in private practice. As payer, the NHS pays general practitioners through purchase of services.[81] In looking at how different types of hospitals and hospital beds are distributed in major OECD countries, we can see that the distribution of public hospitals, private not-for-profit hospitals, and private for-profit hospitals is fairly balanced, and the share of medical services that each supplies is also not dissimilar (see Table 3.2). With a multiplicity of types of suppliers, these countries and regions have been able to form a social transaction model (commercialized, i.e., non-government controlled) that is based on competition in how they pay hospitals and doctors.

7.1.4 Constructing a payment system for the services of hospitals and doctors that is based on equivalent transactions

China's system for paying doctors and hospitals has inherited and continues the system put in place during the planned-economy period. It is an 'administered' system, yet it is embedded in a system that is already a market economy. The conflict

Table 3.2 Distribution of Public Hospitals and Beds in Some OECD Countries (2015)

	Distribution of Hospitals			*Distribution of Beds*		
	Public Hospital	*Private Non-profit Hospital*	*Private For-profit Hospital*	*Public Hospital*	*Private Non-profit Hospital*	*Private For-Profit Hospital*
Australia	52.7%	8.0%	39.3%	67.1%	14.4%	18.5%
Austria	55.0%	15.1%	29.9%	69.2%	17.2%	13.5%
France	45.0%	22.4%	32.7%	62.1%	14.1%	23.9%
Germany	25.9%	31.5%	42.6%	40.8%	29.1%	30.1%
Greece	43.8%	1.4%	54.8%	65.0%	1.9%	33.1%
Italy	41.0%	3.0%	56.0%	67.6%	3.9%	28.5%
ROK	5.8%	94.2%	0.0%	10.4%	89.6%	0.0%
New Zealand	51.5%	17.0%	31.5%	84.4%	3.6%	12.0%
Portugal	50.7%	24.0%	25.3%	68.9%	20.0%	11.1%
Spain	44.8%	15.6%	39.6%	68.7%	12.1%	19.2%
U.S.A.	25.2%	53.1%	21.6%	22.7%	60.4%	16.9%

Source: OECD Stat, https://stats.oecd.org/Index.aspx?DataSetCode=SNATABLE5#

80 Fu Mingwei, Zhu Hengpeng and Xia Yuqing. NHS reforms in the UK and enlightenment to China. *International Economic Review*, 2016 (01).

81 Zhu Fengmei. GPs in the UK. *Health Newspaper*, 2015 (06).

between this administered system and its market-economy environment has dictated the main course of 40 years of reforms in the medical sphere, ever since the start of Reform and Opening Up. The condensed expression of this conflict is the practice of 'subsidizing medicine through selling drugs,' and the resulting distortion in drug prices. Because of this, behind any reform of pricing mechanisms lies the crux of the matter, namely reform of the payment system for hospitals and doctors.

China set out on the course of creating a medical insurance system in the country at the end of the 1990s. From then on, it was in fact decided that payment of doctors and hospitals would be commercialized, a system based on transactions with the purchase of services. In 2018, the National Health Security Administration was set up with the aim of establishing a universal medical insurance system, and in fact this too reconfirmed that the goal of reform was to institute the transaction-based purchase of medical services. The relationship between medical insurance and medical services providers, as well as pharmaceutical supply companies, would become one of the commercial transactions.

Having a commercialized payment system for hospitals and doctors means that the monopoly position of China's public medical and healthcare organizations must change, and the staffing system of public institutions must be reformed. A commercialized (socialized) and diversified supply pattern must emerge. As things stand now, the following several reforms have either taken place or are in the process of taking place.

The first has to do with reform of the pension system that applies to government organs and public institutions. Such reform began in October 2014, and put pensions on the same track as the system that applies to employees of corporations, namely a 'basic pension insurance system.' This broke through one of the primary obstacles that had prevented doctors from moving freely between public and private institutions.

The second has to do with reform of the system that designates the professional titles of doctors. Progress to date indicates that the specifying of titles of medical personnel has basically already been 'socialized' (that is, not set by administrative fiat). Medical personnel may themselves participate in the designation of their professional standing, whether in public or private hospitals, as carried out by the local human resources department and healthcare administrative authorities.

The third has to do with pushing forward reforms that allow doctors to work in more than one location. Such ability to work in multiple locations has been one of the crucial parts of the New Medical Reform. In 2017, the National Health and Family Planning Commission issued the *Administrative measures for registering the professional status of doctors*. This relaxed restrictions that had applied to working in more than one place, and also allowed doctors to be registered in different administrative jurisdictions. In 2018, the same Commission issued a notice called *Notice on further reforming the licensing process (review and approval process) whereby doctors work in medical institutions*. This explicitly said that a single registration permit (or license) is valid at both the provincial and county levels.

The fourth has to do with encouraging private investment in the medical sector. Encouraging such investment has also been a key policy measure since the New Medical Reform began. In 2019, further steps were taken to relax restrictions in regional healthcare plans that had not allowed private (commercial, 'social') interests to operate medical businesses. Under the impetus of these policies, private investment in the medical sector has developed quickly in recent years. Its share of the supply of medical services is not yet dominant but it already constitutes close to one half of all institutions in terms of numbers.

The fifth has to do with medical insurance and agreements with designated medical providers. By now, the insurance system deals with both public and private medical institutions on an equal basis.

The sixth has to do with reform of the payment methods by which medical insurance reimburses for hospital services. Reform in this regard has been put on the agenda. It will gradually progress in the direction of advance payments for Diagnosis Related Groups.

Nevertheless, China still needs to break through the following hurdles as it sets up a transaction-based payment system for doctors and hospitals.

First, on the supply side, we must continue to push forward reform of the staffing system in public institutions and government organs. This includes peeling away the policy protections and public benefits that accrue to the staffing system. Even though some things that were originally part of the system have been changed, such as the pension system and professional ranking, many other hidden policy protections and benefits still apply. As examples, it is hard to fire an employee under the staffing system, and there are safeguards on the type of wages that come from public-finance pockets. The goal of reform should be to enable the staffing system to become no more than a tool used in hospital management. Doctors should be able to make their own decisions on where to work based on their risk and income preferences and their professional interests. They should not be influenced by the policy protections and discriminatory benefits that lie behind the staffing system of public institutions.

Second, with respect to insurance as the payer side, we must break through limitations on what the insurance fund is allowed to pay for. According to regulations set forth in the *Social Insurance Law*, the health insurance fund may only reimburse for expenses that are directly medical treatment related. The fund is not allowed to make payments for indirect costs or for doctor's remuneration. In theory, this regulation is aimed at public hospitals that operate under 'administered' management, because in theory such hospitals are already being funded by the government for investment in fixed assets and the costs of personnel.

In practice, however, the main income of doctors and hospitals does not come from public finance. It comes from medical insurance funds and the self-paid costs of patients. In reality, in line with the principle behind advance payments that are made by the Diagnosis Related Group, namely that 'hospitals keep any surplus while paying for any cost over-runs,' we have already deviated from the regulation.

The next step must be to carry out reform of public-finance allocations. Currently, allocations are paid to both supply and demand sides. We should move to methods that primarily subsidize the demand side.

The second breakthrough we need to achieve involves gradually setting up payment systems and payment standards for doctors. To date, there are no such standards, whether the money comes from public-finance allocations or via medical insurance transactions. This is the main reason for the radical disorder in the sphere of medicine, pharmaceuticals, and healthcare in China. Doctors are the primary actors and absolute core of medical services. Without getting a reasonable amount of compensation, any 'payment method' that is set up is bound to be ineffective. Reasonable pay should reflect the true value of doctors, which can only be determined by setting up a professional model of practicing medicine and setting up channels that enable doctors to move from one position to another. Right now, the most feasible way to do this is to set up a fee schedule that lists the value of doctors' services and thereby arrives at payment standards for reimbursement by medical insurance. This would be the (initial) basis for formulating compensation for doctors. The second part relates to setting up contractual relationships directly between doctors and health insurance, so as to encourage the mobility of doctors.

7.2 Payment standards of drugs that are reimbursed by health insurance

7.2.1 Incentive mechanisms

While pushing forward the separation of the practice of medicine and the business of selling drugs, we must at the same time speed up the process of setting reimbursement standards, so that insurance can moderate drug prices through applying these standards. In countries and regions that have a universal healthcare system, this is an indispensable component of pricing mechanisms.

What we are calling 'payment standards' for drugs covered by insurance are in fact the same thing as the 'reference price system' commonly practiced in the United States and European countries. Reference prices have an impact on actual price-formation by applying the principle, '[hospitals] keep any surplus, but have to pay for any amounts beyond what is covered by insurance.' While containing medical expenses, this leaves more price margin between the seller of drugs and the medical services provider. If a medical institution (or the seller of drugs) buys in drugs at a price that is lower than the insurance payment standard, then the hospital retains the difference in price. If the actual purchase price is higher than the insurance payment standard, then the hospital bears the burden of covering the loss (see Figure 3.12). Given this incentive, medical institutions (or drug sellers) are motivated to keep purchase prices of drugs low. The health insurance fund, as payer for the drugs, can influence actual buying and selling prices of drugs through dynamic adjustment.

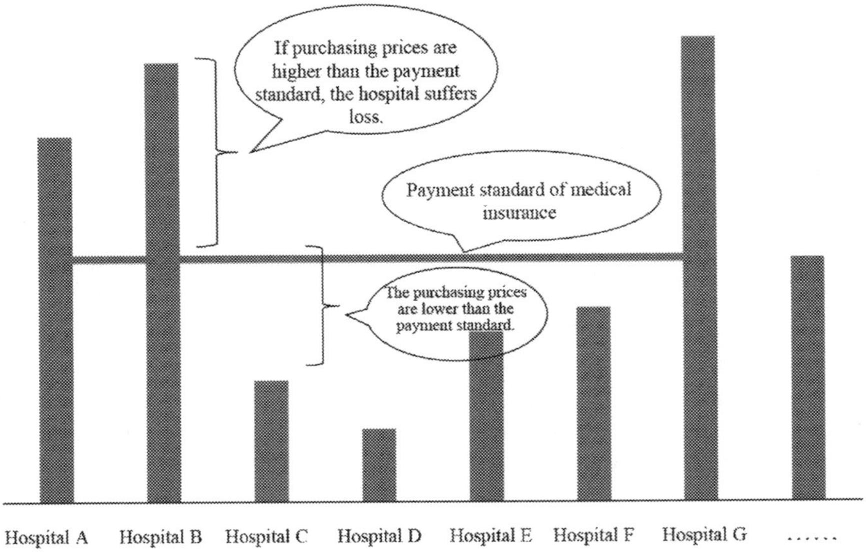

Figure 3.12 Incentive Mechanisms Relating to the Payment Standards (for Reimbursement of Claims) for Medical Insurance

7.2.2 Institutional prerequisites for setting up incentive mechanisms that enable the proper functioning of drug payment standards

In the United States and European countries, as well as the Taiwan (China) region, there is a precondition for enabling reference prices to actually work. This is that medical institutions are the primary entity doing the buying but independent commercial pharmacies are the primary entity doing the selling of clinical drugs. This is the 'institutional prerequisite' for a workable system of reference prices. Medical institutions carry on negotiations with drug suppliers through Group Purchasing Organizations or some other method, in order to determine reasonable drug prices. Hospitals and commercial pharmacies are able to be the primary buying and selling entities since they are independent operating entities, making their own decisions. Whether public or private, for-profit or not-for-profit, they take on the burden of potential losses and they also benefit from potential surpluses. Given this, it is possible that hospitals and commercial pharmacies will use the differential in drug prices to seek excessive income. An example is the 'black hole in drug pricing' in Taiwan (China).[82] Generally speaking, however, chaotic drug pricing is rare.

82 Chen Jing, Zhao Xizi, Zhao Liang and Shi Luwen. Experience and enlightenment of drug price regulation in Germany, Japan and Taiwan area of China. *China Pharmacy*, 2017 (25).

Two structural conditions lie behind this rationale. The first is the constraining effect of having multiple parties competing on the supply side. The best win, others lose out. The second is that both medical services suppliers and drug suppliers are independent legal entities, and any supplier who cannot provide qualified services is eliminated from among the market of suppliers. If there is only one medical services supplier and that supplier does not have to exit the market if it fails to deliver, then the structural (or institutional) preconditions for having a payment standards system do not exist. Incentive mechanisms cannot play their intended role.

In China right now, hospitals are the primary entities selling drugs. However, the authority of public hospitals to make autonomous decisions in buying and selling drugs was removed back in the late 1990s. Government-led centralized procurement of drugs was the method by which hospitals were deprived of this authority. In the 1980s and 1990s, hospitals were the primary buyers and sellers of drugs, but not only did hospitals not keep prices down but the more drugs they bought, the higher prices went. Underlying this phenomenon was the way drug sales subsidized hospitals, and also the control system that placed a fixed limit on markups as a percentage of price. Under both of these inducements, hospitals were fully motivated to buy in high-priced drugs.

In order to 'straighten out' drug pricing, all parts of China began to promote the centralized procurement of drugs after 2000. Such procurement was first done at the prefectural level, that is, within the jurisdictional bounds of the prefectural level of government, and later this progressed to being government-led procurement at the provincial level. The reason it was necessary to remove hospitals' authority to make independent decisions on drug procurement was not just that drug selling was subsidizing hospitals, or that money was being made off higher markups on high-priced drugs. In addition, there was a deeper-level cause that had to do with the administrative monopoly on hospitals in China. This was true particularly in the local supply of medical services – administrative monopolies were formed through administrative protectionism. This led to the inability to make comparisons among medical suppliers or to engage in competition.

Given administrative protection, public hospitals had both the incentive and the ability to make use of their monopoly standing. They combined this with their authority to use public resources (funds), to 'seek illicit gains,' and they did this by making money off exorbitant drug prices. In the design of policy, therefore, depriving hospitals of their authority over buying and selling drugs had a certain rationale. However, it also had the potential to make hospitals even less motivated to try to control drug prices.

Before the National Health Security Administration was established, centralized drug procurement for public hospitals was under the guidance of healthcare administrative departments. Once the NHSA was set up, responsibility was shifted to the new entity and the NHSA began to play the leading role in centralized drug procurement as the representative of payers for drugs. The current trend in policies say that centralized procurement is not just about price negotiation but also about quantity-based procurement. In theory, the incentive mechanisms behind centralized procurement and reimbursement prices are different and even in conflict with one another. This is indeed one of the central conflicts that China faces as it develops drug-pricing mechanisms.

7.2.3 Conflicts in the course of implementing payment standards (reimbursement prices) for drugs

In international practice, there are two main types of reference prices for drugs. One is external, in that it looks at prices in other countries and regions (either singly, or as a group), and then links the average of those to prices within the country. The second is internal, in which case the reference price is determined through negotiations (for innovative drugs) or price surveys (for generic drugs). In 2015, the National Development and Reform Commission determined that the prices of drugs on the reimbursable drug list should be used as the payment standard for medical insurance, and after this various parts of China began to experiment with different ways to implement this. There were two mainstream approaches: one determined the payment standard through a bidding and procurement process (for example, as in Anhui and Fujian). Generally speaking, the lowest winning bid became the standard. The second approach links prices to the lowest bid in other areas, which then becomes the payment standard in the home territory.[83]

Both of these mix up the relationship between the standards by which medical insurance reimburses for drugs, and centralized procurement. Centralized procurement means that the primary buyer and seller of drugs (the government) reach agreement with drug suppliers on the ultimate price of a drug. Medical insurance standards are merely the reference prices that medical insurance funds use to reimburse for medicines – they are not the ultimate price. Centralized procurement makes use of its advantage as monopoly buyer in making strategic purchases of drugs – this is the 'incentive mechanism' it has at its disposal. The concept of exchanging greater quantity for lower price is a distillation of that strategic kind of buying. In contrast, the payment standards of medical insurance are meant to take into consideration such things as the ability of insurance funds to pay, and average prices of drugs. The incentive mechanism in this case is to encourage the entities actually buying and selling drugs (hospitals) to act on their own in holding down the actual prices of drugs. However, linking prices to the lowest prices is the epitome of administratively dictated prices: the lowest price is unrelated to sales quantity, and it also is unrelated to the clinical value of drugs. It is definitely unrelated to the ability of the insurance fund to pay for drugs.

83 Li Jingjing, Kang Qiafu, Ding Rongfang, Huang Shaozhong and Huang Xianxiang. The impact of medical insurance payment standard reform on clinical drug use in designated medical institutions: Based on Fujian provincial level, Fuzhou medical insurance insured personnel empirical evidence. *Chinese Journal of Health Policy*, 2017 (11).

Once the NHSA was established, it focused strongly on centralized procurement, which was seen as the primary method by which excessive drug prices would be lowered. This naturally was because of the group buying advantage of health insurance as a strategic buyer. However, if one looks at the deeper levels of operating mechanisms, payment standards of medical insurance and the centralized procurement mechanisms of health insurance are in conflict with one another. Medical insurance *payment standards* operate by giving sufficient autonomy to medical institutions and commercial pharmacies so that they can make their own buying decisions. It incentivizes medical institutions and commercial pharmacies to try to control the actual price at which drugs are bought and sold. Controls over the total costs of drugs and the prices of medical insurance are mainly achieved through payment standards – they are not achieved through interference with the buying and selling behavior of medical institutions and commercial pharmacies. This same principle has given rise to highly developed Group Purchasing Organizations in the United States and Europe. In contrast, *centralized procurement* in China is carried out by medical insurance itself, and not only requires that medical institutions buy and sell drugs at centrally procured prices, but even at mandated quantities. This actually deprives medical institutions of their power to make their own decisions on buying, selling, and using drugs, and is equivalent to having medical insurance take on the functions of managing a hospital's drug business. At the same time, it reduces the authority of doctors to prescribe drugs. This approach is fundamentally at odds with payment standards.

Naturally, at the current time in China, medical insurance cannot help but rely on centralized purchasing as a way to try to control drug prices. Given the powerful administrative monopoly position of hospitals and the way hospitals and doctors are managed as an integral unit, medical insurance is fundamentally unable to use payment standards to keep hospitals and doctors from seeking personal interest. Hospitals use their authority to buy drugs and doctors use their authority to write prescriptions; both engage in behavior that pushes up drug prices and the total cost of drugs.

However, such centralized purchasing can only be a short-term solution. In the long run, it will be hard to control drug prices and drug costs by limiting the authority of hospitals to manage their own drug matters and interfering in the prescribing authority of doctors. This has been proven time and again over the past several decades of trying to enforce administrative controls over drug prices. Part Three of this chapter makes this crystal clear – not only does such intervention not produce the desired results, but it introduces new ways of distorting prices.

With respect to reforming drug pricing, our orientation must therefore return to using the market as the basis for price-formation. Payment standards must be the way that China manages to control drug prices and costs, which is also consistent with current reforms on methods of reimbursement. China is right now in the midst of reforms that launch reimbursement by Diagnosis Related Group (DRG) on a nationwide basis. Other countries have broadly adopted DRG payment for hospital services and its core incentive mechanisms are in line with those of payment standards for drugs. By design, the package of DRG payments includes drug expenses. This is basically equivalent to allowing hospitals to handle their own businesses and make their own decisions on drug prescribing. Meanwhile, as China sets up a system whereby doctors are contracted by medical insurance, and are doctors are increasingly allowed to work in multiple locations, the country will gradually establish a payment system for doctors. These things all provide the conditions for launching medical payment standards on a nationwide basis.

7.2.4 Formulating and implementing payment standards (reimbursement prices) for medical insurance

Reference prices for innovative drugs in other countries are mainly arrived at through negotiations. In recent years, the mainstream way of doing this is to base negotiations on the clinical value of innovative drugs, and to arrive at that clinical value by using pharmaco-economic evaluations. As for generics, the mainstream method is to determine a reference price that is based on the average market price of similar drugs, and to get that average market price through price surveys. These methods require a degree of systemic prerequisites, however. First and foremost, existing prices cannot incorporate payments to doctors and hospitals. If such payments are indeed contained in existing prices, this betrays the existence of 'drugs subsidizing medicine.' Not only are price surveys then inappropriate, but using them will serve to solidify the high levels of exorbitant prices. Second, such methods require a market for the supply of drugs and medical services that is competitive and has multiple suppliers, or it will be hard to curtail the opportunistic behavior of hospitals and drug suppliers. Third, they require a sound foundation for pharmaco-economic evaluations that can make comparative judgments about the clinical value of drugs. Fourth, they require that generics are as consistent in quality, safety considerations, and clinical results as original-research drugs. This last point is of supreme importance in setting payment standards for generics and enabling them to be substituted for other drugs. Although China has begun the work of promoting consistency in generics, the great majority of generic drugs have not been evaluated and quality is uneven.

At the present time, these four prerequisites would be hard to implement in China's medical, pharmaceutical, and healthcare arena. This is yet another main reason the NHSA has chosen to focus on centralized procurement as the way to push down drug prices. From the standpoint of feasibility, we should achieve progress in the following four areas in order to build and launch payment standards by which insurance reimburses hospitals. These take into account the actual situation in medical care and drug supply in China, and the policies that China has already launched in this regard.

First, link and coordinate the various reforms, that is, methods by which medical insurance reimburses hospitals, reform of public hospitals, and the centralized procurement of drugs. In parts of China where reimbursement to hospitals is already being made according to Diagnosis Related Groups and is operating in a stable manner, gradually transition from centralized procurement to using payment standards for drugs that are reimbursed by health insurance. First confirm the payment standards in the initial period by using such methods as bidding and procurement. At the same time, via payment-method reform in hospitals, and by instituting payment standards for drugs, push forward reform of public hospitals.

Second, devise payment standards for health insurance according to two categories: drugs for inpatients, and drugs sold in clinics. Given that 'medicine' and 'drugs' are still a combined business, first launch payment standards for drugs that are used for inpatients in hospitals, but incorporate those in the DRG-based payments that insurance makes to hospitals and establish a unified payment standard. As for payment standards for clinics, these should depend on the extent of progress in separating out 'medicine' from drug sales, and the extent of progress in setting up a compensation system for doctors and commercially run pharmacies. Right now, China has already eliminated the drug markup income to hospitals, and hospitals are less enthusiastic about establishing their own outpatient pharmacies. This creates the necessary conditions for hospitals to allow prescriptions to be fulfilled outside their own jurisdiction. From the standpoint of medical insurance, we should gradually bring commercially run pharmacies within the scope of reimbursements for prescriptions. At the same time, we should strengthen regulatory controls over pharmacies and include pharmacies within the supervision network of health insurance. In this regard, we should set up a system of accredited pharmacists and payment for such pharmacists.

Third, we should attempt to set up a system of monitoring and surveying prices of drugs, in order to lay the foundation for establishing payment standards for medical insurance that are based on price surveys. The scope of this monitoring and surveying should not be limited to the mainland part of China but should include all major drug markets as well as the Taiwan, Macao, and Hong Kong regions. In the early period of establishing payment standards, we can also set up an external price reference system. This would compare prices with drugs in countries and regions with similar economies and level of social development. The price monitoring and examination systems can also build a foundation for price negotiations and centralized bidding and procurement.

Fourth, given the current negotiations to include certain drugs in the reimbursable drug list, we should sum up our experience and use what comes out of these negotiations as the basis for negotiations on insurance payment standards for innovative and high-priced drugs.

8 Conclusions and policy recommendations

Distorted drug prices are a condensed expression of the primary problems in China's medical, pharmaceutical, and healthcare arenas. Medicine in China has been plagued by these distorted prices ever since the start of Reform and Opening Up. The root cause of the phenomenon is on the supply side of medical services – that is, the problem of drug prices 'lies with medicine, not with drugs.' Prices of drugs in China incorporate payments for the services of doctors and hospitals, in addition to the normal production, distribution, and a margin of profit on drugs. This leads to the so-called 'subsidizing medicine through drugs.' Meanwhile, in order to circumvent all kinds of administrative attempts to control distortions, hospitals and doctors have resorted to further distortions as they take income out of drug sales to cover expenses. These additional distortions have also been incorporated in the actual prices of drugs.

Part of the reason China 'subsidizes medicine through drugs' relates to the way in which drugs and medicine have traditionally been combined as a profession. In addition to this, however, are institutional causes. The first is the unfortunate legacy of the way public medical organs were governed through administrative fiat under the planned economy. Under such administered governance, the expenses of hospitals depended on public-finance allocations – including the cost of personnel and investment in fixed assets. Because of this, fees taken in by hospitals did not include any payment for hospitals and doctors themselves. In order to provide incentives to medical institutions and doctors, starting in the 1980s, (authorities) expanded the independent operating authority of hospitals. Hospitals and doctors were then in a quandary – administrative governance of hospitals requires control of expenses, but greater autonomy requires sufficient incentives. Using drug pricing as a source of income became the only feasible option. The second institutional cause of distorted prices relates to administrative protectionism and the public-institution staffing system in China (the *bianzhi* system). Administratively determined controls meant that it was impossible to curtail the opportunistic behavior of doctors and hospitals, since there was no competition and no means of comparison with alternative suppliers of medical services. Under the protection of administrative monopolies, 'the best do not rise to the top and the worst do not get washed out.' Instead, opportunistic behavior flourishes.

Under the model of administrative governance of medical institutions, payment standards for drugs – the reimbursement prices paid out by insurance – cannot play their role as an inherent incentive mechanism. That mechanism normally would allow hospitals to retain surplus income and to absorb excess expenses. Instead, surplus cannot be retained and it is also hard for the institution to cover excess costs. Given this situation, payment standards fail to function as incentive and constraint mechanisms. This is one of the main reasons China's National Health Security Administration has decided to adopt centralized procurement in lieu of adopting payment standards as a way to control drug prices.

Over the long run, however, in view of China's already determined model of social medical insurance and the fact that China has already realized universal medical insurance, the goal of China's drug-pricing reform should be to develop price-formation mechanisms that are market based while using payment standards as a means of adjustment. Drug prices in China should be able to reflect the true supply and demand situation. They should help encourage innovation, while at the same time ensuring that prices are affordable and that insurance funds are sustainable.

To achieve this goal, we first must realize separate systems for the payment of doctors' services and those of hospitals. Payment for such services should be removed from payment for drugs. In setting up such independent systems, the overall orientation should be to establish a supply of medical services that is commercialized (socialized), competitive, and that allows for comparisons among suppliers.

Given the monopoly position still held by public medical institutions, from the standpoint of feasibility, the first step is to launch nationwide reform of payment methods for medical institutions. That is, set up payment methods that pay for services on the basis of Diagnosis Related Groups. The second is to set up a fee schedule for payment for doctors' services. Initially link pay scales to average wages in society, then, through reform of the employment model for doctors and on the basis of making mobility the norm, gradually transition to a value-based system for paying doctors' fees. Meanwhile, set up a system whereby insurance pays doctors directly based on contractual arrangements. In this process, public-finance subsidies to public hospitals should also go from subsidizing the supply side to subsidizing the demand side. Subsidies for public medical institutions should be reduced, to the point of being eliminated altogether.

With respect to setting up payment standards by which insurance pays for drugs, reform should proceed according to the principle of moving forward gradually in the proper sequence and according to categories. In this case, the sequence is to reform payment standards for drugs used by inpatients in hospitals first, and then later those used by outpatients in clinics. The reform should be integrated with reform of public hospitals and the centralized procurement of drugs.

First, set up payment of fees for inpatient services that are by Diagnostic Related Groups. Do this in coordination with reform of the payment methods of medical insurance, and include the cost of drugs in the package of any specific DRG. The hospital itself is then responsible for procuring and managing the drugs that are used by inpatients. Medical insurance pays a unified sum for the package at fixed payment standards.

Second, gradually remove outpatient pharmacies of hospitals from the jurisdiction of hospitals, and loosen restrictions on buying drugs from pharmacies outside hospitals. Prior to doing this, strengthen regulatory management of social (private) pharmacies, and set up a mandatory system that requires open dissemination of price data on drugs being sold in pharmacies. Establish the profession of 'medical pharmacist' and then incorporate licensed pharmacists into the contracted management system of medical insurance.

Gradually set up payment standards for those drugs that are reimbursed by medical insurance, with standards to be based on price surveys and commercial negotiations. With respect to innovative and high-priced drugs, primarily establish payment standards via negotiations and quantity-based procurement. Speed up the process of conducting pharmaco-economic evaluations on innovative drugs, so as to establish the basis for negotiations on price standards. With respect to generic drugs, first promote consistency evaluations and make every effort to upgrade the quality of generics. Based on results, speed up the process of substituting generics for patented drugs. Use average market prices as the basis for payment standards for generic drugs, and adjust as necessary depending on the payment capacity of the medical insurance fund. In the beginning stage, we recommend using the drug prices in other countries that are at the same economic and social-development level as China, as reference for China's payment standards.

4 Research on payment for and usage of drugs

Zhang Yuhui and Wang Rongrong

Since the New Medical Reform (2009), but particularly since the 18th National Congress of the Communist Party of China, governments at all levels have continued to invest in building up healthcare to the extent that a universal medical insurance system has basically been established. The affordability of medical and healthcare services has improved, enabling more equitable access to health. Overall, the health of the population has shown constant improvement. At the same time, however, such factors as industrialization, urbanization, and the aging of the population are accelerating and affecting health in increasingly complex ways. Such things as malignant tumors and cardiovascular and cerebrovascular diseases are now hitting people at a younger age. Meanwhile, attitudes toward consumption are changing in both urban and rural areas as incomes continue to rise, and people are upgrading the structure of what they consume. For now and the foreseeable future, China will continue to face fairly strong momentum behind the growth of its total demand for healthcare.

Unfortunately, the increase in spending out of China's medical insurance funds is outpacing the increase in money coming into the funds. Substantial deficits are appearing in some parts of the country. On a nationwide basis, effective cost-control mechanisms have not yet been established, and some areas still make insurance payments in a singular and inflexible way. These things are all posing a challenge to the sustainability of insurance funds. Given the attempt to control costs of insurance funds, lowering drug prices has become the overall focus (of policy makers). Innovative drugs are clearly effective in treating diseases, relieving symptoms and improving people's quality of life. They are irreplaceable. At the same time, though, innovative drugs generally hold a market monopoly due to their exclusive patent protection and can be obtained through limited channels. Given these attributes, their prices remain high and they cannot meet the medical needs of most of those who are insured.

What follows is therefore a systematic study of how to balance the relationship between using innovative drugs and needing to control the costs of medical insurance. This study looks at the role of payment methods in controlling costs and analyzes the entire process of how drugs that are covered by insurance enter into and are used by hospitals. It looks at the policy requirements for the current

DOI: 10.4324/9781003325345-4

round of deepening medical reform, and it makes policy recommendations on the prescribing of and payment for drugs.

1 How to balance the relationship between paying for new drugs and holding down the costs of the medical insurance system

In 2018, the *China Statistical Yearbook for Health and Family Planning* revealed that malignant tumors, heart disease, and cerebrovascular disease are the three leading causes of death among Chinese people. As the spectrum of disease changes in China, and as its residents enjoy more disposable income, the greater demand for innovative drugs with a clear therapeutic value is becoming apparent. Such drugs can play an enormous role in treating disease and improving patients' quality of life, but their high prices, enabled by exclusive patent protections, carry the risk of pushing up medical costs. From the perspective of controlling costs and controlling spending out of insurance funds, it is necessary to study how to balance the cost of new drugs and their cost to medical insurance.

1.1 The increase in expenditures out of China's medical insurance funds

China's medical insurance system is an important component of the country's social security system. The system is an effective means of pooling funds in the service of public healthcare. As of now, China has already built up a multi-layered system of medical insurance that includes basic medical insurance, supplementary medical insurance, critical illness insurance, and medical relief programs, as well as commercial health insurance and various forms of social philanthropy.

In terms of the institutional framework for these programs, China has been pushing forward the integration of the urban and rural parts of 'basic medical insurance' for some years. In January 2016, the State Council issued an opinion called *Opinion on consolidating the basic medical insurance systems for China's urban and rural residents*. State Council Document #3 of 2016 was released and noted the decision to 'consolidate the two systems of the "basic medical insurance program for urban residents" and the "new-style rural cooperative medical program for rural residents," and thereby to establish a unified basic medical insurance system for urban and rural residents.' The effect of this was to launch a move to unify the situation in which urban and rural programs have been separately designed, with dispersed funding and fragmented management. The institutional structures that manage the basic medical insurance program are now constantly being improved upon.

In 2018, the State Council set up the National Healthcare Security Administration. This unified the various duties and responsibilities for managing medical insurance systems. It changed the way fragmented funds had been managed by different administrative departments, and the way responsibilities and authorities were separate. In terms of the target population, the rate of participation in China's basic medical insurance reached 96.36% in 2018, meaning that the country has basically realized universal coverage of its basic medical insurance. In terms of the actual level of safeguards, fiscal subsidies into the fund are being upgraded every year. In June 2020, the notice by the State Tax Administration of the Ministry of Finance and the National Healthcare Safeguards Administration, *Notice on the proper handling of the work of the urban-rural residents' basic medical insurance safeguards*, noted that the per capita subsidies into the fund had increased by RMB 30 over the 2019 base and had reached a level of no lower than RMB 550 per person per year. However, the pooling of funds in different places shows quite large discrepancies due to different systems. In 2019, estimates indicate that per capita amounts in urban areas reached RMB 4530, while in rural areas the figure was RMB 847.

1.1.1 Social basic medical insurance

1.1.1.1 INPUTS INTO DIFFERENT TYPES OF MEDICAL INSURANCE AS A PERCENT OF TOTAL HEALTHCARE COSTS

Between 2009 and 2014, the absolute value of China's basic medical insurance funds for covering urban workers went from RMB 342.03 billion to 756.68 billion. The funds increased at an average annual rate of 13.31%. Inputs into these funds constituted roughly 19% to 20% of total healthcare costs, and this rate stayed fairly stable. This was prior to the implementation of the 'urban and rural medical insurance system.'

Meanwhile, the income of the medical insurance funds for 'urban residents' went from RMB 25.16 billion in 2009 to RMB 59.42 billion in 2012, which represented an increase in percentage of healthcare costs from 1.4% to 2.4%. Given statistical limitations, between 2012 and 2014, the income into urban residents' medical insurance funds was included in income into the funds for the 'new-style rural cooperative medical fund.' Income into this combined fund rose from RMB 94.44 billion to RMB 444.09 billion, or an increase of 7.2% as a percent of total healthcare costs. Inputs going into commercial insurance funds were quite notable, and went from RMB 57.4 billion to RMB 158.72 billion. Such funds went from representing 3.3% of total healthcare costs to representing 4.5% (Tables 4.1 & 4.2).

In 2015, China began to integrate two major insurance systems, the 'urban residents basic medical insurance,' and the 'new-style rural cooperative medical fund.' China thereby began the establishment of a unified medical insurance system that covers both urban and rural residents. At present, all 31 provinces in the country (regions, municipalities) and the Xinjiang Production and Construction Corps have issued documents as required by Central arrangements, and done the initial planning work to integrate these two systems. Meanwhile, the four cities under direct jurisdiction of the central government and 85% of China's prefectural cities have already established unified systems for urban and rural residents.

Table 4.1 Income from Different Insurance Programs as a Percentage of Total Health Expenses, from 2009 to 2014

Year	*Basic Medical Insurance for Urban Workers*		*Basic Medical Insurance for Non-working Urban Residents*		*New-Type Rural Cooperative Medical Insurance*		*Commercial Health Insurance*	
	Incomes (100 mln Yuan)	*Proportion in Total Health Expenses (%)*	*Incomes (100 mln Yuan)*	*Proportion in Total Health Expenses (%)*	*Incomes (100 mln Yuan)*	*Proportion in Total Health Expenses (%)*	*Incomes (100 mln Yuan)*	*Proportion in Total Health Expenses (%)*
2009	3,420.3	19.5	251.6	1.4	944.4	5.4	574.0	3.3
2010	3,955.4	19.8	353.5	1.8	1,308.3	6.6	677.5	3.4
2011	4,945.0	20.3	594.2	2.4	2,038.2	8.4	691.7	2.8
2012	5,908.9	21.0			3,262.4	11.6	862.8	3.1
2013	6,613.7	20.9			3,855.4	12.2	1,123.5	3.5
2014	7,566.8	21.4			4,440.9	12.6	1,587.2	4.5

Note: Insurance incomes include government subsidies, individual (employers) contributions and interest incomes among others.

Table 4.2 Income into Different Insurance Programs as a Percent of Total Health Expenses from 2015 to 2018

Year	*Basic Medical Insurance for Urban Workers*		*Basic Medical Insurance for Non-working Urban Residents*		*New-Type Rural Cooperative Medical Insurance*		*Basic Medical Insurance for Urban and Rural Residents*		*Commercial Health Insurance*	
	Incomes (100 mln Yuan)	*Proportion in Total Health Expenses (%)*	*Incomes (100 mln Yuan)*	*Proportion in Total Health Expenses (%)*	*Incomes (100 mln Yuan)*	*Proportion in Total Health Expenses (%)*	*Incomes (100 mln Yuan)*	*Proportion in Total Health Expenses (%)*	*Incomes (100 mln Yuan)*	*Proportion in Total Health Expenses (%)*
2015	8,926.1	21.8	671.7	1.6	3,111.2	7.6	1,621.8	4.0	2,410.5	5.9
2016	9,733.0	21.0	410.3	0.2	1,894.4	4.1	3,711.5	8.0	4,042.5	8.7
2017	11,604.6	22.1	199.6	0.1	692.7	1.3	5,878.5	11.2	4,389.5	8.3
2018	13,358.6	22.6	191.3	0.1	713.0	1.2	7,063.6	12.0	5,448.1	9.2

Source: China health expenditure reports (2016–2019) and national social insurance funds revenue (2015–2019)

1.1.1.2 RATE OF INCREASE OF INCOME IN DIFFERENT TYPES OF MEDICAL INSURANCE

Figure 4.1 shows the rate of increase in income for three types of insurance between the years 2009 and 2018, namely basic medical insurance for urban workers, basic medical insurance for urban residents, and commercial insurance. The first grew at a rate of 8.2% in 2010 but that increased to 16.8% in 2012, then dropped to 9.6% in 2013. After 2013, it maintained a steady rate of increase until it peaked at 17.9% in 2015. In 2016, the rate of increase again fell to 7.9% but in 2017 it returned to an increase of 14.8%. In 2018, it fell yet again to 11.8%. The urban residents' medical insurance funds in Figure 4.1 include income from the 'urban residents basic medical insurance,' the 'new-style rural cooperative medical insurance,' and the 'urban and rural residents medical insurance.' The rate of increase of this category of insurance showed a declining trend with some fluctuation. It rose from 30% increase in 2010 to 46.6% in 2012, but then declined to 14.3% in 2014. In 2015, however, it again increased to 21.6% and for the following two years it declined before turning up again in 2018, to 14.3%.

1.1.1.3 INTERNAL COMPOSITION OF MEDICAL INSURANCE

In 2018, the 'basic medical insurance for urban workers' took in 49.89% of all insurance-fund income in China. Next was the 'basic medical insurance for urban and rural residents' at 26.38%. The 'new-style rural cooperative medical insurance' funds took in 2.66% of all insurance-fund income, and the 'urban residents' basic medical insurance' funds took in 0.71% of insurance income. Meanwhile, commercial medical insurance took in premium income that constituted 20.35% of all insurance income (Figure 4.2).

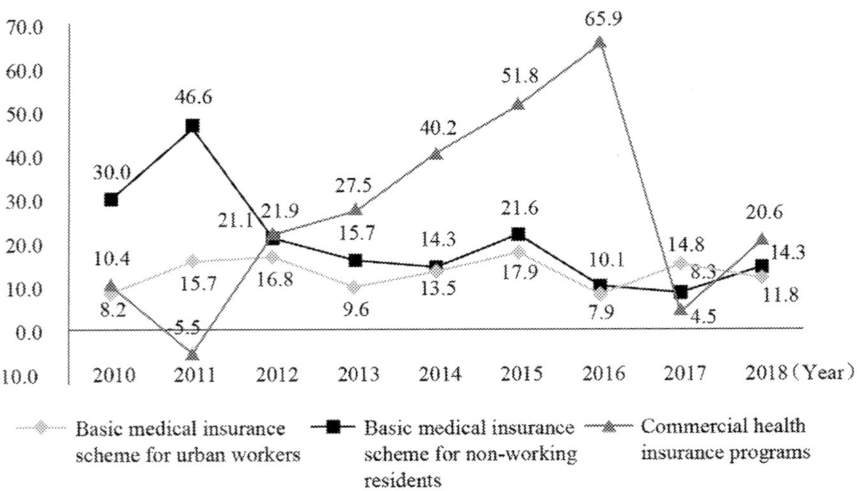

Figure 4.1 Changes in the Growth Rates of Income Going to Major Healthcare Insurance Programs in 2018 (%)

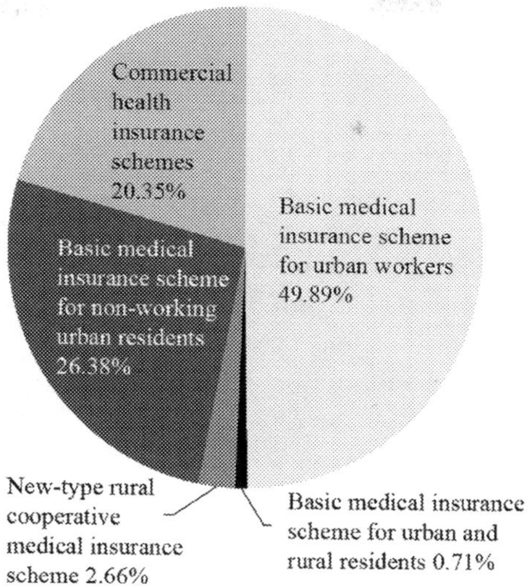

Figure 4.2 Income into China's Major Healthcare Insurance Funds in 2018, as Percent of Total

1.1.2 Forecasting China's medical costs and analyzing the sustainability of China's medical insurance funds

The fifth plenary session of the 18th Central Committee of the Communist Party of China declared the need to 'push forward the building up of a healthy China.' This stemmed from the worthy desire to protect people's health and realize the ability of society to achieve growth over the long run. As economic and social levels rise in China, attitudes about consumption are changing in both urban and rural areas and people are rapidly upgrading what they buy. At the same time, there is substantial momentum behind an increase in total demand for medical and healthcare in the country, given accelerating urbanization, accelerating aging, and the change in the spectrum of illness. This is already occurring and will go on for some time. Medical costs relating to older age groups will be rising quickly, as this segment of the population expands and as services are upgraded in terms of both quality and quantity.

Given the previously mentioned contributing factors and the ways in which each will evolve, we have forecast the medical costs of different groups (costs include inpatient costs in hospitals and outpatient costs in clinics). We have estimated the scope of medical services that groups will require and the potential cost burden on pooled healthcare funds. This is to provide supporting evidence for policy adjustments and policy formulation, so as to ensure better use of medical services and improvement in people's health. In what follows, we have adopted a 'compositional model,' commonly used in other countries, to predict medical costs. In combination with potential situations in the operations of medical funds in the future, we have made a predictive judgment about the sustainability of China's medical insurance funds.

1.1.2.1 PREDICTING THE MEDICAL COSTS OF DIFFERENT GROUPS IN 2030

1.1.2.1.1 Major contributing factors and trends

Population aging

In 2017, people age 65 and over constituted 11.4% of China's population. This was 4.4% more than the figure had been in 2000. It is predicted that around 255 million people in China will be over the age of 60 in the year 2020. These people will then constitute around 17.8% of the population.

By 2020, there will be around 29 million 'very' elderly people in China. Some 118 million older people will be living alone or will be 'empty nesters.' The old-age dependency ratio will be around 28%. Social security spending that goes toward older people will continue to increase and the problems of people who are aging in rural areas will continue to deepen.

According to the 5th National Health-Services Survey, the two-week treatment rate is 26.4% for seniors age 65 and over, and the two-week hospitalization rate for the same is 19.9%. These rates are respectively 13.4% higher and 10.9% higher than the population in general. In terms of the cost per visit, in 2016, the average cost of people over 65 visiting a clinic was RMB 176, and the average cost of a hospital stay was RMB 9,267. Both of these were 1.2 times what they cost for the public at large.

Shift in the spectrum of disease

The prevailing diseases in China have changed precipitously as the country's society has developed. Chronic diseases are now the dominant health problem. Such things as cardiovascular and cerebrovascular diseases, diabetes, chronic obstructive pneumonia, and cancers are having a major impact on the population. Between 1973 and 2009, chronic non-contagious diseases went from being 53% of the cause of death to 85%. In 2017, this figure continued to rise and reached 89.5%. In 2017, chronic diseases constituted 82.6% of the burden of illness in the country. At present, over half of the elderly population has some form of chronic disease – given the stimulus of aging, this will lead directly to an increase in the incidence of such age-related diseases as cancer and cardiovascular disease. Within the next 20 years, the number of people suffering from chronic disease among the elderly will double or triple. Changes in the age structure of the population and changes in prevailing diseases are mutually interactive, and the results will stimulate an even faster increase in medical needs and medical costs in the future.

Changes in socio-economic structure

Urbanization is a key factor behind changes in socio-economic structure. Levels of medical and healthcare spending increase as the 'urban' percentage of population increases. Meanwhile, the urban population in China is steadily rising as people flow into cities. Demand for healthcare services is only going to keep going up as China urbanizes.

Upgrading of the structure of consumption

The path that other countries have taken indicates that consumption moves from a focus on sufficient food and clothing to a focus on living quarters, and then to a focus on health and enjoyment as GDP per capita rises. Once GDP per capita goes over USD 3,000, the percentage of personal consumption spent on services goes up quickly, and the components of 'health and enjoyment' that rise the fastest relate to medical care, insurance and financial services, and the entertainment industry.[1] In 2019, GDP per capita in China broke through the figure of USD 10,000, which is regarded as entering territory that leads to a fast upgrading of consumption. Not only do people require a greater quantity of medical services, but they demand higher quality. In China, this is going to put pressure on the sustainability of the country's healthcare funding.

Advances in medical technology

'Medical technology' includes the drugs, medical devices and equipment, medical procedures and post-treatment support systems, as well as the administrative and governmental organizations that are used to prevent illness, diagnose and treat illness, restore health and promote wellbeing. Advances in medical technology contribute substantially to increases in medical costs. The most commonly quoted estimate is that of Newhouse, from 1992, which puts the contribution at 50% to 75%.

Increases in the level of medical safeguards

Research indicates that there is a positive correlation between levels of medical insurance, extent of coverage in a population, and the demand for medical and healthcare services. China's system of providing universal safeguards is the 'basic medical insurance,' which already covers more than 95% of the population and levels of subsidies are gradually going up. The demand for healthcare services is in the process of being 'released,' as more and more services are being used. On the other hand, health insurance in China has *de facto* destroyed the relationship that prices play in adjusting market supply and demand. As a result, the price sensitivity of the demand for medical services is going down.

1.1.2.1.2 Levels and composition of medical costs of different groups in 2030

1.1.2.1.2.1 Predicting the total medical spending of different groups of people

Compositional models predict the following results: at 2017 prices, China's total medical spending will be RMB 4.2 trillion in 2020. In 2025, it will be RMB 6.5 trillion, and in 2030, it will be RMB 8.8 trillion. This represents an increase of RMB 4.6 trillion over the decade. Over ten years, therefore, spending will increase by 105.6%, which means an average annual growth rate of 7.7%. In terms of relative levels, the predicted annual medical spending of groups is relatively stable as a percent of total healthcare costs, and stays at around 68–69% of the total.

If the future growth of GDP uses the benchmarks described in the report *Strategy and Approach: China Strides Forward to 2049*, then between 2016 and 2020, GDP rose at an average annual rate of 6.5%. Between 2020 and 2035, it averages

1 Zhang Yingxi and Xia Jiechang, Experience of foreign countries in service consumption upgrading. *Chongqing Social Sciences*, Issue 11, 2011.

Table 4.3 An Estimate of China's Total Medical and Healthcare Expenses in 2030, and Percent of GDP in 2020, 2025, and 2030

	Unit	*2020*	*2025*	*2030*
Medical expense	100 mln yuan	42,006.64	64,976.00	88,449.56
Total healthcare expense	100 mln yuan	61,361.00	94,418.00	129,539.00
Proportion of medical expense in total healthcare expense	%	68.46	68.82	68.28
Proportion of medical expense in GDP	%	4.23	4.88	5.17

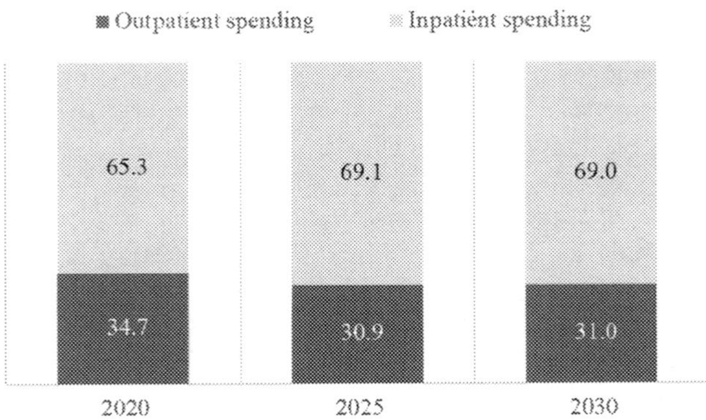

Figure 4.3 An Estimate of the Composition of China's Medical Expenses from 2020 to 2030: Percentages Incurred by Inpatients and Outpatients (%)

5%, and between 2036 and 2050, it averages 3.5%. Using these GDP figures as the basis, in 2020, medical costs as a percent of GDP come to 4.2%; in 2030, they rise to 5.2%.

1.1.2.1.2.2 Structure of future medical costs

The main component of medical costs in China is the cost of hospital stays. Specifically, hospitalization was 65.3% of total medical costs in 2020, and in 2025 and 2030 it will approach 69%. This fairly high level is expected to continue. (See Figure 4.3.)

In terms of the distribution of costs by different groups in the population, costs are mainly concentrated on the elderly, and this group is expected to use an increasingly larger percent of the total. In 2020, people over the age of 65 took up 40.9% of total medical spending; in 2030, this figure is expected to reach 50%. This group consumes a far higher percentage of medical resources than any other group – to take the forecast for 2030 as an example, despite constituting just 17.1% of the population, the elderly is expected to consume nearly one half of medical costs. (See Figures 4.4, 4.5.)

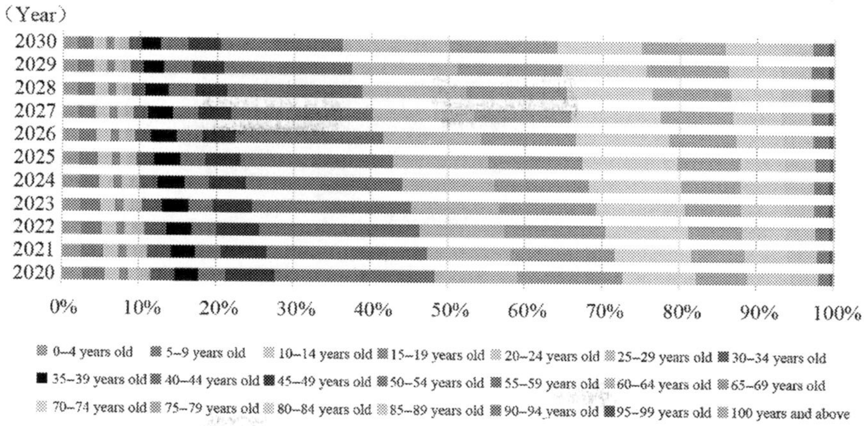

Figure 4.4 An Estimate of the Medical Expenses of Each Demographic Group in China from 2020 to 2030

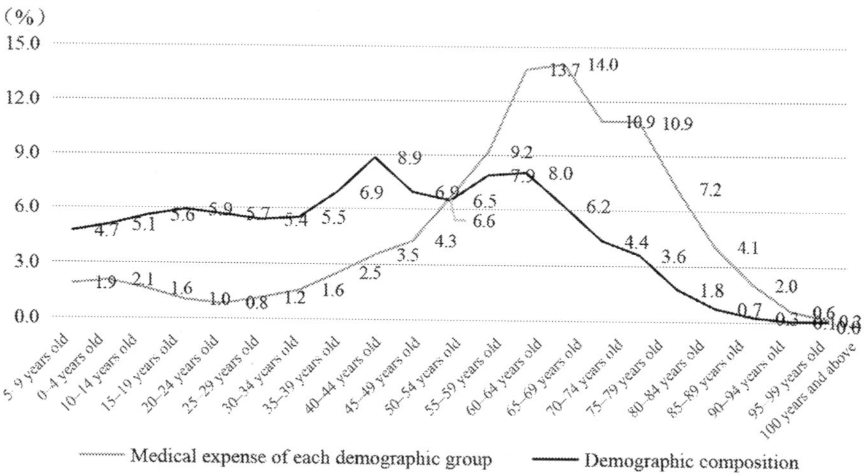

Figure 4.5 An Estimate of China's Demographic Composition and the Medical Expenses of Each Demographic Group, 2020–2030

In order to evaluate the effect that the changing spectrum of diseases in China will have on medical costs, this study first evaluated the costs of different kinds of illness. In overall terms, treatment costs are gradually rising for all of the following main chronic conditions: circulatory system diseases, respiratory system diseases, malignant tumors, and digestive system diseases, as well as endocrine disorders and problems relating to nutrition and metabolism. In 2020, costs for treating these diseases came to around 65.2% of total medical costs, and in 2030 they are expected to constitute 67.7% of total costs. Within these categories, circulatory system diseases will take up 30–33% of total medical costs in the decade between 2020 and 2030; respiratory diseases will require close to 14%, while malignant cancers will require between 7% and 8% (see Figure 4.6, and Table 4.4).

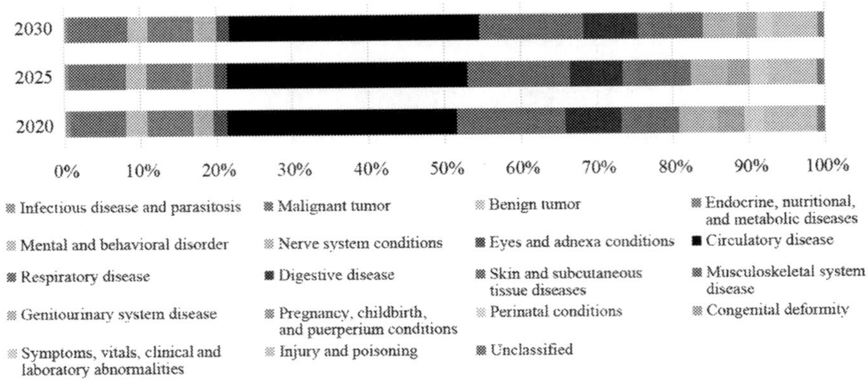

Figure 4.6 An Estimate of the Medical Expenses for Different Diseases as a Percent of Total Medical Expenditures in China, from 2020 to 2030

Table 4.4 An Estimate of Medical Expenses for Different Diseases as a Percent of Total Medical Expenditures in China from 2020 to 2030 (%)

Type of Disease	*2020*	*2025*	*2030*
Infectious disease and parasitosis	0.71	0.56	0.48
Malignant tumor	7.34	7.54	7.98
Benign tumor	2.89	2.75	2.66
Endocrine, nutritional, and metabolic diseases	6.02	6.02	5.98
Mental and behavioral disorder	0.51	0.41	0.39
Nerve system conditions	2.14	2.42	2.62
Eyes and adnexa conditions	1.82	1.75	1.65
Circulatory disease	30.24	31.58	32.98
Respiratory disease	14.23	13.48	13.58
Digestive disease	7.35	6.97	7.20
Skin and subcutaneous tissue diseases	1.67	1.80	1.76
Musculoskeletal system disease	5.93	7.15	6.83
Genitourinary system disease	4.81	4.61	4.27
Pregnancy, childbirth, and puerperium conditions	0.06	0.05	0.04
Perinatal conditions	0.08	0.06	0.05
congenital deformity	3.61	3.10	2.73
Symptoms, vitals, clinical and laboratory abnormalities	2.47	2.29	2.02
Injury and poisoning	7.06	6.48	5.92
Unclassified	1.08	0.97	0.86

1.1.2.2 FORECASTING MEDICAL INSURANCE COSTS IN 2030, AND A COMPARATIVE ANALYSIS

1.1.2.2.1 Forecasting future income and spending of medical insurance According to the 2017 edition of the *World Population Prospects*, put out by the UN's Department of Economic and Social Affairs, China's population is projected to reach 1.405 billion in 2020, 1.419 billion in 2025, and 1.421 billion in 2030. If you combine that with the percentage of the total population that has been covered by insurance under China's 'urban employee medical insurance' program for the past few years, and take into consideration expected changes in that figure as well as other factors, the number of people that this program should expect to cover in the future will be 325 million in 2020, 359 million in 2025, and 393 million in 2030. With respect to what this will cost, we used the average funding per person in this program between 2006 and 2016 and applied an exponential smoothing method to project future costs. In 2020, the per person funding level will be RMB 4,695 in 2020, RMB 6,284 in 2025, and RMB 7,872 in 2030. We therefore calculate that the total funding required for China's urban employee medical insurance will be RMB 1.5258 trillion in 2020, RMB 2.2548 trillion in 2025, and RMB 3.0932 trillion in 2030.

The next step involves calculations of the funding required for China's 'basic medical insurance for urban and rural residents': in 2020, 1.08 billion people are expected to be covered by this program. In 2025, 1.06 billion should be covered, and in 2030, 1.028 billion should be covered. We estimate the per-person level of funding at RMB 870 in 2020, RMB 1,270 in 2025, and RMB 1,670 in 2030. At these figures, the total amount of funding required for this program will be RMB 939.5 billion in 2020, RMB 1.3464 trillion in 2025, and RMB 1.7174 trillion in 2030. Adding up the funding amounts for the two programs, the total funding requirements for China's basic medical insurance will be RMB 2.47 trillion in 2020, RMB 3.6 trillion in 2025, and 4.81 trillion in 2030.

In 2017, spending out of the basic medical insurance program funds for urban employees came to 80.1% of the total amount of pooled income that came into the funds. Spending out of the funds for the basic medical insurance for urban and rural residents came to 90.4% of total pooled income. If these percentages hold steady for China's two main basic medical insurance programs, total spending out of the combined programs in the future will be RMB 2.1 trillion in 2020, RMB 3 trillion in 2025, and RMB 4 trillion in 2030.

In 2017, nearly 18.5% of the spending by the basic medical insurance program for urban employees was used to purchase drugs from pharmacies at the retail level. An additional 35.9% was spent on services at clinics, and 45.5% was spent on services during hospital stays. Meanwhile, 15.8% of spending by the medical insurance for urban and rural residents was spent on services at clinics, and 84.2% was spent on services during hospital stays. If we assume that the composition of spending and usage does not change in the future, we can estimate the future spending that will be required by basic medical insurance for clinics and hospital stays.

Table 4.5 An Estimate of the Total Pooled Funding in China's Basic Medical Insurance Funds from 2020 to 2030

Year	*Urban Worker (10,000)*	*Payment per Person (Yuan)*	*Total Fund (100 mln Yuan)*	*Urban Non-working Residents Covered by Healthcare Scheme (10,000)*	*Payment per Person (Yuan)*	*Total Fund (100 mln Yuan)*	*Total Healthcare Fund (100 mln Yuan)*
2020	32,500	4,695	15,258	107,990	870	9,395	24,653
2025	35,885	6,284	22,548	106,014	1,270	13,464	36,012
2030	39,293	7,872	30,932	102,837	1,670	17,174	48,106

Table 4.6 An Estimate of the Total Pooled Funding in China's Basic Medical Insurance Funds from 2020 to 2030

Year	*Basic Medical Insurance for Urban Workers*		*Basic Medical Insurance for Urban and Rural Residents*		*Basic Medical Insurance*	
	Scheme Fund	*Expenditure*	*Scheme Fund*	*Expenditure*	*Scheme Fund*	*Expenditure*
2020	15,258	12,221.658	9,395	8,493.08	24,653	20,714.738
2025	22,548	18,060.948	13,464	12,171.456	36,012	30,232.404
2030	30,932	24,776.532	17,174	15,525.296	48,106	40,301.828

Table 4.7 Object of Expenditure of China's Healthcare Fund from 2020 to 2030 (100 mln Yuan)

Year	*Basic Medical Insurance for Urban Workers*			*Basic Medical Insurance for Urban and Rural Residents*	
	Outpatient	*Inpatient*	*Retail Pharmacies*	*Outpatient*	*Inpatient*
2020	4,383.58	5,564.15	2,273.93	1,481.35	7,913.65
2025	6,477.98	8,222.60	3,360.38	2,122.93	11,341.07
2030	8,886.67	11,280.00	4,609.86	2,707.90	14,466.10

1.1.2.2.2 Analysis of the sustainability of insurance funding in the future If we deduct the portion of medical expenses that are subsidized by public finance, in 2020, China's pooled insurance funds will be able to reimburse 41.9% of clinic costs and 51.5% of hospital stays. On an overall basis, it will be able to reimburse 48.1% of medical costs. In 2025 and 2030, the levels of reimbursement for clinics are projected to rise slightly, while those for hospital stays are expected to decline.

In overall terms, reimbursements for medical treatment will be declining. If we assume that China eliminates the program of 'personal accounts' for its urban employee basic medical insurance program, and uses funds only for reimbursing the services of clinics and hospitals, in 2020, the level of reimbursements for medical treatment as a whole is expected to be 54%. In 2025, it should be 51.6%, and in 2030 it should be 50.5%.

Given an aging population, change in the spectrum of disease, and advances of medical technology, China can expect to see a powerful increase in the medical spending required by its population. In addition, however, the percentage of people paying into the basic medical fund for urban employees will go down as people retire. We should be forewarned that income into insurance funds will be declining and expenditures will be increasing as the population ages. Meanwhile, the basic medical insurance for urban and rural residents operates on the basis of a fixed amount of funding per person. Increases in this amount will find it hard to catch up with the pace at which medical costs are rising. The bottom line is that medical costs will be rising faster than the speed at which medical insurance funds can be assembled.

Medical insurance is one major means by which to ensure people's right to health and to mitigate their economic risk from medical causes. It is imperative

Table 4.8 Estimated Reimbursement of Insurance Claims for Medical Expenses from 2020 to 2030

Type	*Unit*	*Individual Account Kept*			*Individual Account Canceled*		
		2020	*2025*	*2030*	*2020*	*2025*	*2030*
Outpatient reimbursement	100 mln yuan	5,722.72	8,397.10	11,334.62	6,724.76	10,210.29	13,802.38
Outpatient expense	100 mln yuan	13,669.96	18,829.77	25,750.20	13,669.96	18,829.77	25,750.20
Outpatient reimbursement ratio	%	41.86	44.59	44.02	49.19	54.22	53.60
Inpatient reimbursement	100 mln yuan	12,718.08	18,474.92	24,357.35	13,989.98	20,354.51	26,935.82
Inpatient expense	100 mln yuan	24,703.20	40,430.70	54,924.30	24,703.20	40,430.70	54,924.30
Inpatient reimbursement ratio	%	51.48	45.70	44.35	56.63	50.34	49.04
Total reimbursement	100 mln yuan	18,440.81	26,872.03	35,691.97	20,714.74	30,564.80	40,738.20
Medical expense	100 mln yuan	38,373.16	59,260.47	80,674.50	38,373.16	59,260.47	80,674.50
Medical reimbursement ratio	%	48.06	45.35	44.24	53.98	51.58	50.50

that China have sufficiently effective medical safeguards if the country is to realize its goal of a moderately prosperous society for all. (In what follows), this study analyzes the scale of funding that will be required for China's medical insurance funds. It looks at pressures on those funds by using three scenarios that assume three levels of reimbursement. In 2020, China (will be) achieving the status of a 'moderately prosperous society for all.' Its basic healthcare systems are continuing to improve and actual reimbursements for medical costs are continuing to rise. At present, the country has not yet set target goals for specific reimbursement percentages, but we use the standards of 60%, 70%, and 80% for purposes of our analysis.

Assuming the reimbursement level is raised to 60%, in 2020, 93% of the total pooled funding in that year will be paid out in costs. The sum paid out will come to RMB 2.30239 billion. In 2025, the amount paid out will come close to the amount paid in – RMB 3.555628 will be spent and RMB 3.6012 will come in. In 2030, the amount being spent will exceed the amount coming in by RMB 29.87 billion – RMB 4.84047 billion will be going out versus RMB 4.9106 billion coming in. If the reimbursement level is raised to 70%, then there will be deficits in 2020, 2025, and 2030, and they will come to RMB 220.821 billion, RMB 547.033 billion, and RMB 836.615 billion. If the reimbursement level is raised to 80%, then deficits in those three years will come to RMB 604.553 billion, RMB 1.139637 trillion, and RMB 1.64336 trillion. (See Table 4.9.)

1.1.2.2.3 Policies and measures to contain (control) medical insurance costs China's medical insurance fund is facing fairly substantial pressures in order to be sustainable. Medical costs are constantly rising, given that the country is implementing better safeguards through its basic medical insurance program, and given that levels of coverage are rising. In addition, urbanization and the aging of the population are both speeding up, the spectrum of diseases is changing, and medical technologies are improving – all of this impacts sustainability of funding. In order to reduce unreasonable waste and satisfy the healthcare demands of a broader segment of the population, and still ensure the stable operations of medical

Table 4.9 Deficits in Insurance Pension Funds that may be Incurred Depending on Different Reimbursement Levels, 2020 to 2030 (RMB 100 Million)

Item	*2020*	*2025*	*2030*
Medical expense	38373.16	59260.47	80674.50
Total healthcare fund	24653.00	36012.00	48106.00
Reimbursement ratio at 60%	23023.90	35556.28	48404.70
Deficit	-	-	298.70
Reimbursement ratio at 70%	26861.21	41482.33	56472.15
Deficit	2208.21	5470.33	8366.15
Reimbursement ratio at 80%	30698.53	47408.37	64539.60
Deficit	6045.53	11396.37	16433.60

insurance funds nationwide, controlling the costs of medical insurance has become a key part of controlling unreasonable increases in medical expenses. To deal with this, policy measures are constantly being improved.

In October 2015, a group of key government departments jointly issued a Notice called *Notice on various opinions on controlling the unreasonable increase in medical expenditures of public hospitals*. The departments issuing this *Notice* were the former National Health and Family Planning Commission, the Ministry of Finance, the Ministry of Human Resources, and the National Administration of Traditional Chinese Medicine. (Directive #89, 2015, of the National Health Restructuring.) This characterized the goal of controlling medical costs and the unreasonable rise in medical insurance costs as being 'a key goal and task of the process of deepening medical reform.' In overall terms, measures to do this include the following two main categories. The first is aimed at the demand side of medical services and includes such things as a mechanism for sharing insurance costs, limiting insurance liability, and incorporating health management by the insured into insurance plans. The second is aimed at control measures that deal with the supply side of medical services. It mainly includes reform of the payment methods of medical insurance, and it includes strengthening regulatory controls over medical services suppliers.

1.1.2.2.3.1 Policies to control medical insurance costs that are aimed at the suppliers of medical services

Policies to control the costs of medical insurance focus primarily on the supply side, and mainly include reform of payment methods used by medical insurance, regulatory supervision over the suppliers of medical insurance, and strict control over drug prices through the use of centralized drug procurement and a zero-markup rate on drugs.

1 Payment methods for medical insurance (that is, methods by which insurance funds pay hospitals)

Finding reasonable ways for insurance to reimburse medical providers can play an important role in constraining and guiding behavior of providers. Different methods can influence the allocation of resources and the control of costs. In overall terms, they can be divided into post-payment and pre-payment categories.

China's medical insurance funds use two different settlement procedures to pay for medical services. The post-payment method refers to payment after a hospital has provided services, and it pays designated medical facilities according to a specific standard for specific services. Pre-payment is when medical insurance pays contracted (designated) facilities for services in advance, according to specific standards which have been arrived at through negotiations. This type of payment includes payment per headcount, payment per service, per type of illness, and full payment of total budget. Each type of payment has its advantages and disadvantages in the course of actual implementation. Right now, the great majority of insurance funds in China adopt a combination of the two. Most costs of outpatient clinics are reimbursed according to itemized services. Settlement (payment) for hospital stays is primarily paid according to headcount with the total amount being capped at a certain limit. The second most common method is to pay according to type of illness, again with a control on the total amount. Payments made to clinics for certain special types of illness can be paid according to a single service unit or according to type of illness and service unit. A more detailed discussion of China's payment methods is below, in the section of this report called 'Research on how reform of payment methods can control costs.'

2 Strengthening management controls and regulatory supervision over medical institutions and medical staff

China's medical insurance system operates a control system with respect to designated hospitals and pharmacies. Designated medical institutions must strictly abide by the system of standard fees for drugs and medical services that are determined by government. They must abide by treatment protocols as formulated by health-care administrative departments, and by quality standards for medical care and for technical procedures. Departments in charge of medical insurance implement administrative control and regulatory supervision over such things as scope of business, types, quality, and prices of drugs, as well as the fulfilling of prescriptions and their fees. They can issue warnings to designated institutions if they break rules, or they can cancel their qualified status, depending on the severity of the infringement. This is done to manage and control the quality and effectiveness of services.

Based on this supervisory control over designated medical institutions, the behavior of medical personnel is included within the scope of regulatory oversight. Both the diagnosing and treating of patients are evaluated. Medical insurance departments formulate a list of key items to be under supervision. If any behavior is found to be breaking laws and regulations, then the medical institution can have its contract temporarily rescinded or terminated, and the doctors or pharmacists who have broken rules can have their ability to be reimbursed by insurance taken away. Such behavior can include things like faking the number of visits to a clinic or the number of hospital stays, faking emergency visits, deceptively separating out fees, duplicating charges, keeping false accounts, misusing social security cards to garner profit, opposing and finding ways around supervisory investigations, and refusing to abide by administrative punishment. By investigating and regulating the behavior of medical institutions and personnel, the aim is to standardize services and better protect the health rights and interests of people who are insured, and to protect the steadiness and security of the health insurance fund that insures them.

1.1.2.2.3.2 Policies aimed at controlling the supply side of medical insurance costs

In its 2017 audit of medical insurance funds, the National Audit Office discovered that there had been 923 cases of fraudulent withdrawal of funds in just the provinces and cities where audits had been conducted. The amounts withdrawn came to a total of RMB 207 million, of which individuals had fraudulently cashed out RMB 10 million. Methods used to control costs on the supply side mainly include cost-sharing of medical expenses, strengthening demand-side group health management, strengthening incentives and punishments on the demand side.

1.1.2.2.4 Cost-sharing on the demand side Cost-sharing on the demand side, whereby the institution bears some of the cost burden, is beneficial in that institutions voluntarily reduce unreasonable and unnecessary costs. At the same time, this mechanism can be used as a form of leverage to guide demand in the direction of grassroots-level medical institutions, which thereby lowers the risk of abusing medical funds. Ways by which cost-sharing is achieved mainly include a threshold and a ceiling for cost-sharing by the institution, the scope of things medical insurance will reimburse for, and percentage of costs that will be reimbursed. The weighting of costs that the demand side has to cover depends on the level of economic development of both the country and its regions, and the state of medical insurance funds. Cost-sharing takes a compound form, depending on the region, in terms of minimum and maximum amounts that must be paid as well as reimbursement percentages. The scope of what will be reimbursed, however, is extremely clear, since it is set forth in explicit regulations with regard to drugs, treatments, and medical facilities. These have been specified in three 'catalogues': the *Interim regulations on managing the scope of drugs that are covered under the urban employees basic medical insurance*, the *Opinion on (Guidelines on) administering the list of diagnostic and treatment items that are covered under the urban employees basic medical insurance*, and the *Opinion on (Guidelines on) confirming the scope of medical facilities that are covered under the urban employees basic medical insurance, as well as payment standards for the insurance*. (These are abbreviated to 'the three catalogues' later.) These provide clear regulatory descriptions of the items that will be covered. Items included in these catalogues are either fully covered or partially covered. Anything not included must be paid for by the individual. That is, this program aims to guarantee basic medical and pharmaceutical services, and to exclude from reimbursement what is not 'basic' but instead is high-cost medical and pharmaceutical services.

More specifically, the catalogue describing drugs that basic medical insurance will cover is divided into Part A and Part B. Part A is a nationwide standardized list which guarantees basic drugs needed for clinical treatment. The cost of these is included in the scope of payment by medical insurance funds, and payment is made according to specific standards. Part B lists optional drugs for clinical treatment. These are more effective but also more expensive than similar drugs in Part A. Basic Medical Insurance only covers a portion of the cost.

1.1.2.2.5 Strengthening health management Enhancing health management is an effective way to reduce medical outlays and save on medical insurance costs. Kaiser Permanente (KP) has adopted policies that encourage those under its coverage to voluntarily undertake physical examinations. It has increased its investment in having such people manage their own health – for example, it offers higher reimbursement rates to those who get diagnosed and treated at the early stages of a disease. This achieves several objectives at the same time – on the one hand, it improves the overall health of the insured, and on the other it achieves the goal of lowering medical costs. In September 2019, China's National Health Security Administration noted, 'China has not yet expanded the scope of insurance coverage to include non-treatment related expenses, such as preventive-medicine and health checkups.' However, some parts of the country are already exploring this idea. In 2005, Suzhou City for the first time introduced physical examinations into the scope of coverage by clinics, and Zhenjiang City announced that people who are insured and have 'personal accounts' may use these to pay for the cost of physical examinations. The aim is to encourage people to get examined, diagnosed, and treated at an early stage.

1.1.2.2.6 Policies to do with incentives and punishments that are targeted at the supply side People who have not visited a doctor within a given year, or who have visited rarely, and who thereby have accumulated a fairly large balance, are rewarded appropriately for their contribution to saving resources on the supply side. For example, in Zhenjiang City, people whose personal medical insurance accounts have more than RMB 3,000 may use that as premium contributions toward supplementary insurance programs. They are incentivized to set up such things as supplementary insurance accounts, family accounts, health maintenance programs, and so on. Meanwhile, there are explicit measures to punish any person whose illicit behavior causes insurance funds to lose or waste resources. For example, in Tianjin City, anyone who breaks the rules is told to rectify behavior but also has his or her name put on a list of untrustworthy people and is subject to follow-up monitoring. Funds that were taken by fraudulent means are tracked down and returned as per legal procedures. In serious cases, the person is deprived of medical insurance coverage.

1.1.2.2.7 Innovative drugs and controlling medical insurance costs In order to ameliorate the problems of affording medical care in China, in April 2018, Premier Li Keqiang made a formal announcement to the Standing Committee of the State Council. He said that innovative drugs, but particularly anticancer treatments that are urgently needed by people suffering from cancer, will be subject to a zero tax rate. At the same time, medical insurance departments have been proactive in pushing to include anticancer drugs in the list of drugs that are reimbursed by insurance. Between 2015 and 2019, nearly 50 such drugs were incorporated into the list and these have already come down substantially in price, tremendously lowering an individual's burden of paying for these drugs. Even with price reductions, however, high costs for innovative drugs are still putting pressure on the sound operations of China's medical insurance funds.

1.1.2.2.7.1 The impact that the cost of new drugs may have on medical insurance spending

1 New drugs have both positive and negative impacts on increases in medical insurance spending

Drugs are a key component of medical insurance costs. Research indicates their combined cost comes to some 43.34% of total medical insurance costs for all categories of reimbursements. Such high costs are one of the main factors driving up medical insurance costs. The National Health Security Administration has released a notification on cancer drugs that are now included in Type 2 of the reimbursable drugs list (*Notice on including seventeen types of drugs into the scope of China's basic medical insurance, workers' injury compensation insurance, and maternity insurance*). Among these 17 drugs are 12 that treat solid mass tumors and five that treat hematologic cancer diseases. Drugs that treat cancer (including new drugs) typically have extremely high prices. The drug that treats breast cancer, for example, Herceptin, costs between RMB 21,613 and 24,000 per dose. The price of Tasigna, for chronic myelogenous leukemia, is RMB 36,986 per package. The price of drugs for late-stage renal cell carcinoma is RMB 24,192 per package. The average price of most cancer drugs, especially new drugs, is over RMB 10,000. Including such drugs under coverage by insurance implies a certain 'shock' to insurance funds. Controlling the cost of such drugs, and particularly new drugs, is a key aspect to effective control over medical insurance costs as a whole.[2]

On the other side of the equation, savings can be derived from the use of such drugs. Although reimbursements will go up when innovative drugs are covered, it may be possible to lower expenditures in other areas. For example, costs of inpatient stays in hospitals may go down as it becomes possible to avoid the complex interactions that require other treatments. More importantly, however, such drugs can extend the lives of patients, improve their quality of life, and allow them to generate greater social value. Seen over the long term, this contributes to lowering the total burden on society of medical insurance.

2 Unreasonable reimbursement policies indirectly increase risks to the medical insurance fund

A research team working on the topic called 'Improving services for people who suffer from tumors in China' found that, on average, people who are treated for cancer have to pay as much as RMB 140,000 out of pocket after they receive reimbursement from insurance. If they received targeted treatment, their total expenses may reach RMB 220,000. These figures represent 1.75 and 2.7 times the disposable annual income of an average family. The great majority of people with cancer

2 Ma Weishu, Path analysis on affecting factors for healthcare expenditure [J]. *Chinese Journal of Health Statistics*, Issue 2, 2011.

must use innovative drugs to treat it. Some of these are not reimbursable, and when they are, the rate of reimbursement is low. In addition, it is hard to get reimbursement from clinics. The results of the research team on this topic show that 49% of the respondents said they could not get reimbursed, that drugs obtained from clinics were not reimbursable – they could be reimbursed only by being admitted to a hospital. Close to 30% of respondents were (extremely) upset as a result of the way hospitals restrict the use of drugs. For example, they could only fulfill prescriptions at certain prescribed departments of the hospital and only at certain times, or they could only get a small quantity fulfilled at one time. Analysis shows that, first, the medical insurance fund places budget controls on the total amount of medical insurance that a designated hospital can be reimbursed for by limiting the percentage that will be reimbursed. Second, a higher percentage of drug costs can be reimbursed in the case of hospital stays. Many patients who would have had drugs fulfilled at a clinic instead go through the process of being admitted to a hospital. Not only does this waste medical resources, but it greatly increases medical expenses and thereby poses a grave risk to medical insurance funds.

3 Recommendations on how to balance the need for new drugs with the need to control medical insurance costs

1 Establish reasonable mechanisms that allow new drugs access to reimbursement by insurance

China's medical insurance system features low levels of coverage in terms of reimbursable amounts but very broad coverage in terms of numbers of people. Because of this, the extremely high prices of innovative drugs pose a major challenge to the ongoing sustainability of the country's insurance funds. Any innovative drug coming into the market must take into consideration the limited pricing capacity that is caused by having a single payer. The new drug must accept the challenge of the pricing of the China market. At present, the market share that commercial insurance holds in China is fairly small – commercial insurance is not in fact the primary payer. Instead, the country relies on social insurance as its core pillar, and social health insurance cannot shift the onus of paying onto others. In negotiating prices for new drugs, therefore, insurance funds must focus on their ability to bear the cost. They will find that reference prices become critical in determining payment standards for health insurance.

2 Develop generic drugs as a way to open up space for the introduction of innovative drugs

We recommend learning from the experience of Germany, Japan, and other countries with respect to how to balance the need to incentivize innovation with the need to make drugs affordable. These countries have improved pricing mechanisms that manage innovative drugs and generics by category and that thereby lower the price of generics in order to carve out space for innovative drug prices. This thereby stimulates greater vitality in pharmaceutical markets. In 2018, China's

National Health Security Administration explored a drug procurement model that was aimed at lowering the prices of original-research drugs and substituting in generics when possible. This was the 4+7 model of centralized procurement. Original-research drugs and generic drugs competed in the same bidding group and the lowest bid won the procurement contract. This model was successful in lowering the prices of 25 drugs by an average of 52%. It lowered the spending on drugs on which patents had expired, and opened up space for new drugs that have clear therapeutic value. We should, therefore, fully implement the policies recommended in the opinion issued by the State Council in 2018 (No. 20, 2018): *Opinion of the General Office of the State Council on reforming and improving policies to do with the supply and use of generic drugs*. We should speed up development of generic drugs, and ensure their reliable quality, adequate supply, reasonable price, and therapeutic efficacy.

3 Improve the results of negotiations for admitting drugs into the reimbursable drug list

The idea of managing drug procurement by category began to take hold after 2017, when the reimbursable drug list was readjusted. What this means is that common new drugs, with just the normal level of innovation and affordable prices, were procured by using the traditional 'batch' method. High-priced and highly innovative new drugs, for which there was clear clinical demand, but which were not competitive pricewise, were procured based on evidence-based negotiations. Since there were not many of this kind of drug, it was possible to use negotiated access mechanisms that were both detailed and evidence-based.

In order to improve the negotiating effectiveness of allowing drugs entry into the reimbursable drug list, we recommend as follows. First, adhere to the rules of the market and comply with supply and demand relationships and the laws of value. Create an environment of fair play so that the market can play the decisive role in allocating resources. Second, select types of drugs to be negotiated in a scientific manner, and focus on those that should be and can be negotiated. Use reasonable evaluations to generate payment standards. Third, use new-age information tools, make use of big data analysis and other measures to improve the effectiveness of evidence-based decisions. Fourth, set up a conceptual framework that allows for win-win solutions, that both seeks to balance interests and also encourages and supports technical innovation – that is, ensure that policies for negotiating access are prudent and moderate. Fifth, adhere to the principles and procedures that are described in shorthand as 'open but strict,' and that include fairness, transparency, and integrity but also rigorous and serious focus. Separate procedures into three stages: application filing by enterprises, review of qualifications, and then price negotiation. Sixth, improve access standards and negotiating procedures by strengthening the professional level of personnel through human resource training.

4 Promote rational drug use (prescribing behavior), adjust compensation structures, increase room for growth

(We recommend) launching reforms that address the entire pharmaceutical process, from production to distribution to prescribing and use. This includes wringing out exorbitant prices, reforming payment methods of medical insurance, getting hospitals and medical personnel to prescribe drugs more rationally, and controlling the inherent drivers behind costs. Second, use the space that is generated by lowering drug prices and standardizing medical behaviors to adjust prices of medical services as a whole. That is, create a situation in which the technical expertise of medical personnel is more valued and improve the compensation structures of hospitals.

5 Increase the level of funding for medical insurance funds, and find more space in the budget

In 2019, the subsidy standard at which public finance funded the medical insurance of urban and rural residents came to no less than RMB 520 per person per year. Half of the new increase in public-finance subsidies was put to improving the safeguards for major diseases (this was increased by RMB 15 per person over the standard funding amount in 2018). At the same time, the new increase in the individual premium amount was RMB 30, which brought individual's contribution up to RMB 250 per person per year. However, the level of individual contributions to basic insurance for urban and rural residents was not linked to the economic standing of those who are insured and it also did not take into consideration the ability of people living in impoverished regions to pay costs. Meanwhile, in 2018, total income into the basic medical insurance funds on a nationwide basis came to RMB 2.1384 trillion. Within this amount, income into the basic medical insurance funds for urban employees came to RMB 1.3538 trillion, and income into the basic medical insurance for urban and rural employees came to RMB 697.1 billion. However, total costs of healthcare that same year, nationwide, came to RMB 5.9122 trillion. To a certain degree, this reflects the fact that levels of funding are inadequate, and there is an urgent need to find more space in the budget for healthcare.

Some regions in China are already exploring ways to do this. Zhejiang province is an example. Since 2015, it has incorporated rare diseases into its 'major disease safeguards' category and been fairly successful in maintaining stable budgetary management over spending on medical insurance for major diseases and on special drugs (including new drugs) for rare diseases. According to a notice that the Zhejiang Provincial Department of Human Resources and Social Security, together with four other departments, put out on the system of insuring major diseases, in 2018, the reimbursement percentage for major diseases went from 50% to 60%. As a result, the additional reimbursements came to RMB 270 million. In addition, 21 additional special drugs (including new drugs) were incorporated into insurance for major diseases, which meant that another RMB 800 million in reimbursements went to patients. In total, the insurance funds in Zhejiang province increased their expenditures on major diseases by RMB 1.07 billion. In terms of what came into the funds, per person contributions were raised from RMB 25 per year to RMB 40 per year, which added RMB 776 million to the funds. Meanwhile, 11 special drugs were incorporated in the national basic medical insurance drug list and were then removed from the insurance for major diseases – this freed up RMB 400 million. By taking these actions, Zhejiang province basically achieved a balance in payments in 2018 and even showed a slight surplus. In order to generate more funding for new medicines, therefore, we can learn from the experience in Zhejiang.

6 Take full advantage of the role that commercial health insurance can play in covering the cost of new drugs

China's public health insurance provides a low level of safeguards to a broad number of people and is centered on the basic medical insurance system. Its catalogue of coverage includes strict regulations on the type and scope of things that will be reimbursed, and it mainly provides safeguards for basic medicines and the medicine needs of low-income people. It generally will not reimburse for new drugs that are higher priced but also are more effective, or it will reimburse only at a low rate. This limits the clinical use of new drugs to a degree, and shrinks their potential market. Commercial health insurance, in contrast, is not limited by the restrictions of national health insurance funds, including the reimbursable drug list. Supplementary types of insurance are mainly commercial in nature, and they are well suited to extending the reach and usage of innovative products. Commercial insurance can deal with pharmaceutical companies in a much more flexible way as they conduct negotiations and mutually reach agreement on prices. They can lead the way in introducing certain high-quality but highly priced new products to a broader audience, to segments of the public that need high-end medical services and pharmaceuticals.[3] At the same time, we must strengthen policy guidance as well as macro-adjustment measures that guide different commercial insurance companies to develop insurance products aimed at different types of diseases. We have to avoid ethical risk, and the possibility that companies will take on too high a risk as they incorporate any particular new drug into their insurance plans.

7 Consider setting up a special medical insurance fund that is targeted specifically at covering drugs that treat cancers and rare diseases

This fund would be funded by multiple sources. Participation could include the National Health Security Administration (more than 60% of the funding would be supported by the basic medical insurance), as well as participation by others (public finance, civil affairs, public forces). Funding from public finance may consider using the tobacco tax, and civil affairs funding may consider using the substantial existing funding platforms such as the China Welfare Lottery Fund, with participation by social forces. We may also consider encouraging corporations and

3 Zhao Lili and Ma Aixia, Reflection on improving medical insurance policy to encourage innovation of pharmaceutical firms [J]. *China Licensed Pharmacists*, Issue 7, 2012.

individuals to make donations as a part of their social responsibility, and we may even consider preferential tax treatment on business taxes in return.

2 Research on how reform of payment methods can control costs

Reform of the payment methods by which health insurance reimburses costs is a key component of China's overall reform of the medical system. Such reform plays a critical role as an economic lever in several ways – it reduces the cost of accessing medical care for patients, helps control medical costs, helps change the behavior of medical services, and improves the allocation of medical resources. The essence of the task here is to achieve a balance that ensures the quality of medical safeguards while at the same time controlling costs.

2.1 Analysis of the impact that such reform has on the behavior of the supply side of medical services

The supply side of medical and healthcare services essentially means medical institutions and medical personnel. They make the final determination on what diagnosis and what treatment patients should receive. Different payment methods, however, can have an impact on their decisions by applying different incentives and benefit risks. Different payment methods can make providers adjust medical services in terms of quantity, and also in terms of quality, and they can provide options that are in between 'treatment-type services' and 'preventive-type services.' At the same time, medical services providers are 'rational actors' and, as such, will seek their own maximum interests. They will avoid behavior that puts them at risk with respect to certain payment methods – an example would be in how they choose patients for medical services or adjust the types of drugs that they prescribe.

2.1.1 Payment by service item

Under a payment-by-services model, the size of a hospital's 'surplus' or profit depends on the quantity of drugs or services being supplied times the surplus per each drug or service. This kind of payment method occurs after the fact so is less able to restrain behavior. On the contrary, it creates conditions that are conducive to over-prescribing drugs or supplying unreasonable services. Meanwhile, the medical provider does not need to take the cost of services into account – the provider can gain an ever larger surplus simply by extending a hospital stay or prescribing more drugs. This may lead to prescribing highly expensive drugs that a patient does not need, and indeed it unavoidably leads to unreasonable inflation of costs for the patient. An analysis of this type of payment method on the prescribing of drugs is as follows.

In Figure 4.7, the horizontal axis represents the quantity of drugs that are provided (Q), and the vertical axis represents the price of drugs (P). Fixed costs

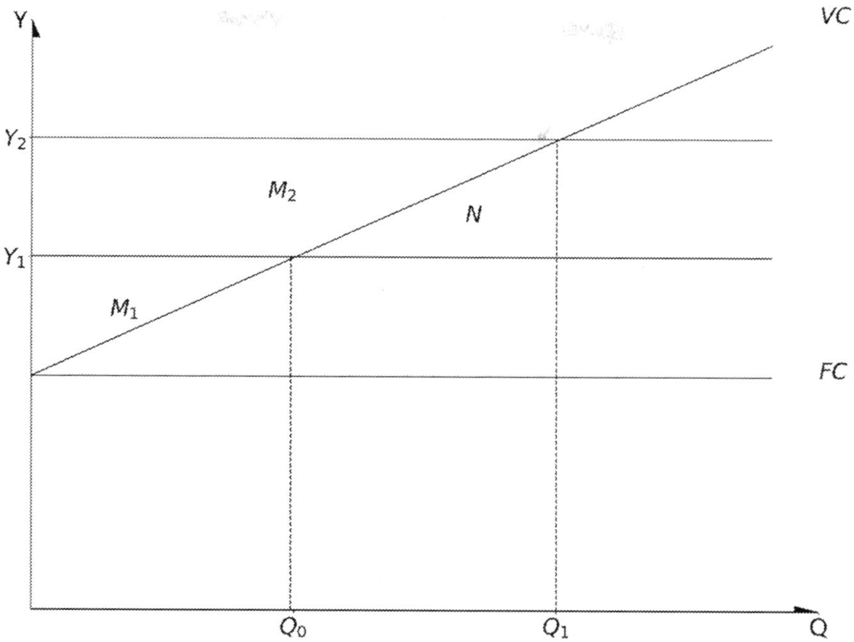

Figure 4.7 Behavior of Medical Services Providers if Payment is by Type of Itemized Services

(*FC*) include such things as the doctors' labor, the infrastructure of the hospital, equipment, and so on. Variable costs (*VC*) include such things as materials used in treatment, such as drugs and injections. Variable costs increase as the number and price of drugs increase. The income of a doctor is represented by line (*R*) under the itemized-services method of being reimbursed by insurance. When the quantity of drugs that a doctor prescribes is precisely at point Q_0, then the income of the hospital cancels out the cost to the hospital and, at that point, the profit to the doctor is 0. When the quantity of drugs goes above Q_0, for example when it reaches Q_1, the income of the provider rises as the quantity of prescribed drugs goes up.

2.1.2 *Payment by unit of service*

This payment system operates by setting a fixed amount of reimbursement for each time a person visits a clinic or each day that a patient stays in a hospital. The actual cost of the visits is unrelated to the amount the institution is reimbursed by insurance. As the per-unit number of services goes up, the income of medical services also goes up. This can motivate doctors to try to increase the number of units by intentionally shortening the average time of a hospital stay, or the time at a clinic. Through such improper means as writing more prescriptions for smaller amounts, redundant registration of inpatients, having patients divide up

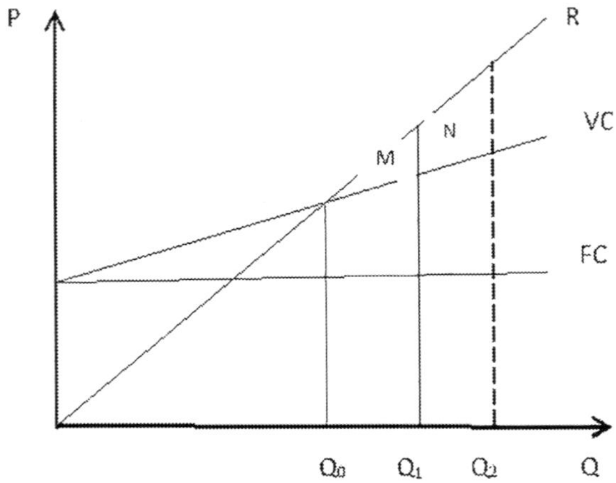

Figure 4.8 Behavior of Medical Services Providers if Payment is by Individual Unit of Services

their hospital stay into segments and come to the hospital twice, and so on, doctors may try to increase the quantity of service units. The aim is to increase income. From the perspective of rational prescribing of drugs, this method of payment has a strong restraining effect. In this regard, it promotes rational behavior, but there is also the chance that an insufficient amount of drugs will be prescribed. The influence of this per-unit of services model of payment is as follows:

In Figure 4.8, under the system of paying insurance according to units of services, line Q is the number of service units and P is price. As both go up, a hospital brings in income, line R. The segment M reflects profit given a certain number of units that are supplied, after subtracting fixed and variable costs (FC and VC). However, medical facility and doctors may attempt to gain more profit, as represented by the segment N. They may make one two-day visit to a hospital into two one-day visits, for example, and thereby earn twice the income. The profit motive encourages providers to divide up hospital stays, but it also encourages them to lower their expenses on hospitalization per day or outpatient services provided per patient.

2.1.3 Payment by headcount

Under the system of payment by headcount, payment is made in advance for a specific contracted period. The medical institution or doctor is then responsible for providing all medical services as per contract, and is not to charge any extra fees. This system provides an incentive for medical providers to launch preventive medicine programs, health education, exercise programs, and so on, in order to maximize their own benefits. In so doing, they hope to lower rates of illness and reduce medical expenses as a way to put more of the contracted income into their own pockets. The payment by headcount method therefore strengthens awareness on the part of medical providers of the need to provide preventive services and the need to control costs. Providers focus on reasonable use of healthcare resources and can thereby prevent excessive prescribing of drugs by doctors. However, this system may also lead to having doctors under-prescribe drugs or lower the quality of drugs that they supply. Another problem occurs when a designated medical institution does everything possible to increase the number of people it provides services to prior to signing a contract – but as soon as the contract is signed, it then lowers the number of people it services as well as the quality of services. An analysis of the impact of the headcount method of payment on providers' behavior is as follows:

In Figure 4.9, the horizontal axis represents quantity of services provided, and the vertical axis represents income received by providers as according to headcount. When charges by the institution are at Y1, and the quantity of medical services is controlled within point Q0, then the medical institution is profitable and the amount of profit is M1. If the medical institution constantly increases the headcount that it services, from this base, then its income as per headcount increases to Y2. If the corresponding quantity of medical services is controlled within Q1, the medical institution's profit will then increase from the base of M1 and go to M2. That is, within the costs of the medical services, as head count increases, the medical institutions' profit from services will constantly increase. This will incentivize the institution to be provide coverage to even

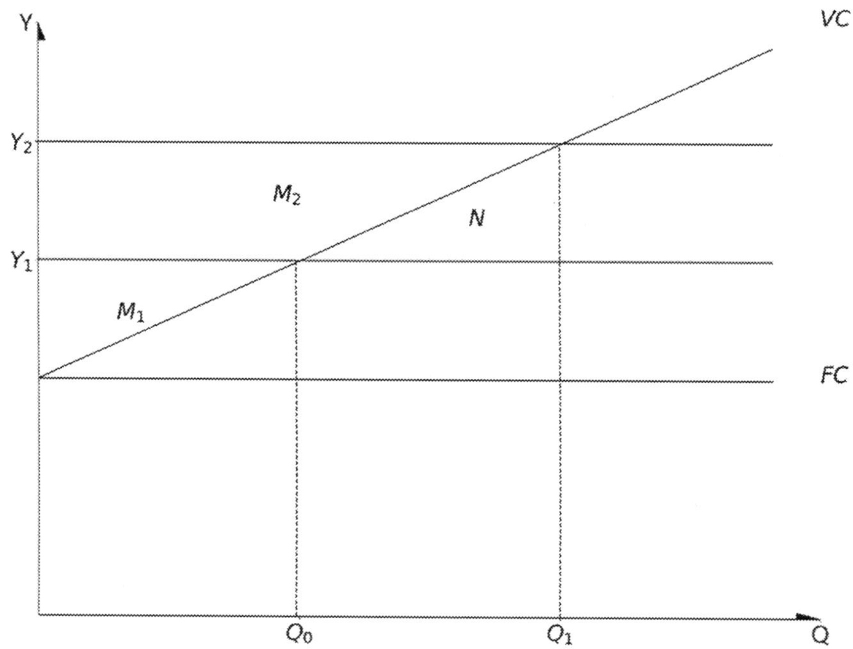

Figure 4.9 Behavior of Medical Services Providers if Payment is by Headcount

more serviceable groups, and it will encourage medical resources to flow more toward preventive type healthcare services.

If Y1 is fixed and unchanging, that is, the income received by medical services institutions according to headcount, then within a services quantity of Q0, the medical institution is profitable and the profit is the M1 portion. Once the medical services quantity exceeds Q0 and goes to Q1, then the medical institution will start to lose money and the loss is represented by N. That is, under the method of payment according to headcount, the quantity of medical services and income of the medical institution are negatively correlated. The more services are provided, the less the income of the medical services provider, even to the point of loss. This spurs the provider to do its best to adopt all kinds of means to lower medical costs, even to the point of decreasing services provided or lowering quality.

2.1.4 Advance payment of the total amount

The essence of having a total sum paid in advance is to transfer the power to control medical consumption and expense from health insurance payer to the providers of medical services. The economic risk of expense losses is shared at the same time. Under the model, medical service providers must provide services to patients as agreed, but their revenue doesn't increase as more services are provided. If the expense of all services provided surpasses the total annual budget, the losses will be assumed by medical facilities. Therefore, under such a model, medical facilities and doctors have a greater awareness of the need to control expenses. They will voluntarily strengthen their cost accounting and control over medical expenses by strengthening management, rationally using healthcare resources, and by controlling medical consumption. They will not oversell drugs to patients, and will use cheaper drugs if the efficacy is the same. However, doctors may overdo their cost controls and harm patients' benefits by reducing medical services and drugs and service quality.

In addition, this particular model means that the income of a hospital is at most the total amount budgeted under an agreement with insurance. Insurance will not reimburse for costs that go over the budgeted amount so those must be borne by the institution itself. As a result, when there is still budget left to be absorbed, this payment method may lead to the designated institution's intentionally promoting consumption by patients in order to use up the total guaranteed amount. When the budget is insufficient, institutions may choose to reduce their quantity or work and lower the quality of their services. They may reject patients so as to avoid overspending, or to try to overspend less.

In Figure 4.10, medical insurance organs pay medical institutions a total sum as per an annual budget, and this is indicated by line B. Medical institutions must complete all medical services at a cost that comes to under this line. If their services quantity is within the line Q0, then the institution makes a profit. If services go over Q0, then the medical institution must pay the costs of the additional amount, even if it puts the institution at a loss.

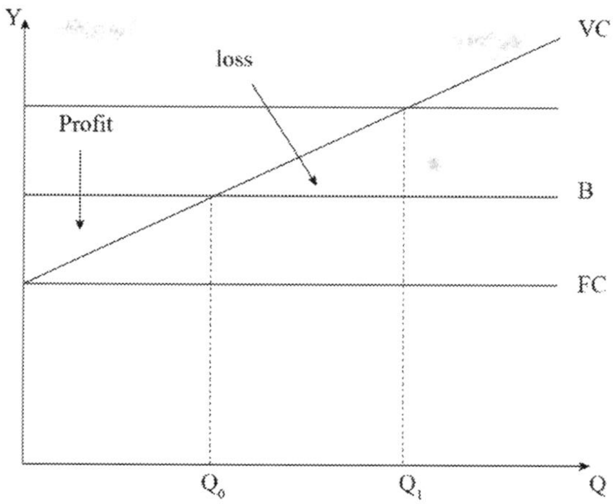

Figure 4.10 Behavior of Medical Services Providers if Payment is by Advance Payment of a Total Fixed Amount

2.1.5 Payment by type of disease (by Diagnosis Related Group)

In this model, prices are first set for the various medical services that each kind of illness or procedure will cost. Insurance pays for these services according to a preset standard. Under this model, the medical provider will voluntarily adopt cost-control measures. It will provide the most effective treatment possible for patients by improving medical services, shortening length of stay in order to prevent contagion within a hospital, using reasonable pricing and appropriate drugs and materials in order to lower per-unit medical outlays. It will do its best to avoid having patients undergo unnecessary medical procedures or take unnecessary drugs. It will have its doctors prescribe drugs in a reasonable manner. However, this payment method can also lead to irregular behavior and practices, such as dividing up hospital stays into shorter 'units,' reducing the amount of reasonable medical procedures that are on offer, and so on. To save on their costs, hospitals can also reduce supply of drugs to patients or can prescribe unreasonably if a diagnosis is upgraded. Diagnosis Related Groups are paid according to the number of times of hospitalization, so this payment method can also induce hospitals to trick patients into coming into hospitals for unnecessary procedures. When a diagnosis is not particularly clear, a hospital may adopt expensive diagnostic procedures in order to clarify the diagnosis and upgrade it to a worse scenario. That is, they will make an insignificant problem into a serious one in order to get more reimbursement. Another problem is repeating hospital admittances while at the same time shortening length of stay in order to increase number of hospital visits. Sometimes the expenses that should normally be applied to a hospital are shifted over to an outpatient clinic, which is done to increase the income of the hospital.

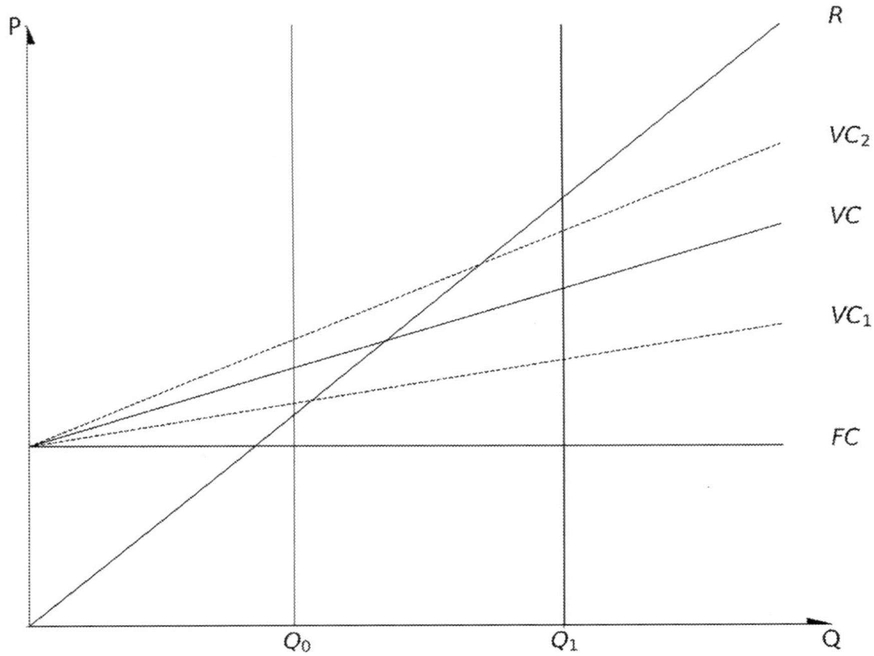

Figure 4.11 Behavior of Medical Services Providers if Payment is by Type of Disease

In Figure 4.11, the horizontal axis represents the total services that a medical provider must provide for a given type of illness, Q. The vertical axis represents the price of these services, P. The area between Q0 and Q1 represents the services that must be provided for this particular disease, that is, the quantity under the fixed payment scheme. When the level of services supplied is at Q0, income and costs equal one another and profit is 0. If the supplier wants to increase profit, it must increase awareness of costs and raise efficiencies, and it must use medical resources reasonably. If it does this, costs can shift to the position VC1 and the profits of the medical institution will increase. If the provider does not focus on cost control but instead raises the price of drugs to extreme levels, the cost line will shift to VC2, in which case profits will be reduced.

The results of different reforms that are aimed at controlling costs are shown in Figure 4.11. Different types of payment methods have either a direct or an indirect impact on both the ability to control medical costs and the quality of services. The payment method that involves paying for service items after the fact produces less favorable cost-control results. Paying in advance provides better results. In terms of the quality of medical services, quality appears to benefit under the payment method of according to items, paid after the fact. Paying in advance for service items shows that quality suffers somewhat. In terms of efficiency of services, better results come from payment for service items after the fact as opposed to paying in advance.

Table 4.10 Influence of Different Payment Systems (Methods of Calculating Insurance Reimbursement) on the Behavior of Medical Services Providers

Payment	*Incentive Mechanism*	*Behavior of Service Providers*	*Patients' Choice*	*Drug Use*
Payment by service item	Improving internal efficiency of medical facilities and the productivity of medical workers, ensuring medical service quality, having weak control on medical expense and service	Increasing service amount and input; some service input is necessary	Discriminating no patient	Pushing patients to buy unnecessary drugs
Payment by service unit	Encouraging medical facilities to reduce daily hospitalization expense or cost per outpatient visit	Extending hospital stay, reducing daily service input, dividing prescriptions, and increasing revisit times	Rejecting patients with critical conditions	Promoting rational drug use, and leading to shortage of drugs supply
Payment by headcount	Encouraging medical facilities to lower cost, preventing them from providing unnecessary services and expensive treatment service, improving the efficiency of service input; placing attention on health promotion and disease prevention programs with higher input-yield efficiency	Maximizing patient numbers, and reducing service input and amount	Selecting service targets, or preferring to those with normal conditions	There is rarely situation when drugs or medical services are insufficient
Total amount prospective payment	Giving medical facilities motivation to control expense, and yielding better cost control effect	High or low total amount budget will lead to service surplus or shortage	When total budget is insufficient, medical facilities may transfer patients to other facilities	Reducing drug supply, quality and level
Payment by disease type	Encouraging medical facilities to improve medical input structure, shortening hospital stay and reducing unnecessary medical service and drugs	Increasing number of patients including unnecessary hospitalization, and reducing service input per patient; possible upgrading of diagnosis	Rejecting patients with critical conditions	Promoting national use of drugs; there is possibilities that medical facilities cut down drug supply for cost control, or abuse drug prescriptions due to upgrading of diagnosis

Table 4.11 Comparison of Different Methods of Reimbursing Health Insurance

Payment	*Expense Control*	*Service Quality*	*Service Efficiency*
Payment by service item	Poor	Relatively good	Good
Payment by service unit	Moderate	Moderate	Relatively good
Payment by headcount	Good	Poor	Poor
Total amount prospective payment	Good	Poor	Poor
Payment by disease type	Good	Relatively good	Relatively good

2.1.5.1 PAYMENT BY SERVICE ITEM

Under a payment method by which medical providers are reimbursed by insurance for service items, the providers and doctors do not have to carry the burden of sharing costs of overspending. They therefore are not obliged to pay attention to controlling costs. Administering this type of method involves more expense since it is easy for problems to occur. These include an unwarranted increase in examinations, drug prescribing, and treatments, as well as the practice of extending hospital stays for more days than necessary, excessive use of expensive new medical procedures, purchase of high-end diagnostic equipment, and prescribing expensive drugs. This method carries a high risk of having providers make improper choices. As medical and healthcare institutions seek their own greatest profit, they may provide an excess of services, which wastes medical resources and makes it hard to control costs.

2.1.5.2 PAYMENT BY SERVICE UNIT

Under a payment method that pays by unit of services, the principle is that the medical provider 'may retain any surplus but does not pay for overspending.' Within a given contracted period, medical costs are no longer affected by the behavior of medical personnel (in terms of over-diagnosing or over-prescribing drugs), but instead are mainly determined by such things as the diagnosis of the patient's disease, the ranking of the medical institution, and the number of days a patient spends in the hospital. The income that would be derived from these things is now transformed into 'costs.' This forces medical institutions to cut down on unnecessary losses by carrying out self-constraint and self-examination in order to raise their own benefits. Evidence from this model shows that medical institutions do increase their income by standardizing their behavior. They try to increase the number of patients and to shorten their length of stay in a hospital as much as possible. They thereby improve the 'usage rate' of hospital beds and increase the frequency of the cycle in order to maximize benefits. This forces medical institutions to cut down on costs and it results in control over medical costs as a whole.

2.1.5.3 PAYMENT BY HEADCOUNT

Under the payment method by headcount, the motivation to control costs is shifted from medical insurance departments to medical institutions themselves. By such means as linking doctors' compensation for performance to the profit or loss of the institutions, the motivation to control costs is in turn shifted to doctors themselves. Doctors are the ones who actually implement medical insurance policies. By increasing the number of patients they see and the time spent, they improve communication channels with patients and can carry out health advice and effectively lower the costs of medical care for patients. In addition, this payment method can encourage medical hospitals and doctors to shift their focus forward and pay more attention to preventive medicine, as well as doing more screening of early-period symptoms. In the long run, they can achieve tremendous savings in future medical expenses.

2.1.5.4 PAYMENT IN ADVANCE OF THE TOTAL AMOUNT

This method of payment makes medical institutions aware of the need to control costs themselves. It also saves on administrative costs and is beneficial to macro-controls over medical and healthcare costs. By shortening the average length of stay in a hospital, medical providers speed up the bed-use cycle, increase the number of times beds are used and thereby improve the efficiency of bed usage. Not only do they achieve the objectives of controlling medical costs and raising operating efficiency but they lower the economic burden on patients. This method of payment began to be implemented in 2010. Shanghai City simultaneously began a program of payment in advance for general costs and drug costs, which made medical institutions in the city strengthen their controls over such costs. In 2008, the percentage of drug costs to total costs in Grade 3 hospitals (Grade 3 is the top rank of hospitals) went from 47.81% in 2008 to 43.3% in 2012. In general hospitals, this percentage also declined every year, from 45% in 2008 to 40.68% in 2012.

2.1.5.5 PAYMENT BY DISEASE TYPE

To a certain degree, payment by disease type can moderate the speed at which medical costs rise and thereby control costs. To a certain degree also, however, this keeps a hospital from setting up its own items of service and from improving how services are delivered. Hospitals go from being 'an income center' to 'being a cost center' in terms of management model. This method of payment puts very explicit guidelines and rules on all the stages a patient might go through, from examinations to diagnosis and treatment. It can effectively avoid excessive medical behavior and can thereby reduce what the patient has to pay for medical services. Payment by disease type not only is beneficial in controlling total medical costs but it also can strengthen incentives for the hospital to lower costs by raising efficiency, on a voluntary basis. It helps to curb the occurrence of such things as inducing (unwarranted) demand as a way to generate more profits.

3 Analysis of the progress China has made in reforming the way insurance pays for medical services

Depending on when payments are made, China's payment methods can be divided into pre-payment and post-payment systems. Post-payment refers to a method by which insurance reimburses for the services of designated medical institutions after services have been provided. Pre-payment refers to reimbursement of costs that are determined by negotiations with the medical institution prior to the services being provided. Beyond that main distinction, payment methods can be further subdivided according to the specifics of medical services, that is, payment by headcount, payment by unit of services, payment by type of illness, and total payment in advance.

3.1 Implementing diversified and compound medical insurance payment methods

Since the start of the New Medical Reform, China has been promoting the development of a diversified compound payment system. It has been promoting reform that allows for different types of payment depending on the specifics of hospital services. For hospital stays, for example, payment is mainly made by type of illness as grouped into Diagnosis Related Groups. For a longer hospital stay, hospital services for chronic conditions can be according to number of bed-days. For basic-level medical services, payment is made according to headcount. Active attempts are being made to integrate these last two items, payment by headcount and the management of chronic disease. For complex cases that cannot be packaged as one thing or another, and for clinic's costs, payment is made by item of service. In accord with the unique nature of traditional Chinese medicine services, new payment models should be explored that allow for the provision and use of appropriate Chinese medicine services. Pilot-program attempts are going on in various regions to allow for multiple kinds of payment methods, while still controlling the total amount of pooled medical insurance funds. The various kinds of payment methods are being broadly applied in these explorations, including payment by type of illness, payment by headcount, payment by bed-days, and so on. The scope of pilot programs using Diagnosis Related Groups is expanding and innovative methods in certain places are proceeding. By now, diversified and compound methods of payment are being broadly implemented in the country.

3.2 Promoting payment according to type of illness

Most parts of China have adopted payment according to type of illness as their main payment method. By the end of 2017, 78.6% of areas putting a basic medical health system in place, that is, pooling funds for the purpose of health insurance, had launched payment systems according to type of illness. The percentages of all municipal-level areas that adopted the reform of payment method by type of illness and by headcount for different types of insurance were as follows: 94.4% adopted these two payment types for the medical insurance for employees, 96.8% for the medical insurance for urban and rural residents, 88.6% for the medical insurance for urban residents, and 87.5% for the new medical cooperative insurance. The number of public hospitals in urban areas that adopted payment by type of illness increased by 3.6% between 2016 and 2017. By the end of October 2017, 89% of pilot-program cities had applied this method of payment to more than 100 diseases. While exploring how to improve this method, some places came up with a method of accounting that values different disease types, under controls over the total amount. This kind of accounting is simpler relative to total-budget management by region. Payment systems by Diagnosis Related Groups are already being implemented in more than ten places nationwide.

3.3 Implementing pilot programs to pay according to Disease Related Groups

The payment method by Disease Related Group (DRG) is developing rapidly. Sanming City in Fujian province has fully implemented C-DRG, and Yuxi City and Chuxiong Yi Autonomous County in Yunnan province have fully implemented DRG. In Liaoning province, the new cooperative medical insurance program has implemented the practice at the county and provincial levels of public hospitals and has also come up with something called the Liaoning Model. In brief, the number of hospitalized patients who are covered under this model is on the rise. Correspondingly, income from DRG payments is increasing as a percentage of the medicine-and-drug income of hospitals. In Yunnan, for example, in 2016, 3.09% of medicine-and-drug income of hospitals was from DRG payments, whereas in 2017 it was 4.84%. In Shanxi province, the percentage of medicine-and-drug revenue that came from DRG payments was 21.29% in 2017.

3.4 Improving the payment-by-headcount method and other methods such as paying by number of bed-days

Payment by headcount has been widely adopted by medical institutions and clinics at the grassroots level. Local areas have combined this with a process of making the initial diagnosis at the grassroots level and then either doing pilot programs on a widespread basis or fully implementing paying by headcount. In some areas, clinics are going a step further in their pay by headcount and are combining this with having family doctors and clinics manage patients' chronic conditions. In Zhejiang province, for example, 11 counties mobilized to sign contracts with household doctors that combine this model of pay by headcount. Jiangxi province is also exploring methods that combine chronic illness management with pay-by-headcount methods.

3.5 Having medical insurance strengthen regulatory controls over the medical profession

Improving the administering of the service agreements of medical insurance requires shifting the focus of regulatory controls, that is, it requires shifting focus from controls over costs to controls over both costs and quality of medicine. Depending on the specific circumstances of the functions and services of hospitals at all levels, (we must) improve the performance evaluation system in reasonable and scientific ways, and link up the results of performance reviews with payment by medical insurance funds. The target criteria by which performance reviews of Chinese traditional medicine facilities are evaluated should include the percentage of Chinese traditional medicine services that are to be provided. Those places that qualify can have the entities that operate medical insurance pay them a portion of insurance in advance, by agreement, to lessen pressures on their operating funds. The organizations that operate medical insurance should open up monitoring of their functions. With respect to the settlement of medical costs, they must move from having just a portion of costs be audited to having their entire costs be audited, from being reprimanded after a problem to being warned before the problem and supervised during the problem, and from having one single regulatory control system to having a combined system that involves regulatory oversight, management procedures, and services. Organizations that operate medical insurance should constantly improve medical insurance information systems, and ensure that information is secure. They should actively explore effective methods to extend regulatory management of medical insurance to the medical-services behavior of personnel in medical institutions. They should explore making the results of regulatory performance reviews known to the public at large, in order to strengthen management of medical personnel by medical institutions.

China is currently involved in promoting the building of medical alliances. The country needs a scientific method of insurance payment to serve as a support in this effort. These alliances, as a completely new mechanism, will change the economic relationships among different medical and healthcare institutions, as well as their behavior. At the same time, the establishment of medical alliances will be useful to the central medical authorities in calculating the total amount of advance payments (they need to make). Given this situation, local areas have launched a series of reform measures that have to do with payment methods and have gained experience as well as results. Fujian, Qinghai, Zhejiang, and other provinces have launched reforms that may be appropriate for the medical alliances to use as payment methods. Sanming in Fujian Province has promoted a total-amount payment system whereby a 'tightly-knit' form of medical alliance undertakes to perform all services for a lump sum amount. In the first half of 2018, Huzhu county in Haidong City in Qinghai launched a similar pilot program of total-amount payment by the healthcare fund. It is expected to be implemented in four county-level public hospitals under a provincial demonstration program. Zhejiang Province has set up a an incentive-and-constraint mechanism that features 'total-amount budgetary management, surplus to be kept and used as appropriate, overspending to be shared in a reasonable manner.'

4 How best to achieve policy objectives at the hospital level, with respect to prescribing drugs from the reimbursable drug list

4.1 Analysis of the process by which drugs enter hospitals and are prescribed to patients

China formulated its first list of insurance-covered drugs in 2000, and since that time the list has been revised three times, in 2004, 2009, and 2019. Each revision has included a broader scope of drug coverage. After each revision of the national list, China's provinces have then also carried out additions and amendments to the 'B' part of the nationwide list, in order to form their own provincial list of reimbursable drugs. The list that each province comes up with must align with the information systems of the local health insurance bodies and the HIS (Hospital Information Systems) of hospitals. Given the impact of bidding and procurement procedures, the timing of the release of products is different in each province.

4.1.1 The national list of drugs that are covered under insurance

Since the first list was formulated in 2000, China's national reimbursable drug list has been revised three times, as noted earlier, with the intervals in between revisions being four years, five years, and eight years. During this process, the scope of covered drugs constantly increased – details are described in Table 4.12. In the new round of revisions, in 2017, new drugs that came to market after 2009 were the focus of evaluations. The great majority of new chemical drugs and biological products that had received approval between 2008 and the first half of 2015 were incorporated in the 2017 list or were included in the scope of drugs to be negotiated. In March 2019, Hu Jinglin, head of the National Healthcare Security Administration, took questions from reporters at the so-called Minister's Corridor during the 'Two Meetings.' He said the Administration would be setting up a dynamic adjustment system for the reimbursable list of drugs as fast as possible. At the same time, the work of adjusting the 2019 list was being mobilized with an emphasis on basic drugs, drugs for cancer and rare diseases, and drugs for chronic diseases and critical illnesses of children. On September 28, 2019, the National Health Security Administration held a press conference and announced the conclusion of the largest round of negotiations on the drug list since the insurance system began. Ninety-seven drugs came into the list as a result of negotiations. Among them, eight had come to market in recent years and were ranked among the top nationally produced innovative drugs. This gave a clear signal of government support for pharmaceutical innovation. According to the Administration, 70 out of the 119 newly added drugs on the negotiation list were included in the final list.

Table 4.12 Revisions of China's National Drug Reimbursement List, and Features of Each Revision

Healthcare Drug Catalogue	*Characteristics*
National healthcare drug catalogue (2000)	Total drugs involved number 1,535. The scope of drugs paid by the healthcare program is determined. Catalogue A and B are made for western medicine and Chinese patent drugs.
Drug catalogue for national healthcare program and employment injury insurance scheme (2004)	Total drugs involved number 1,854. Drugs with expenses reimbursed expand from those covered by the healthcare program to those under employment injury insurance scheme. The classification is adjusted with some drug types merged. Payment standards for some drugs are determined.
Drug catalogue for national healthcare program, employment injury insurance and maternity insurance schemes (2009)	Total drugs involved number 2,151. The maternity insurance scheme is included. Some drugs are removed from the catalogue including those proved to be ineffective by evidence-based medicine, those with serious untoward effects, and those failing the evaluation of pharmaco-economics, as well as drugs rarely used in clinical treatment or replaceable by more effective and cheap ones.
Drug catalogue for national healthcare program, employment injury insurance and maternity insurance schemes (2017)	Total drugs involved number 2,535. It is made eight years after the last revision. New drugs included are new drugs with high clinical value, widely included in provincial catalogue B, and used for major diseases, children diseases and occupational diseases. The majority of new chemical drugs and biological products approved from 2008 to the first half of 2016 were included in the catalogue or negotiation list.
2019 edition of drug catalogue for national healthcare program, employment injury insurance, and maternity insurance schemes	There are 2,643 drugs admitted in a regular basis. Compared with the 2017 edition, the total number of drugs is stable, but the drug structure changes tremendously as many are included and others are removed. New drugs cover basic medicine necessary to be prioritized, as well as drugs for cancer, rare diseases, children's diseases, and chronic diseases. A total of 74 basic drugs are adjusted from catalogue B to catalogue A. The inclusion method for TCM decoction pieces is adjusted. In addition, localities are required not to adjust catalogue B. By principle, previously added drugs should be handled gradually in three years with those included in the national monitoring program as the priority.
The circular by the National Healthcare Security Administration and the Ministry of Human Resources and Social Security on the scope of drug catalogue B for national healthcare program, employment injury insurance, and maternity insurance schemes	A total of 97 out of 150 drugs on the negotiation list are included. Among them are 70 newly included drugs. The prices are down 60.7% on average. Also, 27 out of 31 drugs remain on the catalogue and the prices are lowered 26.4% on average.

Prices were down 60.7% on average. Prices negotiated for such drugs as tumors and diabetes dropped by an average of around 65%. Negotiations were successful on 27 of 31 drugs that were being continued from the previous list and their prices dropped by an average of 26.4%. By conservative estimates, as a result of negotiations as well as the ability to be reimbursed for drugs, the cost burden to patients came down to below 20% of what it had been, and on some drugs it came to below 5% of what it had been.

4.1.2 Adjustments to the reimbursable list of medical insurance at the provincial level

In August 2019, the National Healthcare Security Administration and the Ministry of Human Resources and Social Security jointly issued a notice on the *Reimbursable drug list for basic medical insurance, workers' injury insurance, and maternity insurance*. This document pulled back the authority of local areas to adjust lists on their own. It explicitly required strict adherence to the national list of basic medical insurance. In principle, local governments were not allowed to formulate their own lists or add drugs to the national list through camouflaged means, and they were not allowed to change the restrictions on scope of payment for drugs in the list. Provinces were given three years to eliminate any drugs that had been added to B lists according to regulations in the past. During this process of elimination, provinces were to give priority to drugs subject to key national regulatory controls and to eliminate them from the scope of payment. At the same time, some room to maneuver was granted to drugs developed by minorities. The document stated that with respect to minority-produced drugs that have been granted approval by relevant national authorities and allowed to come to market, these drugs can be included in the scope of payment by provincial-level insurance funds, depending on the ability of the fund to afford this and the need for the drug. This was to be determined by the health security departments of each province, in concert with the human resources and social security departments of the province. Once each province reported the circumstances on such drugs to the National Healthcare Security Administration, those circumstances were to be made openly available to the public.

Prior to this *Notice*, when each national list of reimbursable drugs was issued, each province faced the task of adjusting its own provincial lists. According to regulations they were limited to adjusting 15% of the number of drugs in the national B list, and that included additions to and subtractions from the list, as well as adjustments to the scope of usage. In making these adjustments, provincial lists had to take three factors into account. The first was the need to fill any gaps in the existing provincial list; the second was to meet local demands for the basic medicines that their doctors needed in clinical practice. The needs of each locality were different, so in adjusting the list, provincial authorities had to localize their lists. Third, in provinces where pharmaceuticals were a major industry, authorities had to localize lists to support the real need for new drugs. Such drugs often had a small market and were not recognized as priority on a national basis, so it was not easy for them to be given consideration in the readjustment of the national list. From the standpoint of the macro-economics of specific provinces, however, supporting these drugs was necessary.[4]

Additions or subtractions to provincial lists had been a major point of reference for readjusting the national list. Reportedly, only once ten or more provinces had included a drug in their lists would the drug be qualified to enter the quasi-list for consideration by the national authorities. Eliminating the ability of provinces to add drugs signifies that decisions on adding to the national list will now go back to being based on clinical demand. This squeezes out the final bit of space that special interests had enjoyed with respect to drugs on the list. It also signifies that the administrative staff positions associated with adding drugs to the list at the provincial level will now either be eliminated or reassigned. In the past, many drugs of the sort that 'bolstered' a person's health were unable to get into the national list but were maintained on a provincial list due to protectionism or some other reason. These drugs appeared in the name list at the provincial level and were thereby able to continue to receive support from medical insurance. This phenomenon will no longer exist once there is only one single national list that insurance payments can use as reference.

Incomplete statistics indicate that at present 23 provinces and municipalities have (nevertheless) already published new provincial-level reimbursement lists. These include Shandong, Shaanxi, and Sichuan. It is believed that the inclusion of drugs in these provincial lists mainly takes into consideration those drugs that were already on the list, and drugs that are reasonably priced and already used widely in hospitals. Those that are removed are done so primarily due either to safety concerns, because there is insufficient clinical demand, production has stopped on the drugs, or registrations have been canceled.

4.1.3 Drug procurement through a bidding process

Centralized procurement of drugs in China has gone through a total of six stages to date. The first stage involved policy preparation (before 2000). Procurement at this time was mainly done by medical institutions in a fragmented way, although some places took the initiative themselves in attempting centralized procurement. The second stage involved improving and finalizing policy (2000–2006). Medical facilities at the municipal level were the primary procuring entity. They commissioned intermediaries to conduct the actual bidding, while the municipality was the administrative unit of procurement. The third stage was a period of testing different models (2006–2010). Systems were promoted that used the province as the administrative unit of procurement and Internet-based procedures, with the government providing guidance. The fourth stage was a period of renewed planning (2010–2015). This period saw the establishment of the basic drugs system, and

4 Ni Huping, Limited space and big demands for adjusting provincial catalogues [J]. *China Health Insurance*, Issue 4, 2017.

new mechanisms were set up for procurement of these basic drugs. The fifth stage was one of changing and improving the model (2015–2018). This period adhered to the orientation of Internet-based procurement and kept decisions at the provincial level. The shorthand description of the process by this time called for 'one platform, with linked action taken above and below, openness and transparency, and procurement by category.' The sixth stage (which dates from the establishment of the National Healthcare Security Administration in 2018) involves centralized procurement of drugs under the guidance of this Administration, with negotiations for anticancer drugs at the national level, with centralized procurement of drugs by the 4+7 cities, and with centralized procurement of anticancer drugs as a single-item program at the provincial level.[5]

In the new round of centralized procurement of drugs, provinces themselves procure drugs by category of drug according to the guiding principles embodied in two documents, the *Guiding opinion on improving the work of centralized drug procurement by public hospitals*, and the *Notice on ensuring the actual implementation of the (previous) Opinion*. Provinces themselves issue plans for the actual implementation by their province. The number of drug categories that each province decides upon varies. Some have only four, some seven, but open bidding is the primary method of procurement. Jilin province is still following its traditional method of bidding and procurement, while Shanghai is leading the way in testing a group procurement model. The procurement by category method includes diverse procedures: competitive price bidding, negotiated-price procurement, Internet-based procurement, procurement from designated producers, procurement of special medicines, procurement by (business) groups, and invitations to bid.[6]

The '4+7 cities initiative for procurement of drugs with specified quantities' was formally launched in December of 2018. This program is under the guidance of the National Healthcare Security Administration. It is mainly aimed at procuring generic drugs that meet consistency evaluations and have the same quality and effectiveness as brand-name drugs, or at procuring brand-name drugs at lower prices. Joint procurement was launched in the four cities under direct jurisdiction of the central government (Beijing and Tianjin among them), and seven cities that are administered as sub-provinces (including Shenyang and Dalian). The results of centralized procurement were as follows: 25 of 31 commonly used brand-name drugs won the bidding. Prices were lower by an average of 52% as compared to the lowest procurement prices of the same drugs in 2017. The highest drop in prices was 96%. A person responsible for the procedures at the pilot locations said that the National Pharmaceutical Regulatory Administration and the Ministry of Industry and Information Technology would be using powerful means to ensure the quality and adequate supply of the drugs that won the bidding, as

5 Wei Wei and Zhang Jian, Analysis on and future of models for centralized procurement of drugs [J]. *Tianjin Pharmacy*, Issue 3, 2019.

6 Xia Yarui and Chang Feng, Study on development trend of centralized procurement of drugs under new circumstances [J]. *Bidding and Tendering*, Issue 3, 2019.

Table 4.13 China's Policies that Relate to Centralized Procurement of Drugs through Bidding

Issuing Date	*Authority*	*Name of Document*	*Content*
February 28, 2015	General Office of the State Council	Guideline for improving centralized procurement in public hospitals (File No. 7)	It functionally replaces the No. 64 document for bid of non-basic drugs released in July 2010 and the No. 56 document for bid of basic drugs released in November 2010, and becomes the pragmatic document for bids of basic and non-basic drugs. **1. Procurement by category (4+1 model)** a. 'large quantity, high price, multiple suppliers,' quantity procurement, and double-envelope bidding and tendering b. 'Exclusivity and patent,' (national and provincial) government-led negotiations c. Procurement information on drugs for women and children, and those urgently needed in clinical treatment are released online and drugs are included on the hospital list after negotiations d. Production of drugs running in shortfall but needing a small quantity is made by designated makers e. Procurement of narcotic and psychotropic drugs, vaccines, biological products, and TCM decoction pieces follow the existing rules **2. Settlement period:** 30 days, shorter than the requirement of 60 days as stipulated in document No. 64 **3. Strengthening management on drug shipment:** enterprises delaying shipment or rejecting shipment to remote areas will have their qualification revoked if they failed to rectify **4. Following supportive medication** and drugs unconventionally used in hospitals **5. Drug price:** cracking down on price-related wrongdoings and monopolies, and illegal activities including fortifying invoices and practicing fraud under the disguise of businesses

June 19, 2015	Then Commission of Health and Family Planning	Circular on implementing the guideline for improving centralized procurement in public hospitals (File No. 70)	It fleshes out document No. 7 and makes specific requirements on double-envelope bidding system, drug payment settlement, drug shipment and building of procurement platforms. **Sticking to double-envelope bidding system:** implementing integrated bidding and procurement, quantity procurement, price varying by quantity systems; announcement of bid winners at various areas will be made in the last 20 days of November; realizing coordination between bidding policies and procurement policies so that enterprises can make rational bids and plan production in advance. **Shipment:** the qualification of enterprises as drug suppliers will be revoked if they fail to ship on many occasions, reject shipment to primary-level medical facilities or refuse to rectify after notification. Supporting measures should be introduced to make former bid winners to assume overspending when hospitals have to use alternative drugs due to the bid winners' negligence. **Pilot cities for public hospital reform:** transaction price in pilot cities is much lower than the tender price at the provincial level and the latter should be adjusted based on the transaction price. Efforts should be made to develop modern pharmaceutical logistics, and explore ways in which private retail pharmacies and designated pharmacies take over the drug-related outpatient services.
November 15, 2018	Office for joint procurement	4+7 cities program for centralized procurement of drugs	On December 6, enterprises made offer and participated in negotiations. The result for quantity procurement was released on December 7.
September 30, 2019	Nine departments including the National Healthcare Security Administration	Suggestion on the implementation of national centralized procurement and expansion of the trial program	After half a year, the '4+7 cities' program will be carried out nationwide. Sticking to the principles of quantity procurement and integration of bidding and procurement; gathering 50 to 70 percent of total drug use in alliance hospitals; the quantity of procurement should be agreed beforehand.

actual implementation went forward. First, they would ensure that drug quality passed regulatory requirements. Second, they would ensure that manufacturers would supply the full amounts as per procurement agreements, and they would ensure that bid-winning drugs would be given prescribing priority by hospitals. Third, they would ensure that payment for the drugs was done on time, and that medical funds would pay no less than 30% as an advance to medical institutions, but they would encourage medical funds to pay advance sums directly to drug manufacturers.

At the same time, to ensure that drugs were indeed up to proper quality standards and hospitals did indeed prescribe the drugs, the National Health Commission and the National Healthcare Security Administration issued a set of affiliated measures. From the perspective of the National Health Commission, relevant measures included the following. First, the Commission will open out a policy channel to ensure that bid-winning drugs will have priority in procurement and reasonable prescribing. Second, the Commission will put bid-winning drugs into the path for clinical use, will formulate guidelines for them and will encourage hospitals to prescribe them, in scientific and reasonable ways. Third, the Commission will introduce the use of bid-winning drugs into the performance evaluation system of public hospitals and will set up incentive-and-constraint mechanisms (for their use by) hospitals and medical personnel.

With respect to the National Healthcare Security Administration, measures included the following. First, the NHSA will incorporate drug-prescribing behavior into agreements signed with medical insurance. Terms will explicitly describe responsibilities and potential violations, together with methods of punishment. Second, the NHSA will issue policies on payment standards for drugs, clarifying that any commonly used drug sold under other brand names will be reimbursed by insurance at the same standard, as per transition policies and detailed operating procedures. This is in order to guide those who are insured to use drugs rationally. Third, the NHSA will strengthen monitoring and regulatory controls over the use of drugs that win bids as well as those that have not yet won bids. In the event anything out of line is discovered, measures will be taken to rectify the problem. Fourth, if hospitals use bid-winning drugs in proper ways and thereby lower the amount of spending out of medical insurance, they may retain the excess in their budgets at the end of the year and use it on reforming such things as the compensation distribution system. This is in order to stimulate the enthusiasm for the whole project by medical personnel (changing the bird in the cage). Fifth, the NHSA will set up and improve upon the system of evaluation standards by which the performance of medical insurance is judged. Information to do with the prescribing of bid-winning drugs will be incorporated into the performance evaluation targets, and a corresponding system of rewards and punishments will be set up.

The pilot-city 4+7 program resulted in a fairly substantial price differential between participating cities and the rest of the country. In order to extend the benefits of this successful program to a broader public, authorities decided to launch the program nationwide. On September 30, 2019, the National Healthcare Security Administration and eight other departments issued an opinion called *Opinion on expanding the regional scope of the pilot program of nationally-organized centralized procurement of drugs*. This said that the estimated amount of centralized procurement will be 50% to 70% of the annual total drug use in all public medical facilities, military facilities, and designated private hospitals that choose on a voluntary basis to join the program. The large quantity is expected to get a favorable price through negotiations between related medical institutions or their representatives with bid-winning companies. This signified that, just one-half year after the start of the 4+7 pilot program, the program was being launched on a nationwide scale.

4.1.4 Alignment with the Hospital Information Systems of hospitals

Generally speaking, after the reimbursable drug list is revised, drugs that come into the list must be aligned with a hospital's HIS system. (In this regard), (we need to) strengthen coordination and the inter-operability of information. The front-end systems of insurance systems and hospitals are mainly operated by staff at medical institutions, as they do claims settlement. For problems with medical insurance systems, or notifications about mistakes, hospitals generally employ professionals to record the issues and report systemic problems on up to social security information departments. After analyzing the record for awhile, the social security departments revise the information on people who are insured in a timely manner. Nevertheless, China's hospital and drug administration technology is fairly outdated. The great majority of hospitals have systems that are closed and independent of other systems. There are no unified standards. The structure of the database of each Hospital Information System is substantially different from others. Statistical discrepancies are common in the data that goes between hospitals and health insurance centers. Transmitting and exchanging data is not easy. In actual operations, most information is not recorded in computer systems, and related management systems are similarly imperfect. As China's medical insurance system undergoes reform, and as reform goes into deeper layers, as claims settlement in different parts of the network becomes more connected, the various structures and varieties of HIS systems in China's hospitals will need to become more aligned with each other. In addition, the systems will soon be facing the need to link up with commercial health insurance organizations (at the current time, claims settlement under commercial health insurance policies is processed manually). These conditions will begin to put increasing pressure on the information systems of hospitals.

In order to meet the needs of reform of China's medical insurance, in June of 2019, the National Healthcare Security Administration issued a guiding opinion called *Guiding opinion on standardizing healthcare safeguards* (Document No. 39 (2019)). This set forth the need to set up basic standards for healthcare security that are held in common and are supported by unified plans, categories, announcements, and administration. These standards would form a 'common language' for the nationwide system of health insurance. They would include coding standards for the information systems of medical insurance, unified identifiers, the standardization of how personal files are administered, and so on. On November

11, 2019, the National Healthcare Security Administration issued a notice called *Notice on publicizing the information on the first batch of drugs included in the healthcare classification and coding database.* Since this has not been met with any objections, the information will be incorporated in the national medical information drug classification and coding database, for use by all medical insurance departments. The classification of drug categories and related codes will become the common language for information exchange that relates to China's national health insurance. This should prove effective in raising the level of how information in health insurance is administered, and in raising the efficiency of making insurance payments.

4.2 Deepening the impact of medical reform policies on the way hospitals prescribe drugs

In order to resolve such key problems as the inability to receive medical care at an affordable price, (China's authorities have issued) a number of policy documents. These have been aimed at deepening reform of the medical and healthcare structures of the country. With a holistic approach to health and the greater wellbeing of the population, (authorities) have worked to maintain the existing base of healthcare, to strengthen grassroots provision of healthcare, to build various mechanisms that allow systems to operate, and to coordinate the work across the medical, insurance, and pharmaceutical arenas. A number of measures have propelled more rational use of drugs and standardized prescribing of drugs in hospitals. Those have included speeding up the process of drug permits, which allows more innovative drugs that are urgently needed for clinical use to come to market. They have included reform of hospitals in order to break down the mechanisms that support hospitals through the selling of drugs, and setting up fees for pharmaceutical services. Pilot programs for the use of Diagnosis Related Groups and the formulation of a nationwide catalogue of supplementary drugs have strengthened the ability of medical insurance to control costs and have lowered prices and taxes on anti-cancer drugs. Other measures have used creative ways to lower prices, including the 4+7 pilot program by which procurement is linked to quantity. All of this has had a profound influence on China's medical and pharmaceutical industries. At the same time, however, they have brought forth new demands on the way hospitals use and prescribe drugs.

4.2.1 Eliminating the markup on drugs

The policy allowing for a markup on drugs was begun in the 1950s and was intended to ensure that public hospitals could continue to operate given that government spending on hospitals was insufficient. The measure was the result of a particular period of history, and it did play a positive role to a degree in enabling China's medical institutions to operate normally. In recent years, however, the problem of using drugs to subsidize hospitals has gradually become more pronounced. In order to break through this drug-related mechanism, in 2012, the

State Council and other departments launched a policy of 'no markups on drugs.' In April 2017, a *Notification on the work of furthering comprehensive reform of public hospitals* noted that 'All markups on drugs in public hospitals are to be eliminated prior to September 30, 2017 (with the exception of those on Traditional Chinese Medicine infusions).' The main positive effects of this policy, once it was implemented, were to lower prices on drugs and lighten the cost burden of medical care for patients. The policy also was helpful in changing the income structure of medical institutions. It gradually broke through the interest chain that had connected hospital results to drugs, and it encouraged more rational prescribing of drugs. It lessened income for doctors and thereby changed the way their services were valued. However, the policy also had negative consequences. Income of hospitals dropped dramatically, which affected the motivation of medical personnel.

In addition, since the policy of a zero markup was instituted, pharmacies quickly went from being profit centers to cost centers for hospitals. To save on costs, hospitals throughout the country started a model of outsourcing pharmacies. What this meant was that hospitals would sign contracts that entrusted other companies with drug transactions in order for them to carry out for-compensation operating and management. The ownership of the pharmacies was still held by hospitals. However, since this practice started, ownership relationships became less clear and problems have arisen relating to how authorized enterprises affect drug prices and how they channel interests in camouflaged ways back to hospitals. The situation did not fundamentally resolve the problem of having drugs pay for medicine. As a result, a number of provinces put a stop to this in 2016, or they called on such outsourced pharmacies to regularize their behavior. In November 2018, the National Health Commission and National Traditional Chinese Medicine Management Administration jointly issued an opinion called *Opinion on speeding up high-quality growth of pharmacological services*. This now forbade public hospitals from outsourcing pharmacy services or 'renting' their pharmacies to profit-oriented companies.[7]

4.2.2 Setting up a fee system for pharmacy services

In April 2009, the Central Committee of the CPC and the State Council issued an *Opinion on deepening reform of the structures that govern medicine, pharmaceuticals, and healthcare*. This explicitly called for gradually reforming or eliminating the markup on drugs by such means as adding graduated fees or charges to drug transactions and pharmacy services. At the same time, it called for rectifying prices of medical services, as appropriate, increasing government inputs, and reforming the payment methods of insurance in order to improve the mechanisms by which public hospitals are subsidized. This was the first time explicit mention had been made of instituting fees for pharmacy services, as a way to compensate for the losses caused by eliminating the markups. In 2010, the (former) Ministry of Health

7 Li Yuqing, Analysis on merits and drawbacks of commissioned pharmacies by public hospitals [J]. *China Market*, Issue 10, 2019.

issued a *Guiding opinion on pilot programs to reform public hospitals*. This again clarified that China should

> gradually eliminate the policy that had allowed markups on drugs, that the loss of legitimate income of public hospitals should be made up for by adopting fees on pharmacy services, as well as adjusting some fee standards on technical services. Lost income should be made up for through increased government investment and by spending out of medical insurance funds.

In 2015, the *Reform plan of the 13th Five-Year Plan on deepening reform of medicine, pharmaceuticals, and healthcare*, noted the need to

> explore setting up a system of Chief Pharmacist in hospitals, improving the management system governing pharmacists in medical institutions and retail pharmacies, and combining that with reform of the pricing of medical services, in order to realize prices of pharmacy services.

Some parts of China did then begin to experiment with taking in fees on pharmacy services. The experience has proven that sound pharmacy services can reduce the adverse effects caused by unreasonable prescribing of drugs.[8] It can help avoid unnecessary economic losses and the waste of resources, and can generate positive economic and social benefits. Charging fees for pharmacy services is a routine practice in the medical industries of fairly developed countries. However, China is still at a very preliminary stage of exploration in this regard. No detailed regulations have been set forth on charges for pharmacy services, and the system awaits further improvement.

4.2.3 Allowing prescriptions to be fulfilled outside of hospitals

Information on prescriptions has always been regarded as one of the core information assets of hospitals. Policies that allow for prescriptions to be fulfilled outside of hospitals are an important way to 'break through the system of having drugs subsidize hospitals.' The goal of these policies is to weaken the monopoly hold that hospitals have on prescriptions, and make hospitals return to their primary function. Policies on zero markup, on controlling insurance costs, and on controlling pharmacies have indeed been one of the most important factors motivating hospitals to give up some of their control over fulfilling prescriptions. In 2014 and 2015, major steps were taken in having prescriptions fulfilled outside of hospitals. These came in the form of initiatives that promoted 'a new model for allowing patients to purchase their prescribed drugs as they wish at either retail pharmacies or within hospitals,' and that 'prohibited hospitals from putting any restrictions on the

8 Leng Jing, Discussions on management of pharmacist services [J]. *Inner Mongolia Journal of Traditional Chinese Medicine*, Issue 7, 2014.

fulfilling of prescriptions outside the hospital.' In 2017, the State Council's Office of Medical Reform released a document on the major tasks in deepening reform of the institutional structures of medicine in 2017. While reiterating the injunction against hospitals' restricting outside fulfillment of prescriptions, this also sought to find ways to sweep away the systemic causes that prevent outside fulfillment. For example, it called for real-time sharing of information and information interconnectedness among hospitals, medical insurance claims settlement, and the retail sale of drugs. In April 2018, an opinion called *Opinion on promoting the development of the 'Internet + medicine and health' initiative* encouraged hospitals to develop Internet-based services. It permitted online tools for treating common illnesses, for prescriptions for chronic diseases, and it allowed third-party organizations to fulfill prescriptions once they had met certain conditions. That is, after a prescription is reviewed and approved by a pharmacist, a hospital or a company in the business of selling drugs may commission an eligible third party to fulfill it.

Allowing fulfillment of prescriptions outside of hospitals involves restructuring the channels through which drugs are distributed. At the present time, the main focus of policies is to guide fulfillment in the direction of retail pharmacies. These policies have become clearer in their orientation in recent years, in terms of having retail pharmacies take on this role. They provide more support by enabling payment by medical insurance, and by allowing retail pharmacies to fulfill prescriptions from multiple sources. The initial batch of drugs that can be fulfilled outside of hospitals will include drugs for chronic illness, anticancer drugs, and new innovative drugs. This will make it more convenient for patients to get such drugs, but it also will help control the way drugs have dominated hospital income. It will also be beneficial in reducing the pressure on the operations of pharmacies that are still within hospitals.[9]

4.2.4 Reform of the methods by which medical insurance pays hospitals

Reforms to do with how insurance reimburses hospitals are putting a certain pressure on how hospitals conduct their internal budgeting. These reforms take full advantage of economic measures, which not only can mobilize the enthusiasm of medical personnel but can also reduce the frequency of such things as over-prescribing drugs, and the unwarranted use of high-tech equipment. They can induce hospitals to take voluntary steps to reduce expenses and reduce avoidable medical costs and expenditures. To a certain degree, they can also induce hospitals to strengthen their cost accounting and cost controls.

4.2.5 Negotiated drug prices

Right now, drugs can be admitted to the reimbursable drug list through normal methods or through negotiations. Specific procedures depend mainly on the prices

9 What business open prescription can bring? www.huxiu.com/article/266029.html.

of drugs that are already in the list. Drugs that have relatively low prices and are similar to low-priced drugs already in the list may go through normal procedures in being granted access to the reimbursable drug list. Drugs that have higher prices or that would have a major effect on insurance funds, such as patented drugs from a sole producer, must go through a negotiated procedure. In this process, health technology assessments, pharmaco-economic evaluations, and analysis of the impact on budgets have officially become a part of the evidence required in evaluations. Companies are required to provide relevant proof as they conduct negotiations with medical insurance departments. In 2017, 44 kinds of drugs were included in the scope of negotiations, of which 36 were successfully entered into the list. On average, prices for these dropped by more than 40%, while the greatest decrease in price was 70%. In 2018, another 17 anticancer drugs were added to insurance coverage. Please refer to Table 4.14 for a detailed listing of policies on gaining coverage by insurance through negotiations.

Negotiations on drugs involve policies regarding reimbursement by insurance, but also the question of the ability of insurance funds to pay for reimbursement. The main device used in negotiations for reimbursement coverage is that of increasing quantity. By granting an increase in sales quantity, drug companies can be forced to lower prices. This is why negotiations were much smoother and more successful once the National Medical Insurance Bureau was set up in 2018, and the bureaus under it became the primary organizations conducting negotiations. At present, drug negotiations can be carried on in a unified manner at the national level, but they can also take place independently at the provincial and municipal levels. Conducting negotiations at different levels has both advantages and drawbacks. Those carried on at the national level benefit from the larger quantity that is ordered, while prices are lower as a result of the price-quantity linkage. Second, the professionalism of the negotiators at the national level is stronger. Third, a company can avoid the trouble and expense of duplicating negotiations in many different provinces. Fourth, a company can avoid the problems of unfair treatment by different regions and excessive difference in price in different provinces. Right now, China's insurance funds are mainly pooled at the prefectural and municipal levels of government. Circumstances differ from city to city within a province, and the differences among provinces are even larger. In some provinces, some insurance funds already have over-drafts given the amount they are required to cover in the reimbursable drug list. This situation means that negotiations at the national level have the potential to put even greater spending pressure on local insurance funds.

4.2.6 The two-invoice policy

The two-invoice policy has been implemented on a nationwide basis since 2017. The form that this policy takes is as follows: only one invoice may be written up for the transaction between a drug producer and a distribution company, and a second may be written up for the transaction between the distributor and the end-user of the drugs. This policy directly confronts the practice in the drug industry of

Table 4.14 China's Policies that Relate to Admitting Drugs to the Reimbursement Drug List through Price Negotiations

Date	*Department*	*Document Name*	*Content*
February 28, 2015	General Office of State Council	Guideline on improving centralized procurement of drugs in public hospitals (Document No. 7)	A transparent and fair negotiation mechanism with multi-party participation for determining the price of some proprietary drugs and exclusively produced drugs should be established. The negotiation result should be released on the information platform for national drug supply and guarantee. Hospitals will procure drugs in accordance with the negotiation result.
May 20, 2016	Former National Commission for Health and Family Planning	Circular on the result of national negotiations for drug price	Negotiation result for the price of first three drug is released.
May 20, 2016	Seven departments including former National Commission for Health and Family Planning	Circular on fully implementing national negotiations for centralized procurement of drugs	Centralized procurement demands will be released online. Delivery and settlement services should be improved (medical facilities should pay for drugs within 30 days after they are delivered and accepted after review. Clinical comprehensive evaluation will be carried out. Administration on healthcare payment scope will be improved and the pilot program of national negotiations for drug prices should be aligned with healthcare payment policies.
September 30, 2016	Ministry of Human Resources and Social Security	2016 work plan for adjusting drug catalogue under basic medical insurance scheme, employment injury insurance scheme, and maternity insurance scheme (draft for public suggestions)	In the first half year of 2017, the selection of drugs for negotiations should be finished.

(*Continued*)

Table 4.14 (Continued)

Date	*Department*	*Document Name*	*Content*
October 14, 2016	Former National Commission for Health and Family Planning	Circular on connecting national drug negotiations with reimbursement policies under the new-type rural cooperative medical insurance scheme	Policy alignment should be finished. Departments should work to include the drugs into the reimbursement catalogue under the new-type rural cooperative medical insurance scheme before the end of October 2016.
November 18, 2016	Former National Commission for Health and Family Planning	Progress of including negotiation drugs into compliance expenditure of healthcare program in localities	There are 20 provincial-level regions including negotiation drugs into compliance expenditure of the healthcare program. In addition, before the negotiation result was released, there have been seven provinces doing so.
July 13, 2017	Former Ministry of Human Resources and Social Security	Circular on including 36 drugs into catalogue B under basic medical insurance scheme, employment injury insurance scheme, and maternity insurance scheme	36 out of 44 drugs under negotiations are included into healthcare catalogue. Among them are 31 types of western medicine and five TCM patent drugs
October 10, 2018	National Healthcare Security Administration	Circular on including 17 anticancer drugs into catalogue B under basic medical insurance scheme, employment injury insurance scheme, and maternity insurance scheme	Releasing negotiation result for 17 drugs

writing out multiple invoices, that is, of concealing *de facto* kickbacks in multiple layers of invoices. One of the objectives of the two-invoice policy is to 'wring the water' out of the system, that is, wringing the cost of kickbacks out of the price of drugs. The policy requires the manufacturer to have the same names of buyer and seller on both the shipping bill and the special value-added tax receipt. When the drug company buys the drugs, it must compare the invoice with that of the manufacturer, and when a hospital enters the drug into its drug-income database, it must ensure that the invoice, quantity, and price are the same as on the first invoice before it can be input into the hospital system. Since being implemented, this two-invoice system has led to a scarcity of some drugs. This has been an inconvenience to patients and hence has affected the demand for medical care.

Table 4.15 China's Policies that Relate to the 'Two-Invoices Policy'

Direction	*Issuing Date*	*Issuing Department*	*Document Name*	*Content*
Changing business tax to value added tax	March 23, 2016	Ministry of Finance and State Taxation Administration	Circular on changing business tax to value-added tax on all sectors	Pharmaceutical circulation sector applies taxation of transportation sector, which means the taxation rate is raised from 5% to 11%.
Cracking down on invoice-related fraud by self-checking	May 3, 2016	CFDA	CFDA rectification action on illegal business operation in drug circulation link (Document No. 94)	The document requires drug wholesales enterprises to conduct self-check on ten illegal activities including fortifying drug sources and voluntarily reporting all involved people and institutions before May 31, 2016.
Promoting two-invoices policy	April 26, 2016	General Office of the State Council	Circular on 2016 key tasks for deepening reform of the medical system	It puts forth quantity-based joint procurement, and requires provinces piloting comprehensive medical reform to implement two-invoices system.
	July 19, 2016	Nine departments including former National Commission for Health and Family Planning	Key work in 2016 to rectify wrongdoings in drug purchase and sales and medical services	Implementing two-invoices system in provincial-level and municipal-level public hospitals in provinces piloting comprehensive medical reform.

(Continued)

Table 4.15 (Continued)

Direction	*Issuing Date*	*Issuing Department*	*Document Name*	*Content*
	November 8, 2016	State Council	Several suggestions of the leading group on medical system reform under the State Council on further promoting experiences in medical reform	Gradually implementing two-invoices system in all public hospitals
	January 9, 2017	Former National Commission for Health and Family Planning	Guideline for implementing two-invoices system in drug purchase and sales in public hospitals (trial)	As a national document for two-invoices system, it defines the system, scope, and implementation.

5 Policy recommendations to do with drug payment and use

5.1 Continue to deepen reform of payment methods by which insurance reimburses hospitals for drugs

Medical insurance payers are the main buyers of the services of medical providers, and they are also the main constraints on those providers. They must now go from their original passive mode of simply paying to an active mode of regulatory supervision.

First, they must continue to push forward reform of payment methods. Instead of paying by service item, they should move to a compound payment system, which means continuing pilot reforms involving payment by Diagnosis Related Group and DIP. Payment for drug fees should be incorporated into this reform of payment methods in the overall design. Second, they should make use of the various policy tools at their disposal, including a dynamic method of adjusting the reimbursable drug list, negotiated prices for drugs, and reimbursement prices, in order to move down drug prices. Finally, in order to implement payment-method reform in an effective way, the most important thing is that medical institutions must shift away from their traditional 'extensive' mode of providing medical services toward a more intensive and more finely tuned way of providing services. This will take place by strengthening investment in information systems that have to do with the hospital's insurance procedures. At the same time, hospitals should improve awareness of the importance of cost control among hospital administrators. They should make use of medical quality control platforms in a reasonable way as they apply quality controls on the hospital costs and insurance costs associated with patients.[10]

5.2 Speed up legislation that establishes a system that administers pharmacists, and formulate standards for related service fees

On June 18, 2020, the National Health Commission released a *Pharmacist Law of the People's Republic of China (Draft, second version, to solicit opinions)*. This explicitly set forth the scope, rights, and obligations of the pharmaceutical industry, and details to do with its examination and registration procedures, accreditation, and training. Article Five of this document specified, 'Pharmacists' practices with respect to the professional technical services they provide to patients are a form of medical treatment, and the price of their labor in supplying that treatment should be recognized by appropriate methods.' This was the first time China had specifically declared, in legal terms, that the country would be setting up a system of managing (administering) pharmacists. In the next stage, (we should) speed up the process of actually enacting this legislation and issue rules and regulations as soon as possible. We should further specify the appropriate methods by which the labor of pharmacists' services is to be priced, in order to have legal guarantees for pharmacists' fees.[11] Meanwhile, given that the allocation of positions of pharmacists is unclear at this time, and training systems are imperfect, and given that the scope of clinical prescribing of drugs and reasonable use of drugs is fairly narrowly defined and also inadequately tied in to clinical practice, we must strengthen the corps of pharmacists who can manage these tasks. We should make plans for the reasonable allocation of pharmacists in all levels of medical institutions. We should set up a reasonable system for compensating pharmacists, and improve upon the system of performance evaluations so that it takes various aspects into consideration. We should emphasize on-the-job training of pharmacists in grassroots medical institutions, as well as continuing education. We should pay particular attention to the role that pharmacists can play in adjusting the medical insurance reimbursement list.

5.3 Strengthen management to induce rational drug prescribing behavior

(We should) strengthen management over the security of drugs in medical institutions, and look into setting up a monitoring system that covers all the processes of drug procurement, storage, fulfillment, distribution, and use, and we should be

10 He Qian, Countermeasures for reform of healthcare payment system in hospitals [J]. *Think Tank Era*, Issue 22, 2019.

11 Zhang Hai, Zhang Wen, et al. Public hospitals' exploration on launching pharmacist charges [J]. *Pharmaceutical Care and Research*, Issue 6, 2018.

able to do real-time monitoring of drug use (prescribing). We should encourage hospitals to undertake investigations that are both scheduled and unscheduled, to evaluate whether or not prescriptions are being made out in a rational manner. Information on the procurement and prescribing of drugs should be an important part of the transparency mechanisms for hospital affairs. Regulations should be actually implemented that relate to how Chinese and western-medicine prescriptions are used for treatment, with a focus on monitoring and controlling the use of antibiotics, supplements, and nutritional-type medicines. Those doctors who are found to be prescribing improperly should be put on public notice. At the same time, we should strengthen performance review components that relate to reasonable prescribing of drugs. Such reasonable use and related performance targets should become a part of the performance review system for all hospitals and medical personnel, and we should encourage all administrative departments in charge of healthcare to make sure this happens. In this regard, we should be more specific in defining the parts of performance reviews that relate to procuring and prescribing drugs. The results of performance reviews should be linked to the total amount of insurance funds that an institution is allocated, as well as the wages of medical personnel.

5.4 Push forward a system of fulfilling prescriptions outside of hospitals, in a stable and secure way

As the 'Internet + medicine' equation advances in China at an ever-faster pace, and as we encourage the fulfillment of prescriptions outside of hospitals, particularly ongoing prescriptions that relate to chronic illness, we need to be aware of two things. On the one hand, prescriptions fulfilled outside of hospitals must be standardized and able to interconnect with Internet platforms – and we should encourage the development and expansion of such platforms. We must guarantee that such outside fulfillment platforms have sufficient capacity to take on the job, in terms of supply-chain capability, servicing, and IT qualifications. On the other hand, we must be sure to strengthen regulatory management over outside fulfillment, to ensure the authenticity, safety, and controllability of the prescriptions.

5.5 Constantly improve regulatory control mechanisms over medical insurance funds

A sound regulatory system for medical insurance must include effective regulatory laws, multiple regulatory bodies whose authorities and responsibilities are clearly defined, and diverse ways to carry out regulatory controls.

First, (we should) push for the passage of laws and regulations relating to regulatory control over medical insurance funds. These should be explicit about the entities that actually regulate, those that are observers, and what the regulation entails. Through bylaws or specific rules, the scope of regulation over medical insurance should be explicit as well as any rewards and punishments, so that there is a legal guarantee behind the work of the regulators.

Second, we should unify and refine systems for regulatory control over medical insurance funds. Performance reviews of funds should be conducted by a group that includes representatives from the relevant departments, with medical insurance departments playing the main role but supported by finance, auditing, healthcare, and development and reform. This group should carry out evaluations of fund operating procedures as well as use of funds.

Third, given that investment in IT by some departments is still minimal, which makes it impossible to have real-time transmittal of medical insurance information, we should greatly increase our efforts in building up information systems. As soon as possible, we must set up a unified nationwide system for claims settlement. All parts of the country should have interconnected claims settlement systems that link medical facilities to medical insurance. At the same time, we must push for the establishment of a medical insurance information system that has greater intelligence capabilities, that can make use of big data analysis and carry out cloud computing. We should constantly raise the level of modernization of insurance, that is, we should set up a whole-process information-based regulatory control system that makes use of IT technology before, during, and after a patient's diagnosis. This should allow examination of a patient's records prior to diagnosis, it should provide advance warning of any fraudulent behavior during diagnosis, and it should be able to analyze medical behavior after a diagnosis.

5 Commercial health insurance in China and its role in the payment of drug costs

Yu Baorong and Jia Yufei

1 Overview of commercial health insurance in China

1.1 General situation

China has already basically realized universal coverage through its system of 'basic medical insurance.' This kind of social insurance can satisfy the needs of people for the most basic medical services, but its role in providing safeguards is facing increasing pressure as medical costs rise. In 2014, the State Council put out *Various opinions on speeding up the development of commercial health insurance*, which called for putting more effort into linking China's basic health insurance system with commercial health insurance. This made it clear that the government feels that commercial health insurance should play an important role within China's New Medical Reform. At the same time, this kind of support gives the commercial health insurance industry an excellent opportunity to develop.

Health insurance insures an individual's physical body. It provides financial reimbursement for medical costs in the event a person gets sick or is injured due to an accident, or suffers the loss of income due to these things, or has costs that may have to be covered in the future for long-term nursing care, and so on. Between 2014 and 2018, premium income in China for commercial health insurance more than tripled, and compensation and payments also basically maintained an increase of more than 30% per year. In 2018, the income of commercial health insurance from premiums reached RMB 544.813 billion, while payments and compensation amounts reached RMB 174.443 billion. These figures were nearly ten times the totals in 2008, which had been RMB 58.546 billion and RMB 17.528 billion respectively.

According to the latest *2018 Statistical Report of the Insurance Industry* published by the China Banking and Insurance Regulatory Commission (CBIRC), China's commercial health insurance industry insured 3.201 billion insurance policies in 2018, which represented an increase of 417.28% over the previous year. The business is clearly growing by leaps and bounds. In the same year, premium income reached RMB 544.813 billion, or an increase of 24.12% over the previous year. Compensation and payments came to RMB 174.434 billion, or an increase of 34.72% over the previous year. Among the indemnities paid by various types

DOI: 10.4324/9781003325345-5

of insurance, including property insurance, life insurance, and accident insurance, those paid out by health insurance are growing the fastest (Figures 5.1 & 5.2).

Nevertheless, China's commercial health insurance industry is still in the early stages of development, as pointed out by *Research Report on China's Commercial Health Insurance Issues and Policy Recommendation*, published by the Insurance Association of China. Given the institutional structures of China's medical system, among other things, its ability to manage medical costs is limited. Meanwhile, the industry is still not providing sufficient services when it comes to health management.

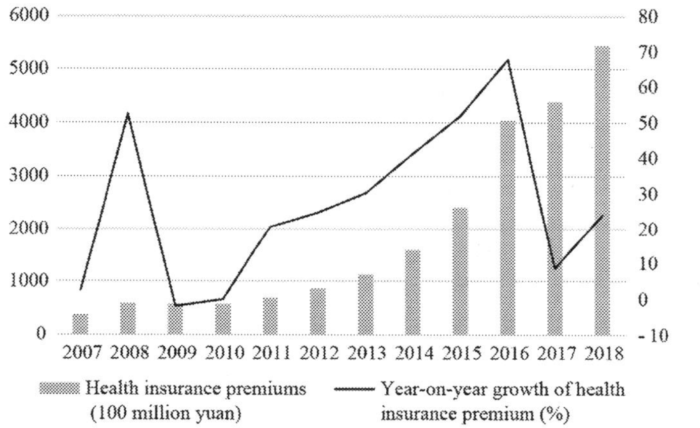

Figure 5.1 Income from Commercial Health Insurance Premiums in China, and Growth Rate from 2007 to 2018

Source: Original CIRC's statistical report of the insurance industry; http://bxjg.circ.gov.cn/web/site0/tab5257/

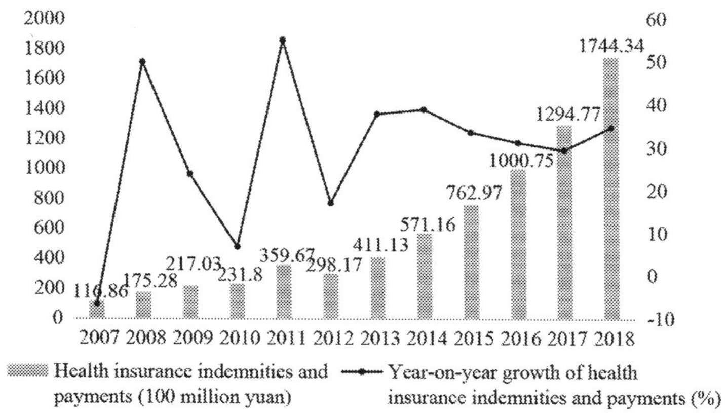

Figure 5.2 Indemnities and Payments Made by Commercial Health Insurance in China from 2007 to 2018, and Growth Rate

Source: Original CIRC's statistical report of the insurance industry; http://bxjg.circ.gov.cn/web/site0/tab5257/

1.2 The 'density' and the 'depth' of commercial health insurance in China

The 'density' of commercial health insurance refers to the average premiums per person in a population (that is, it is the total annual premium income of health insurance divided by total population). This figure can indicate the degree to which a country's population participates in health insurance. The following graph uses statistics on population that China's National Bureau of Statistics publishes to calculate the density of commercial health insurance and its rate of increase (Figure 5.3). Between 2010 and 2016, density maintained a high rate of growth. The rate of growth moderated somewhat in 2017 and 2018. In 2018, per capita health insurance premiums in total came to RMB 390.44, which represented almost a ninefold increase (8.86) over 2008.

Nevertheless, it is useful to look at comparative figures for the United States, France, Germany, and the U.K. In 2015, per capita premiums for health insurance in the United States were USD 3,131. In France, they were USD 1,588, in the U.K., USD 1,007, and in Germany RMB 3,472.[1] The model for health insurance used in the United States is fairly typical. In 2015, the premium density in the U.S. was 110 times that of China (using the average exchange rate in 2015 of USD 1 =

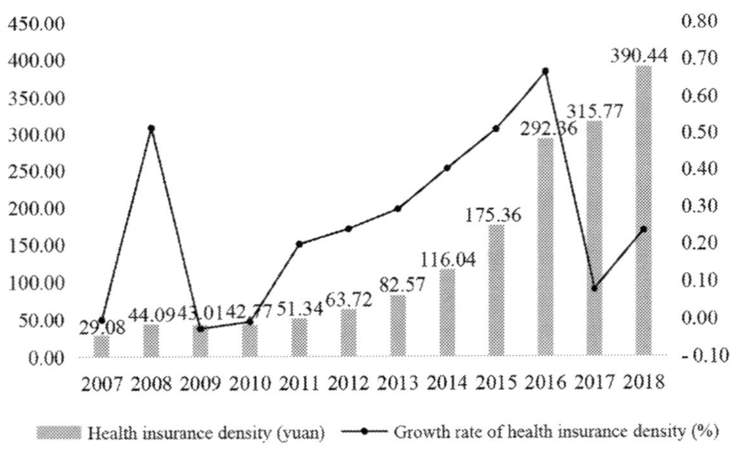

Figure 5.3 The Density and Growth Rate of China's Commercial Health Insurance from 2007 to 2018

Source: CIRC, National Bureau of Statistics (NBS), 132. Statistics source of premium income: http://bxjg.circ.gov.cn/web/site0/tab5257/. Statistics source of population: http://data.stats.gov.cn/easyquery.htm?cn=C01.

1 *Commercial Health Insurance Industry Analysis Report 2018*, published on Apr. 2018, https://wenku.baidu.com/view/0cb3fcdfl62ded630.

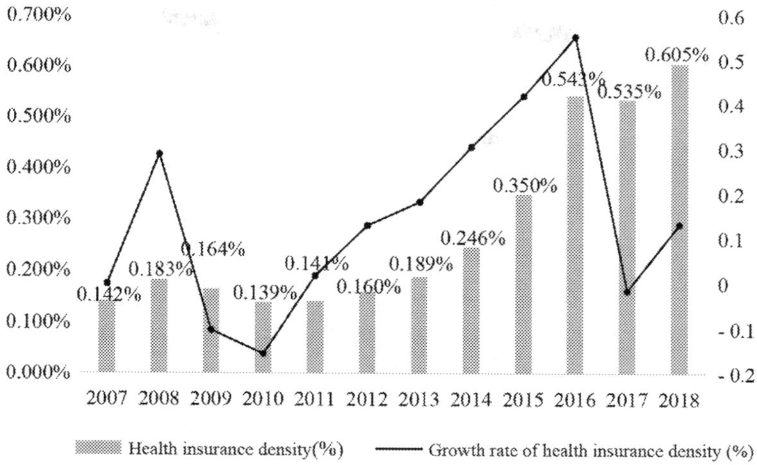

Figure 5.4 The Penetration and the Growth Rate of China's Commercial Health Insurance, from 2007 to 2018

Source: CIRC, National Bureau of Statistics (NBS)

RMB 6.23).[2] Germany uses a social model of medical insurance, but its per capita premiums are still roughly 20 times those in China. Clearly, there is still a certain gap between the density of commercial health insurance in China, and the degree to which its insurance industry has developed, and commercial health insurance in countries where the industry is well developed.

The 'depth' of health insurance, or the penetration, refers to premium income divided by the GDP of a country. This can reflect the status of health insurance within the entire economy. China's rate of penetration showed a rising trend over the ten years, but it is still two times lower than that of either Germany or the United States.[3] (figure 5.4)

1.3 Share of commercial health insurance in China's medical costs

China's total expenditures on healthcare have grown rapidly since the 1990s. From around 3% as a percentage of GDP, they have fluctuated upwards to reach 6.41% in 2017.[4] Meanwhile, with the improvement of the country's system of social safeguards, individual spending on healthcare as a percentage of total spending on healthcare has gone down, from around 60% to 28.77% in 2017. In overall terms,

2 *Average exchange rate of USD to CNY in 2015: Dec. 6.4476*, published on Feb. 11, 2019, www.chinairn.com/news/20190211/145029974.shtml.

3 *In-depth Report on the Insurance Industry: Blue Ocean of the Health Insurance*, published on Mar. 17, 2018, www.sohu.com/a/225770521_620847.

4 Calculated based on statistics.

social spending on healthcare reached 42.32% at the highest point (that is, non-government spending as a percent of total spending on healthcare) (Figure 5.5). This figure includes social medical insurance spending, social donations, commercial insurance spending, and so on.

Compensation by commercial health insurance comes to a tiny percentage of China's total healthcare costs. Statistics indicate that this percentage showed consistent growth between 2013 and 2017, but was still quite small. By 2017, it accounted for just 2.462% of the total (Figure 5.6). This percentage is vastly lower

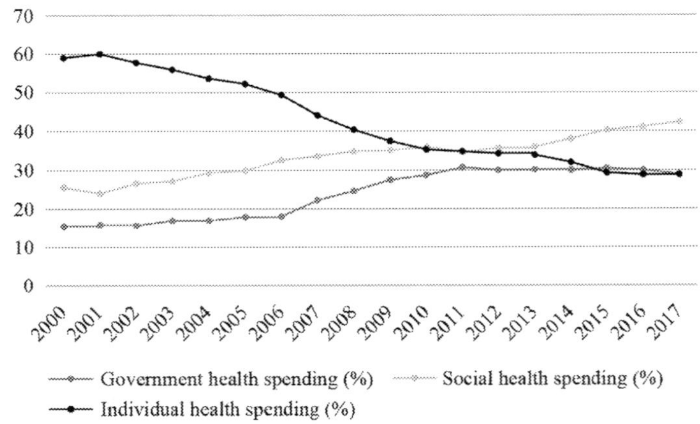

Figure 5.5 Health Spending Percentages by Different Sectors: Government, Society, and Individuals

Source: National Health and Family Planning Commission of the PRC, National Administration of Traditional Chinese Medicine, 137; http://olap.epsnet.com.cn/auth/platform.html?sid=A3E671FBAA 0D710342538857E7

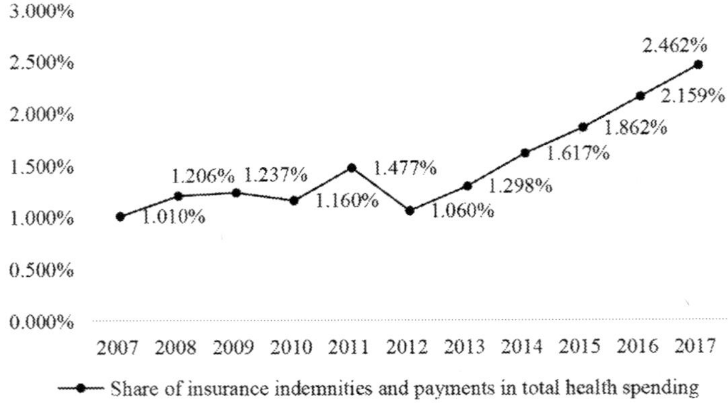

Figure 5.6 Percent of Total Healthcare Spending that is Paid for by Insurance Indemnities and Payments

Source: National Bureau of Statistics (NBS), 139; http://bxjg.circ.gov.cn/web/site0/tab5257/ http://olap.epsnet.com.cn/auth/platform.htm l?sid=A3E671FBAA0D710342538857E7A9F2F7」 pv404848636

Table 5.1 Total and Per Capita Spending on Drugs, 2010–2016, and that Spending as a Percentage of Total Healthcare Costs

	2011	*2013*	*2014*	*2015*	*2016*
Total medical products spending (100 million yuan)	88,35.9	13,113.2	13,925	16,166.3	17,345.9
Per capita medical products spending (yuan)	658.9	963.7	1,018	1,176.1	1,261.9
Proportion of medical products spending in the total (%)	41.6	39.4	37.8	37.7	35.8

Source: 2018 China Health Statistics Summary; http://data.chinabaogao.com/yiyao/2018/10253K1c2018.html

than the amount that social insurance and individuals themselves pay out. In 2015, a statistical analysis showed that the per capita healthcare spending of commercial insurance was not even 6% of total healthcare spending. In the United States, this statistic is over 35%.[5] In other developed countries such as France and Canada, it is generally over 10%.[6]

In recent years, total spending on drugs and per capita spending on drugs have both been rising. In 2016, spending on drugs in China reached RMB 1,734.59 billion. This figure represented 35.8% of all healthcare spending. Using the figure of 2.159% to calculate the share of this paid out by commercial health insurance shows that the total amount of compensation by commercial health insurance totaled just 1/17th of total medical expenditures in 2016. Meanwhile, only a portion of health insurance compensation goes to pay for drugs. It is clear that commercial health insurance makes up a very small share of actual spending on drugs in China (Table 5.1).

Commercial health insurance is affected by such things as levels of economic development and attitudes of people toward commercial insurance, but its coverage rate is still vastly inadequate. The industry also contributes very little to the economy. Among other reasons for this, China lacks ways in which commercial health insurance and medical services providers can cooperate in sharing risk and balancing mutual benefits. In overall terms, commercial insurance occupies a limited percentage of medical spending, and the role that this kind of insurance plays in meeting medical and healthcare needs is still at a low level of development.

1.4 A brief introduction to different types of commercial health insurance

The role that commercial health insurance should play in China's medical safeguards systems is increasingly important. (At present), products are relatively

5 *In 2016, China's pharmaceutical spending reached CNY 1,734.59 billion, 35.8% of total health expenses*, published on October 25, 2018 by www.Chinabaogo.com.

6 Lanjinger.com, *Insurance Association of China: Commercial health insurance is in the primary stage of development and the market size will exceed CNY 1 trillion by 2020*, published on July 27, 2018. http://finance.ifeng.com/a/20180727/16410029_0.shtml

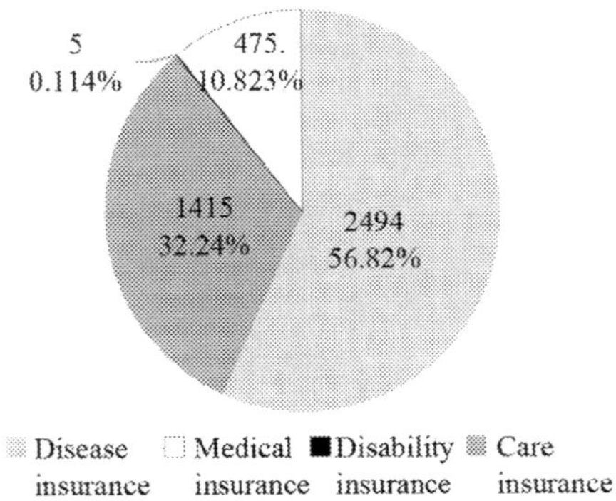

Figure 5.7 Types of Health Insurance and their Share of Total Original Premium Income in 2017

Source: Prospective Industrial Research Institute

simple compared to such things as life insurance and property insurance. The main categories of commercial health insurance include insurance for specific illnesses (critical illness insurance, cancer insurance, the critical illness insurance for other specific diseases, and so on), medical insurance, long-term care insurance, and disability insurance. In the market, the mainstream types of insurance are medical insurance and insurance for specific illnesses. Such things as long-term care insurance and disability insurance have a very small market share and are not adequately recognized as important by insurance companies.

The role that different types of insurance play in covering medical and drug costs can be quite different, given the various payment conditions and methods that each involves. The percentages that each type of insurance held in 2017, together with the original premium income for each, is as follows (Figure 5.7). In general, insurance for specific illnesses and medical insurance constitute nearly 90% of the market for commercial health insurance. The market share of insurance for illnesses is larger, but these two types of insurance are both seeing fairly fast increase in original premium income.

1.4.1 Insurance for a specific illness

This type of insurance pays out for specific illnesses. When a person who is insured under this insurance becomes ill with one of the specified diseases, the insurance company pays as stipulated in a contract, without regard for the actual medical costs that the insured patient may have had to pay. This insurance mainly covers major illnesses and such specific things as anticancer insurance, eye health insurance, dental insurance, maternity insurance, and so on. Generally the contracts for this type of insurance product include a list of types of illness that are covered. When the insured person contracts one of the illnesses on the list, he or she can receive insurance compensation and can then spend that on the medical and drug costs of treating the illness. Insurance for serious illnesses includes commonly

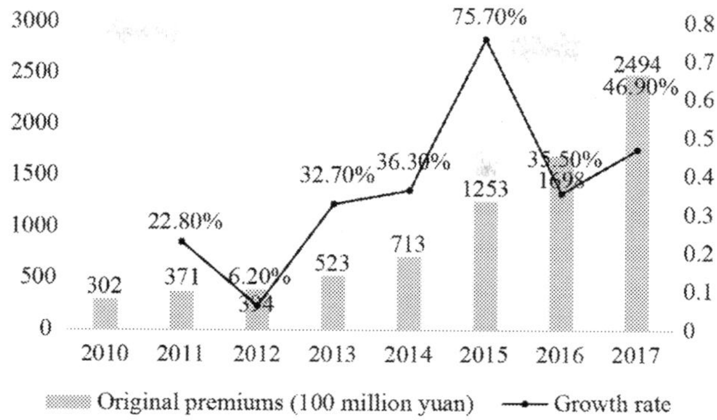

Figure 5.8 Income from and Growth Rate of Original Premiums for Illness Insurance from 2010 to 2017

Source: Prospective Industrial Research Institute; www.qianzhan.com/analyst/detail/220/181211-f5a055ce.html

seen things like malignant tumors (this generally does not include some original-position cancers), acute myocardial infarction, cerebral apoplexy (stroke), major organ transplants or hematopoietic stem cell transplantation (allotransplantation), coronary artery bypass grafting, end-stage renal disease, and so on.

Illness insurance is generally purchased for a long period of time and any compensation also continues over a long period, so premiums are quite high. Given that companies earn the highest income from this kind of insurance in China, illness insurance has developed extremely rapidly in the country. The number of products on offer is also increasing every year – between 2010 and 2018 the average annual rate of growth came to 13.7%.[7] Income from premiums has risen at a commensurate rate – in 2017, income from original premiums came to RMB 249.4 billion (Figure 5.8).

1.4.2 Insurance for medical costs

This type of insurance pays agreed-upon economic compensation to the insured person once that person gets sick or has an unexpected event that leads to medical costs. The coverage of the insurance generally includes reasonable costs of operations, drug costs, nursing costs, examination costs, hospital-stay costs, and so on. This type of insurance pays out on the basis of costs. It usually includes clauses that relate to deductibles, percent-of-payment, and payment limits. The deductible refers to fees that the insured person must pay in advance. Percent-of-payment refers to the percentage of costs that exceed the amount of the deductible – the insured person shares the cost burden by paying a given percentage. 'Payment

7 Official WeChat Account "Chadaoyanshu", *Uncovering China's First Knowledge Map of Disease Insurance Industry*, published on July 30, 2019, https://mp.weixin.qq.com/s/OUkzvoqg2Vcehgdiku58Rg.

limits' refers to the greatest amount that the insurance company will pay to the insured person – any costs over this amount must be borne by the insured person.

Medical insurance compensates for actual medical costs after deducting the subsidies or compensation that the insured person may receive from other sources, and it pays according to contracted terms. Such 'other sources' include things as social medical insurance, public health services, payment through the work unit, or payments received from any other insurance organization. However, spending out of a person's 'individual account' generally is not considered to be medical costs that will not be reimbursed (that is, spending out of these accounts will be reimbursed).

The medical costs that commercial medical insurance generally cover include normal outpatient costs, emergency costs, and hospitalization costs. However, limits are placed on coverage when it comes to major illness. As for drug reimbursements, insurance companies generally do not have a specific list of reimbursable drugs. Instead, they use the social-insurance list of reimbursable drugs as a reference. Different levels of products will reimburse at different rates. Among the conditions of insurance are that the drugs being reimbursed for are both 'reasonable and necessary,' 'prescribed by a doctor,' 'drugs that have a registration number granted by the National Pharmaceutical Regulatory departments or imported drugs with a certificate of authenticity.' Generally speaking, nutritional supplements, immune function regulators, traditional Chinese medicine, beauty-slimming products and preventative drugs are not covered under this kind of insurance. Normally this kind of insurance provides coverage for one year at a time, and there is no guarantee of continued coverage after that. In addition, there is an age limit on people who can buy this kind of coverage (generally around 65). Some products allow preferential policies that allow for extension of coverage once the person has paid premiums for six consecutive years – for example, a person's insurance might be renewed, up to the age of 100.

In recent years, high-end health insurance that is aimed at the market of high-end consumers is expanding, and competition is quite fierce. In contrast to normal health insurance, high-end insurance has higher coverage and fewer restrictions on what a person can have reimbursed. In addition to the normal things like clinic and hospital costs, included now within the scope of coverage can be emergency assistance, dental costs, consultation at the international departments of clinics, and coverage for medical expenses at home but also outside of China. Meanwhile, there are fewer restrictions on the drugs for which one can be reimbursed. The target audience for this kind of insurance is gradually expanding from top-tier cities to second- and third-tier cities. In order to increase competitive advantage, companies are improving their products and going beyond normal medical insurance to include renewal benefits, a broader scope of coverage, and better compensation.

Between 2010 and 2017, premium income of (commercial) health insurance in China has gone up every year (Figure 5.9). Generally speaking, prices of this kind of insurance are low in overall terms, and the percentage of costs that can be reimbursed is fairly high for items within the scope of coverage. This kind of insurance can play a certain supplementary role to China's social medical insurance.

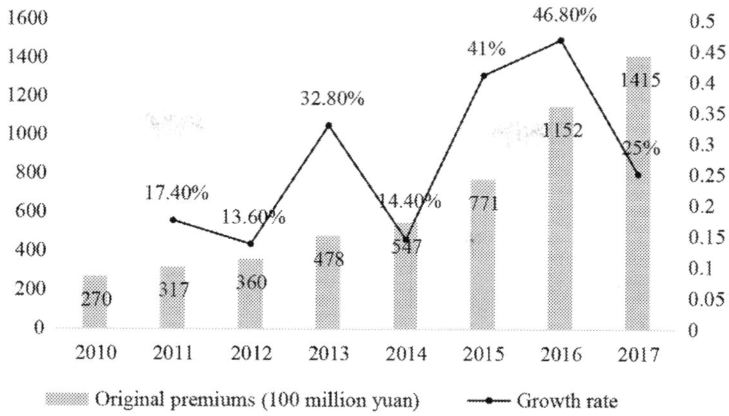

Figure 5.9 Income from and Growth Rate of Original Premiums for Medical Insurance from 2010 to 2017

Source: Prospective Industrial Research Institute, 144; www.qianzhan.com/analyst/detail/220/181211-f5a055ce.html

1.4.3 Long-term care insurance

This is a supplementary kind of insurance that pays for the various costs associated with the need for long-term rehabilitation or nursing care due to a person's inability to take care of themselves. The cause may be old age, or illness, or an unexpected event. This kind of insurance can provide three kinds of coverage, one that pays for actual expenses and reimburses upon receipt, another that pays a certain fixed amount, and a third that pays directly to the provider of long-term care. The coverage generally includes death benefits, care benefits, and benefits on expiration of a policy. 'Care benefits' are directly related to the medical expenses of the insured person and are paid to the person who is deemed to be under long-term care. At the present time, the majority of products offering care benefits in the market are of a universal type. Insurance companies take in premiums and record them into a person's individual account, on which interest accumulates at a specified rate. This kind of insurance generally reimburses at a rate that is a certain percentage of the amount in the individual account, for example, it might be 105% of the value of an individual account. Traditional long-term care insurance generally pays compensation according to a specified and agreed-upon amount of insurance. In actual reality, receipts from this kind of insurance may well be used to make up for care costs, loss of income, and medical costs.

1.4.4 Disability insurance

Disability insurance is also known as coverage for loss of income. This is mainly targeted at people who lose all or some of their ability to work due to some unexpected event or illness. Insurance compensates for a certain portion of the losses caused by such events. The market share of this kind of insurance is extremely small. Insurance amounts are generally tied to the income level of the person who is insured and insurance goes to compensate for income loss – it generally has no direct relationship to medical expenses.

Taken together, long-term care insurance and disability insurance hold a small share of the insurance market. In terms of covering medical costs, the main types of commercial health insurance are medical insurance and major illness insurance.

2 Comparison between commercial health insurance and social insurance

This section looks at the differences between commercial health insurance and social insurance with respect to the following aspects: qualifications of those who are insured, methods of paying premiums, medical services, methods of reimbursement, and payment methods by which insurance reimburses for drugs. Within commercial insurance, we select 'medical insurance' and 'illness insurance' as the types that are directly related to payment for medical costs. Within social insurance, we select the 'basic medical insurance for urban workers' and the 'basic medical insurance for urban and rural residents' as the types for comparison with commercial insurance (Table 5.2).

The primary distinctions between the roles that commercial and social insurance play in paying for medical and drug costs are described later.

2.1 Participants' qualifications and insurance coverage

First, with respect to the groups it covers, commercial insurance is aimed at avoiding risk and making a profit, so it chooses to insure people who are fairly healthy. It can refuse coverage to those people who have a prior history of certain diseases and whose health indications are abnormal. For example, commercial health insurance generally will not insure people in high-risk categories of work, such as mining or blasting with explosives. In addition, if a person is overweight, has high cholesterol, high blood pressure, or other such symptoms, insurance will either refuse to cover or will increase the premium rate. Anyone who is suffering from diabetes, any form of nervous-system disease, and cancer will not be allowed coverage. Meanwhile, premium rates can vary considerably depending on economic constraints, including the level of income of a household and the part of the country a person lives in. Essentially, given the profit-oriented nature of commercial health insurance, groups that are within the bounds of the risk pool that insurance will cover are high-quality groups with low health risks. Those who need insurance the most, due to such factors as health conditions, occupational risk, economic conditions, and so on, are the ones who will not be insured by commercial health insurance.

However, it is worth noting that preferential tax treatment can play a role in determinations. In 2015, the Insurance Regulatory Commission issued a notice called *Interim measures on administering 'preferential-tax-treatment type health*

Table 5.2 A Comparison of Commercial Health Insurance and Social Health Insurance in China

	Commercial Medical Insurance	*Commercial Disease Insurance*	*Basic Medical Insurance System for Urban Workers*	*Urban-Rural Residents Basic Medical Insurance*
Participants' qualifications	Healthy population of prescribed age (e.g., from 28 days of birth to 65 years of age)	Healthy population of prescribed age	Enterprises and their employees; public organs and institutions, intermediary organizations, social organizations, private non-enterprises and their employees; the employing units affiliated to the army and their non-military personnel. No health requirements.	For all urban and rural residents except for those who should be insured by the basic health insurance for urban workers. No health requirements.
Coverage	As contracted, the spending on beds, medical products, meals, treatment, care, examination and surgery operation not covered by social security.	The insurance benefits shall be paid when the insured suffers from illnesses stipulated in policies.	Individual accounts used to pay for the designated retail medical products expenses, outpatient and emergency treatment costs, medical expenses below the maximum line of payment, and unified accounts used to pay for the insured's medical spending on hospitalization, part of the outpatient expenses for critical illnesses, etc.	The medical spending on hospitalization and outpatient services incurred by the insured; the proportion of the payment for hospitalization expenses was maintained at about 75%; the medical products catalogue has extended.
Payment	Voluntary	Voluntary	Employer contributions + individual contributions	Individual contributions + government subsidies
Minimum line of payment	Product deductible	No	Varying from place to place	Varying from place to place
Indemnities and payments ratio	Contracted proportion	No	– –	In general, the reimbursement ratio of hospitalization costs is 75% or so and that of outpatient coordination is about 50%.
Indemnities and payments limit	The amount of insurance	The amount of insurance	3–5 times the average wage of local employees in the previous year	Varying from place to place (e.g., Beijing has a cumulative maximum amount of CNY 200,000)
Insurance period	Generally one year	Generally long-term or lifelong	Lifelong	Lifelong

insurance.' When an insurance company conducts business that involves preferential tax benefits for individuals, the insurance company must comply with certain regulations – the insurance must be long-term health insurance, and it cannot be denied to people who have pre-existing conditions. It must carry a guarantee of the ability to renew coverage. A number of problems still remain to be dealt with in this regard, due to the degree of preferential treatment, implementation procedures, and so on, but preferential-tax-treatment type insurance for individuals is based on principles of fairness and the social obligations of the industry. Its role in lowering the burden of medical costs is worth focusing policy attention on.

China's 'basic medical insurance' provides social security that is of a 'benefits' nature. Different types of safeguards accrue to people who are insured depending on their 'status,' that is, where their household is registered, the nature of their work, and so on. Insurance does not depend on health factors. At present, China's basic medical insurance has basically achieved universal coverage. By the end of 2018, 1.345 billion people were covered under the program. Coverage is stable for over 95% of the population.[8] By way of contrast, commercial health insurance had a coverage rate in 2018 of less than 10%. The great majority of people in China cover their health risks in a form that is fairly singular – they still rely on either basic medical insurance or using their own funds.[9] It is obvious that the contribution commercial health insurance currently makes to covering the medical costs of the population is highly limited.

2.2 *Premiums and 'coverage,' or the responsibilities of insurance*

People decide to be covered by commercial insurance on a voluntary basis. In principle, the reimbursement of claims is determined by the structure of products that people buy, the premiums they pay, and so on. The more complete the safeguards, the higher the premiums. The way in which rates are set is complex and depends on the extent of safeguards, the age and gender of the insured person, state of health, occupation, extent of social security, and also the prices of competitors. In the case of group rates, factors include the age and gender distribution within the group, geographic location, history of routine checkups, and the group's proficiency in using medical benefits. Put simply, rates of premiums take into consideration the various factors that go into measuring the size of health risk, probability of risk occurrence, and market environment.

In addition to this, however, premiums include more than just the costs related to risk. They also include expenses that relate to running the company (such as commissions, taxes, operating costs). As for the coverage of different kinds of insurance, specific details are noted in the section that describes actual cases. In overall

8 *2018 Statistics Express on Medical Security Development*, published by National Healthcare Security Administration, www.nhsa.gov.cn/art/2019/2/28/art-7_942.html.

9 *2018 China (Large and Medium-Sized Cities) Commercial Health Insurance Development Index Report*, by Insurance Association of China, www.199it.com/archives/783975.html.

terms, commercial insurance is positioned as a supplementary form of insurance to social security. It provides coverage for costs that social insurance will not cover. Its main role comes into play in the case of hospitalization and major illness.

The costs of paying for China's basic medical insurance are borne by the individual, the government, and the unit that employs the individual. The system is mandatory and the amount that an individual pays depends on the nature of their employment, personal income, the average income of where they live, the average income of the unit in which they work, and other factors. The focus is on fairness. As a result, health insurance policies are different in different parts of the country due to the various conditions of economic development.

Basic health insurance is divided into two parts, namely 'individual accounts,' and the 'pooled fund account.' The funds in an individual account belong to the individual who is insured and can be used on such things as basic drugs and outpatient clinic's fees. Since commercial health insurance generally requires deductibles, small-sum medical costs are mostly paid for either by the consumer or by social insurance. (Such small things would include non-prescription drugs, outpatient visits for mild problems, or clinic visits.) The pooled funds are generally used to pay for hospital stays for people who are insured, for emergency assistance at non-designated hospitals, for treatment outside of the normal place of residence, and for relocation needs in a new place. There are both minimum and maximum limits on this kind of insurance. What's more, different ranks of hospitals institute different levels of reimbursement percentages. The reimbursement standards used in Henan province for basic medical insurance for urban and rural residents are shown in Table 5.3 as an example, together with the reimbursement percentages and the minimum payments for different levels of hospitals. Percentages of costs that a hospital will reimburse go down as the rank of the hospital goes up (the highest ranking hospitals are Grade 3). The highest total amount that any hospital will reimburse is RMB 150,000.

Social insurance is subject to various restrictions, including a minimum amount and maximum amount of reimbursement, specific reimbursement percentages and the reimbursable drug list. That is, it cannot reimburse for amounts either below the minimum or above the maximum, and it cannot reimburse for costs outside the reimbursable drug list. It does not have any specific restrictions, however, on type of disease. Commercial insurance, on the other hand, is subject to the restrictions of a minimum amount, the total amount of insurance, the reimbursement percentage, the terms of coverage, and the requirement to inform the insured person of any exclusions to the policy. In addition to the restriction on the amount of reimbursement, commercial insurance policies stipulate types of illness, causes of accidents, and whether or not the insured has been fully informed. The conditions for claims settlement of commercial insurance are more stringent than those of social insurance.

With respect to the number of times an insured person can be reimbursed, in the case of basic medical insurance, there is simply a ceiling amount on the total safeguards and an insured person may go up to the ceiling. This kind of insurance has the advantage of insuring even if one is sick, guaranteeing ongoing coverage, and ensuring long-term effectiveness. Commercial insurance, on the other hand, generally makes a one-time payment for something like, for example, a serious

Table 5.3 Percentage of a Claim that will be Reimbursed at Different Levels of Premiums and at Different Levels of Medical Institutions, in Henan Province, 2017

Level	*Hospital*	*Minimum Amount of Payment (Yuan)*	*Reimbursement Ratio*
Township level	Township hospitals (Community medical institutions)	200	70% for 200–800 yuan 90% for over 800 yuan
County level	Level II or below (Including Level II) Hospitals	400	63% for 400–1,500 yuan 83% for over 1,500 yuan
Municipal level	Level II or below (Including Level II) Hospitals	500	55% for 500–3,000 yuan 75% for over 3,000 yuan
	Level III Hospital	900	53% for 900–4,000 yuan 72% for over 4,000 yuan
Provincial level	Level II or below (Including Level II) Hospitals	600	53% for 600–4,000 yuan 72% for over 4,000 yuan
	Level III Hospital	1,500	50% for 1,500–7,000 yuan 68% for over 7,000 yuan
Outside the province		1,500	50% for over 1,500–7,000 yuan 68% for over 7,000 yuan

illness. What's more, after that, if the insurance company does not commit to renewing a policy, it may be hard for the person to get insured for serious illness.

With respect to the medical services that commercial insurance and social insurance cover, commercial insurance generally provides greater choice in medical providers and more convenience, depending on the level of products it offers. For example, a person insured through commercial health insurance can enjoy a 'green channel,' special outpatient services, treatment overseas, and the ability to be reimbursed for special medicines. Basic medical insurance, on the other hand, is mainly aimed at covering routine treatment in public medical institutions. Commercial health insurance can satisfy the demand of consumers who place high demands on their medical services and who have the economic wherewithal to pay for them (Table 5.4).

With respect to the specifics of how insurance pays for drugs, the following describes the components of the reimbursable drug list of China's basic medical insurance.

1 Part A of the list mainly includes drugs that are clinically necessary, broadly used, therapeutically effective, and have lower prices than other drugs of the same type. Regulations stipulate that basic medical insurance funds must pay for these drugs and that payment is guaranteed nationwide in all areas where funding is centrally pooled for the purpose. Except for the deductible portion, 100% of the drug costs are reimbursable.

Table 5.4 A Comparison of Medical Services Provided by Basic Medical Insurance and Commercial Health Insurance

	Hospital	*Time for Queuing*	*Interrogation for Diagnosis*	*Other Services*
Basic health insurance	Only public hospitals and a few private hospitals	Long	Short	No
Commercial health insurance	Besides public hospitals, it includes special outpatient clinics, high-end private hospitals, overseas medical institutions, etc.	Green channel, appointment for medical treatment, short queuing time.	Expert interrogation, online consultation, etc.	Private wards, genetic testing, health management services, etc.

Source: CIRC's official website, Prospective Industrial Research Institute

2 Part B of the list may be adjusted as necessary depending on the economic conditions and prescribing patterns in a given area. The percentage of reimbursement by the medical insurance fund may be determined by each centrally pooled fund jurisdiction. Generally, the percentage of reimbursement from centrally pooled funds for Part B drugs is around 70% to 80%. Drugs that are not included in the reimbursable drug list must be paid for by the individual himself. With respect to new drugs and special drugs, in September 2018, the National Health Security Administration put out a notice saying that 17 such drugs are now incorporated in the list. Of these, 12 treat solid mass tumors, and five treat hematological cancers. As per regulations, these can be reimbursed if they are prescribed in accordance with medical indications. For example, if Gefitinib is prescribed, it will be reimbursed only after genetic testing is performed to confirm EGFR[10] gene mutations, and the reports of the genetic testing must be provided.

In commercial health insurance, the reimbursement of drug costs is directly related to China's medical insurance system. Commercial health insurance will reimburse for drugs that social insurance does not cover due to restrictions on some categories of drugs in the reimbursable drug list. By now, mainstream commercial insurance has broken through the restrictions of the list and will reimburse for the cost of drugs and treatments that are within the disease-related scope of the insurance coverage. At the same time, some insurance products allow for the addition of supplementary drug services and reimbursement of such special treatments as photon and heavy ion therapy, and so on.

To give an example: in one centrally pooled funding jurisdiction, an employee had to be hospitalized and costs came to RMB 20,000, of which RMB 9,000 was for drugs. The drug component included RMB 4,000 of Type A drugs, RMB 2,500

10 EGFR: epidermal growth factor receptor, a member of the HER family.

of Type B drugs, and RMB 2,500 of drugs not on the list. If the reimbursement percentage for Type B drugs is 80%, then the drug costs incurred by this employee are as follows:

1 Self-pay portion: this includes the RMB 2,500 of drugs not on the list, plus 20% of the B drugs, or RMB 500, for a total of RMB 3,000
2 Social insurance portion: for A drugs, this includes a reimbursable amount of RMB 4,000 if all necessary requirements are met, plus 80% of B drugs, or RMB 2,000, for a total of RMB 6,000
3 Commercial insurance portion: if the employee has purchased commercial medical insurance, after deducting the deductible as per the insurance agreement, the insurance will reimburse for the pre-determined percentage.

3 An empirical analysis of the effectiveness of commercial health insurance and social insurance

Commercial health insurance can be divided into group insurance and individual insurance, given the distinct nature of these two categories, and products offered in these categories reflect the differences. Individual commercial health insurance mainly has to do with insuring medical costs and illness.

3.1 Individual commercial health insurance

Products in the market in this category are dominated by illness insurance and medical treatment insurance. Taikang Insurance can serve as an example. Its products mainly include illness insurance and medical treatment insurance, while its share of the total market for long-term nursing care and disability coverage is negligible. In addition, in August 2018, Taikang launched a new insurance product that provides coverage for the 17 new drugs and special drugs now on the reimbursement list.

3.1.1 Insurance that covers medical costs

This kind of insurance generally has a one-year term, but the insured person can frequently extend and continue preferential terms since insurance companies are interested in maintaining their existing base of clients and gaining new clients as they develop their business. For example, if a person has been insured continuously for six years, then the policy will be extended unconditionally whether or not there has been an incident in the previous year, and it can be extended up to the age of 100. To some extent, such renewal clauses can help with the problem of non-renewal due to illness during the term of the insurance.

The market for medical-cost insurance can be segmented by levels of safeguards, which can be described as low, medium, and high.

1 Low-end products: Products on this end of the spectrum provide the same safeguards as social insurance. The difference is that commercial insurance reimburses for the portion of costs that social insurance does not. Premiums of Taikang for this kind of insurance are in the range of RMB 300 per year. Products generally require deductibles and co-pays, and they place an upper limit on reimbursements. Given the restrictions of the social insurance reimbursable drug list, after subtracting the part that social insurance will reimburse and the deductible, this type of product plays a fairly limited role in paying for drug costs. Prior to 2016, this was the main kind of commercial insurance product on the market and it still constitutes the majority of existing policies – it is said to hold about 80% of the total. With the appearance of 'Million Medical' policies in recent years, however, this kind of policy will gradually cease to be offered.
2 Mid-tier products: Taikang Life was the first insurance company to put a 'Million Medical' product on the market. This kind of insurance is a prime example of a mid-tier market product. Its scope of reimbursement goes beyond the limitations of the social insurance reimbursable list. It will reimburse an agreed upon percentage of the costs of such things as costs from hospitalization at a public hospital (including outpatient costs in the seven days before and the 30 days after), special outpatient costs, and so on. The insurance coverage can reach 1 million RMB, hence the name. After Taikang began offering this product in 2016, the product generated more than 50% of the increase in the company's mid-tier policies every year, given market demand and also sales-commission incentives. By now, mid-tier policies dominate the health insurance products that Taikang currently sells. The company's holdings of such policies are continuing to move strongly upward.

Once Taikang offered this product, other similar products sprang into the market. Table 5.5 describes the basic situation. It provides a comparison of the different 'Million Medical' products.

From the previously mentioned, it will be seen that there are only minor distinctions among the coverage and terms of the various Million Medical products. The term of coverage is mostly one year. Insurance generally covers costs in the RMB 10,000 range, and there is generally no deductible in the case of serious illness. Within the prescribed scope of coverage, all costs are reimbursable, and 60% of costs are reimbursed for an insured person who does not have social security. For a person who is 40 years old and wants insurance that will cover between RMB 2 million to RMB 3 million in costs, premiums are in the range of RMB 400 to RMB 500 per year.

This kind of mid-tier insurance product can meet the needs of people who would like to insure the drug costs of hospital stays and the expenses of special outpatient visits that fall outside the scope of the reimbursable list. They represent a great advance over the low-end medical insurance products in terms of the safeguards they offer.

Table 5.5 A Comparison of Several Medical Insurance Products

	Company	*Taikang Life*	*PICC*	*ZhongAn International*
	Product	*Micro-medical Insurance Long-Term Medical Care*	*Good Medical Care and Long-Term Medical Care*	*Enjoy e-Life (Edition 2019)*
Conditions of insurance	Age of the insured	30 days–60 years old	28 days–60 years old	30 days–60 years old
	Waiting period	30 days	30 days	30 days
	Underwriting occupation	No high-risk occupations	No high-risk occupations	Category 1–4
	Time insured	6 years	1 year (6 years with guaranteed renewal)	1 year
	Applicable hospital	General departments of Level II Public hospitals or above	General departments of Level II Public hospitals or above	General departments of Level II Public hospitals or above
Conditions of renewal	Age of renewal	100 years old	100 years old	105 years old
	Health changes or historical claims	no influence	no influence	no influence
Insurance coverage	General medical coverage	CNY 2 million	CNY 2 million	CNY 3 million
	General medical deductible	CNY 10,000	A total of CNY 10,000 for six year	CNY 10,000
	Coverage for malignant tumor (critical illnesses)	100 critical illnesses, CNY 4 million	100 critical illnesses, CNY 4 million	100 critical illnesses, CNY 6 million
	Deductible for malignant tumors (critical illnesses)	Zero deductible for 100 critical illnesses	Zero deductible for 100 critical illnesses	Zero deductible for 100 critical illnesses
	Reimbursement ratio	100% for the insured with social security and 60% the insured without.	100% for the insured with social security and 60% the insured without.	100% for the insured with social security and 60% the insured without.
	Special outpatient and emergency services	Yes.	Yes.	Yes.

	Outpatient and emergency surgery	Yes.	Yes.	Yes.
	Outpatient service and emergency service before and after hospitalization	7 days before hospitalization and 30 days after hospitalization	7 days before hospitalization and 30 days after hospitalization	7 days before hospitalization and 30 days after hospitalization
Value-added services	Hospitalization advance	Hospitalization deposit advance	Yes.	Yes.
	Waiver of premium	Waiver of premium for critical illnesses	/	/
	Reimbursement of proton heavy ion	60% of the treatment fees	60% of the treatment fees	100% reimbursed
	Overseas medical treatment for malignant tumors	/	/	Additional medical treatment in Japan
	Family care after operation	/	/	Yes.
	Does it include accidental death protection	/	/	/
	Service for special medical products	/	/	Yes.
Premium calculation	Premium (with social security)	CNY 405	CNY 229	CNY 306
	30 years old			

Note: 1. Waiver of premium: it means that the insured is exempted from the remaining premium for critical illnesses under coverage in the insurance period. 2. Occupation: Basically, all life insurances will cover categories 1–4 occupations. Specifically, the categories 1–3 include most of ordinary jobs, generally for people engaged in light physical labor, with fixed workplaces and no occupational risks (e.g., teachers, sales and office staff). The category 4 is referred to occupations with certain occupational risks in workplaces or responsibility mainly in machinery manufacturing, forestry, animal husbandry, etc. 3. Guaranteed renewal period: It is guaranteed that during the period, no renewal will be refused due to the health of the insured, historical claims or product suspension.

3 High-end products: high-end medical insurance products satisfy the more demanding needs of high-net worth groups of people by going beyond the limitations offered by other kinds of insurance. These products break through the limitations posed by such things as the reimbursable drug list and restrictions on where treatment can take place. They reimburse the policy holder according to prescribed percentages and for reasonable medical costs, and such costs may now include reasonable costs of being treated overseas. The premiums for this kind of insurance range from RMB 10,000 to 20,000 per year on average, and policies are often sold on a group basis. For example, a company may purchase such insurance for its core team of employees. Since the targeted audience is fairly small, the total inventory of high-end medical policies in the market is also small. Safeguards are quite substantial, but in overall terms, this segment of the market is not representative of the total.

3.1.2 Illness insurance

Illness insurance follows a lump-sum payment model. That is, once a certain illness occurs, the policy holder is paid a certain sum of money and can then spend that as he or she wishes. The policy holder may choose the medical services he or she feels are necessary, which makes it hard to tell how much of the insurance has been spent on drugs.

Insurance for major critical illness is the fastest growing product in this category of insurance. Insurance for major critical illness is one of the types of critical illness insurance. Policies covering major illness and cancer costs are being targeted at such groups as young people, the elderly, students, males, females, and so on, and are developing fairly well.

We selected different types of critical illness insurance in the market to arrive at the following summary.

The waiting period for critical illness insurance is generally 90 days, although it can be 180 days for some products. In terms of coverage, critical illness provides coverage for both major and minor diseases and some products make the distinction of a third category of moderate diseases (Table 5.6). In terms of the effectiveness of this kind of insurance, all types of insurance include within their coverage the 25 types of major diseases that the Insurance Regulatory Commission has determined must be included. These include, for example, malignant tumors (although not some early-period malignant tumors), acute myocardial infarction, cerebral apoplexy, major organ transplants or hematopoietic stem cell transplantation, coronary artery bypass grafting, and end-stage renal disease. More than 95% of all reimbursements in fact fall within covering these 25 diseases. A product that covers 80 types of disease is therefore much the same as one that covers 100 diseases, in terms of the effectiveness of safeguards. In addition to coverage for critical diseases, this kind of insurance frequently also includes death benefits.

Apart from insuring higher amounts and providing one-time lump sum payments that are larger, critical insurance also generally provides coverage over a

Table 5.6 A Comparison of Several Critical Illness Insurance Products

Insurer		*Taiping Life*	*ICBC AXA*	*Ping An*	*China Life*
Product		*Fulukangrui*	*Yuruyi*	*Shouhufu*	*Guoshoufu*
Age of the insured		0–65 years old	0–60 years old	18–55 years old	18–60 years old
Waiting period		90 days	90 days	90 days	180 days
Time insured		Lifelong	Lifelong	Lifelong	Lifelong
Critical illness insurance	Kinds of critical illnesses	100 kinds	80 kinds, 4 categories	80 kinds	80 kinds
	Payment for critical illnesses	CNY 500,000	CNY 500,000	CNY 500,000	CNY 500,000
	Number of claims	once	three times	once	once
Light illness protection	Kinds of small illnesses	50 kinds	33 kinds, 4 categories	30 kinds	30 kinds
	Payment for small illnesses	CNY 100,000	CNY 100,000	CNY 100,000	CNY 100,000
	Number of claims	five times	three times	three times	once
Death	Death compensation	CNY 500,000	CNY 500,000	CNY 500,000	CNY 500,000
Premium		CNY 500,000	20 years of payment	Lifelong	
	0 year old, male	CNY 4,450	CNY 4,430	/	/
	30 years old, male	CNY 11,550	CNY 11,650	CNY 14,650	CNY 14,179

longer term. It might insure, for example, for 30 to 50 years, or till death. Unlike insurance that covers medical costs, when somebody dies this kind of insurance generally returns the unused portion of premiums or advance payments (to heirs). Because of this, premiums are quite high, usually in the range of RMB 1000. Premiums go up as the policy holder ages. In the case described earlier, the annual premium for a product with RMB 500,000 in total coverage can reach RMB 10,000. In recent years, given intensified competition in the insurance market, insurance companies are racing to diversify their critical illness insurance product lines. For example, a given policy can have multiple reimbursements within the term of the policy, that is, a policy holder can be reimbursed three times for critical illness. Some products are beginning to divide illnesses into sub-categories, however, so that one type of illness can only be reimbursed once during the term of the policy.

In terms of how this kind of insurance is sold, Internet sales are still quite modest and the prices of products sold via the Internet are fairly low, so the main channels for growing the business are still insurance agents. The commission income that agents receive is directly related to the premium income from policies they have sold. Since premiums are bound to be higher than those for normal medical insurance, agents focus on promoting critical illness insurance products in order to get that higher commission. People inside the company at Taikang Life have said that critical illness insurance is at the forefront of all their insurance, both in terms of the quantity of policies and the income from premiums.

3.1.3 Insurance that reimburses for the cost of drugs

As a new kind of commercial insurance product that has been put on the market in the past couple of years, insurance that covers drug costs is primarily aimed at providing safeguards to policy holders for the costs of anticancer and special drugs. These policies are sold in the traditional manner, as a supplementary form of insurance, but marketing is also based on Internet models.

3.1.3.1 THE TRADITIONAL MODEL FOR INSURANCE POLICIES

In August 2018, Taikang Life Insurance put out the first insurance policies for individuals that related to ‘special drugs’ inside China. The full name of the initiative was the ‘Taikang medical insurance for the costs of specifically designated malignant tumors,’ or the ‘Taikang special drug insurance’ for short. This covered 17 kinds of commonly used medicines for seven major kinds of commonly seen cancers. It also allowed the insurance to cover costs that were not incurred within a hospital. Insurance that covers the costs of drugs is mainly a supplementary type of insurance, and Taikang also for the first time put out a business model that it calls ‘commercial medical insurance + specialized medical services + specialized drug services.’

Insurance products of this kind are designed to cover seven types of malignant tumors: leukemia, primary hepatic malignancy, primary malignant tumors, primary gastric malignancy, primary breast malignancy, primary rectal malignancy, and primary bronchial malignancy. The scope of coverage includes drugs included on the list of reimbursable drugs: gefitinib, ectinib, erlotinib, sorafenib, imatinib, apatinib, trituzumab and its biological analogues, lapatinib; the off-catalog medical products under coverage include Navumab, Prazopani, Shunitinib, Ibutinib, cetuximab, Rigofini, Ohitigni, Avatini, and Clozotinib. During the term of the policy, drugs that are considered necessary for treatment are reimbursed according to the following percentages: 50% for drugs that are not yet reimbursed by social insurance but are on the list of reimbursable drugs (eight types), 100% for drugs not on the list (nine types). Prescriptions are not to exceed one month's worth of the drug at a time, and a total insured amount for one year cannot exceed RMB 500,000.

These products are designed only for people under the age of 60, but once a person starts the insurance, they can renew the policy until the age of 90. For people under the age of 45, the premium rate is RMB 100 (RMB 95 for the first time). As such, the premiums are in the middle of the cost range. Rates are as indicated in Table 5.7.

This initiative improves the safeguards that commercial insurance can provide to cover the cost of special drugs. It represents a major breakthrough. The hope is that it will lighten the cost burden of policy holders who are suffering from major diseases.

Table 5.7 Premium Rates of Taikang Life's Insurance for Drug Costs in Treating Malignant Cancers, Unit: RMB

Age of the Insured (One Full Year of Life)	*Renewal Rate*	*Rate When First Insured or Re-insured after Interruption*
0–4	78	74
5–9	78	74
10–14	78	74
15–19	86	82
20–24	86	82
25–29	94	90
30–34	94	90
35–39	100	95
40–44	100	95
45–49	204	195
50–54	204	195
55–59	235	225
60–64	235	225
65–69	484	
70–74	484	
75–79	890	
80–84	890	
85–89	1,471	
90–94	2,174	
95–99	3,211	

3.1.3.2 THE INTERNET-BASED MODEL FOR INSURANCE POLICIES

The prime example of Internet-based insurance at the present time, and also the most mature, is the 'Yaoshenbao' product which was launched by Taikang Online in cooperation with (the Internet company) WeSure. This type of insurance is used to supplement the lacunae of social insurance with regard to special drugs for treating cancer. Yaoshenbao policies are offered in two forms, either basic or upgraded. Once a person has been diagnosed with cancer, the individual can be reimbursed for medications for a certain period of time and at the same time can have such value-added services as home delivery. Specific product information is in Table 5.8.

In addition to simple reimbursement of costs, the model for this kind of insurance includes a supply chain that was set up in cooperation with MediTrust Health, which is described as 'policy holder + insurance + drug supplier.' Not only does this product supply safeguards (benefits) to healthy people, but in September 2019 a version was launched that is targeted at sick people. A policy holder who is a patient can pay in installments at no interest charge. If the disease progresses to the point where the person dies, then the remaining amount is repaid by the insurance company – this creates a link among a bank, an insurance company, and a pharmaceutical company. This was an innovative move that integrates healthcare insurance, the drug manufacturing chain, and banks. Meanwhile, it breaks out of the constraints that had formerly bound policy holders – using an Internet-based sales model indicates that it is oriented in the direction of widespread application, which should help resolve the problems that people have in affording drugs to treat cancer.

Table 5.8 Product Information on 'Yaoshenbao'

	Basic Version	*Updated Version*
Insurance period	one year	one year
Waiting period	30 days	30 days
Insurance amount of special cancer drugs	0–18: CNY 1.5 million 19–40: CNY 1.2 million 41–50: CNY 1 million	CNY 3 million
Reimbursement ratio	Excluded from social security: 100% Included in social security: 100%/60%	Excluded from social security: 100% Included in social security: 100%/90%
Age of the insured	30 days–50 years old	30 days–65 years old
Oldest age of renewal	85 years old	85 years old
Amount of medication benefit	CNY 1–1.5 million	3 million
Scope of medication benefit	Special cancer drugs excluded from the social security catalog (12 types)	All cancer drugs on the market
Liability renewal	Two years after diagnosis	Three years after diagnosis
Premium	CNY 1/month	CNY 6–CNY 190/month

3.2 Empirical analysis of claims settlement results in the case of commercial health insurance

3.2.1 Distribution of claims settlement for 2018

According to data on the settlement of claims as reported by all insurance companies in 2018, the overall reimbursement rate is mostly over 95%. Both the reimbursement rate and the efficiency of claims settlement are fairly high (Figure 5.10).

Commercial health insurance is characterized by high total value in claims for critical illness, and by high volume for claims for medical insurance. The annual data released by Taikang Life (Figure 5.11) can serve as an example: in terms of the number of claims, medical insurance brought in far more claims than any

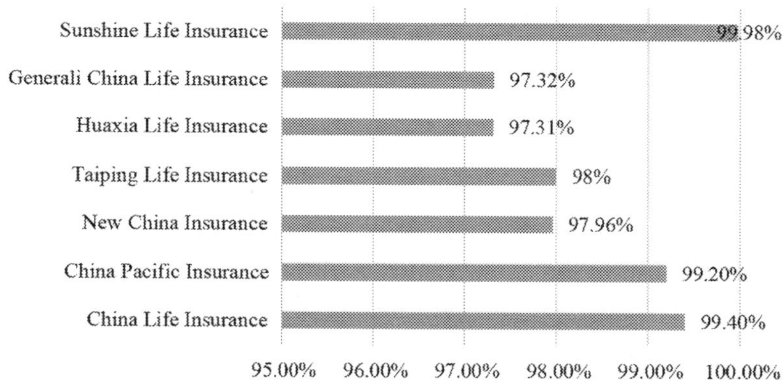

Figure 5.10 Reimbursement Rates of Some Insurance Companies in 2018

Source: 2018 annual claims reports of insurers

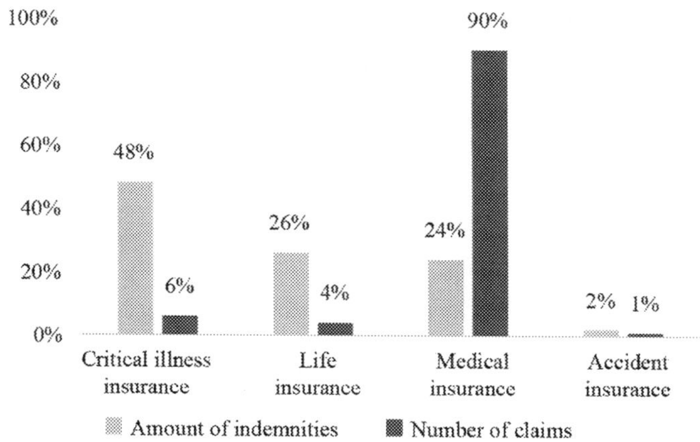

Figure 5.11 Taikang Life Insurance Indemnities and Payments

Source: 2018 Annual Claim Report of Taikang Life

other kind of insurance, constituting 90% of the number of payments in the year. In terms of RMB amounts, however, medical insurance constituted just 24% of total payments. In contrast, insurance for critical illness had just 6% of the total number of claims, but the reimbursed RMB amount was 48% of the total. It is clear that medical insurance is more related to reimbursements for daily medical costs. The per-prescription value is rather small but reimbursements are made for a large number of prescriptions.

The data on insured events shows that death from critical illness leads to higher reimbursement ratios than death from accidents. This indicates that the death rate from critical illness at the present time is higher than the rate of death from accidents. Cancer accounted for the highest proportion of claims due to critical illness, followed by cardiovascular and cerebrovascular diseases, acute myocardial infarction, cerebral apoplexy, and heart valve problems. For example, 71.6% of Taiping Life's claims for critical illnesses in 2018 were for malignant tumors, 9.8% for cardiovascular diseases, and 3.8% for sequelae of cerebral apoplexy. Malignant tumors accounted for 66% and cardiovascular diseases for 17% of the total claims for critical illnesses in Sunshine Insurance Group in 2018. For Ping An Life Insurance of China, malignant tumors accounted for 66.7%, acute myocardial infarction for 11%, and cerebral apoplexy for 5.3%.

Meanwhile, the claims settlement rate for women was slightly higher than that for men with regard to critical illness. In overall terms, the incidence of insurance claims for women was higher than that for men with respect to critical illness, which may be related to gynecological illnesses. There are also gender differences in terms of the distribution of types of illness. Women suffered mainly from breast cancer, thyroid cancer, lung cancer, cervical cancer, and ovarian cancer, while men suffered from lung cancer, thyroid cancer, liver cancer, and gastrointestinal cancer (Figure 5.12).

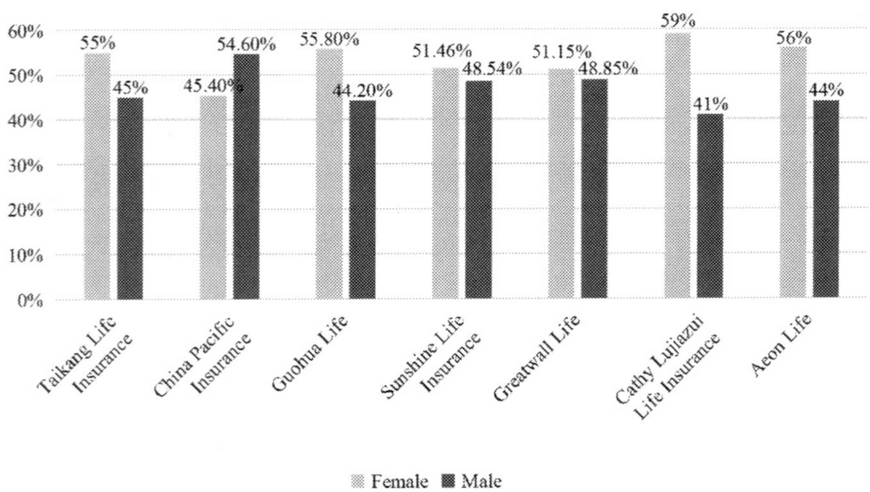

Figure 5.12 Sex Ratio in Critical Illness (or Malignant Tumors) of Some Insurers

Source: 2018 annual claim reports of insurers

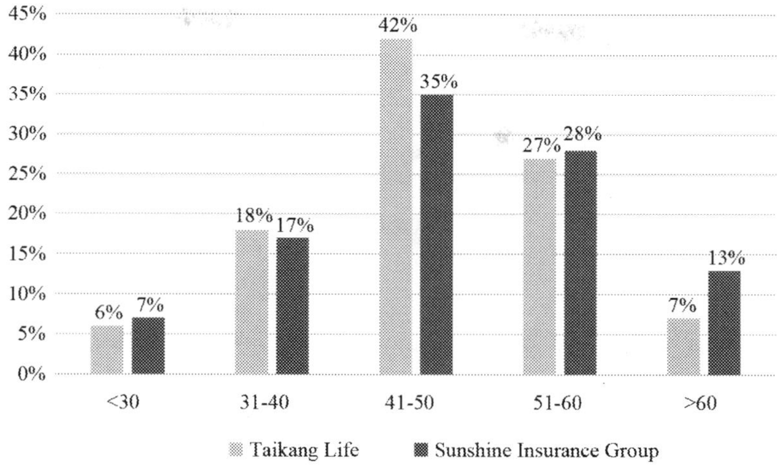

Figure 5.13 Age Distribution of People who are Insuring against Critical Illness

Source: 2018 Annual Claim Report of Taikang Life, 2018 Annual Claim Report of Sunshine Insurance Group

With regard to age distribution, all insurance companies showed that health insurance claims were mainly concentrated in the over-40 age group. After the age of 40, the incidence of critical illness increased noticeably. Sunshine Insurance Group can serve as an example: 63% of clients with claims for critical illness were between the ages of 41 and 60. Among this age group, 35% of claims were from people between the ages of 41 and 50. In Taikang Life, 42% of claims settlements for malignant tumors came from customers between the ages of 41 and 50. In addition, Taikang's statistics indicate that the percentage of claims settlements from people between the ages of 21 and 40 is rising, which means that insurable events are moving in the direction of a younger population (Figure 5.13).

3.2.2 Analysis of the results of claims that are initiated by different groups of people

This section is based on statistics from insurance companies with regard to their settlement of claims. It seeks to examine how complete the settlements are when policy holders initiate claims.

Statistics show that people who have commercial insurance coverage find that social security reimbursements cover only roughly half of their medical costs when they have an insurable event. The remaining portion needs to be covered by their commercial policy. For example, according to statistics on claims settlement from Taikang Life with regard to hospitalization, in 2018, 51.7% of its policy holders who presented claims had less than 50% of their costs covered by social security. Only 13.21% of claimants had more than 70% of their costs covered by social insurance (Figure 5.14).

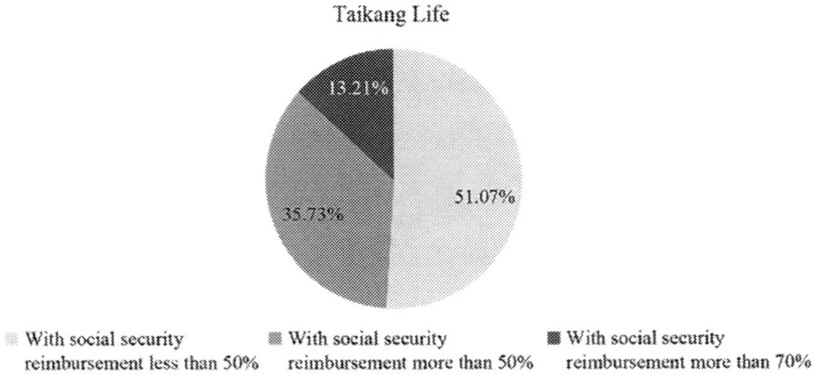

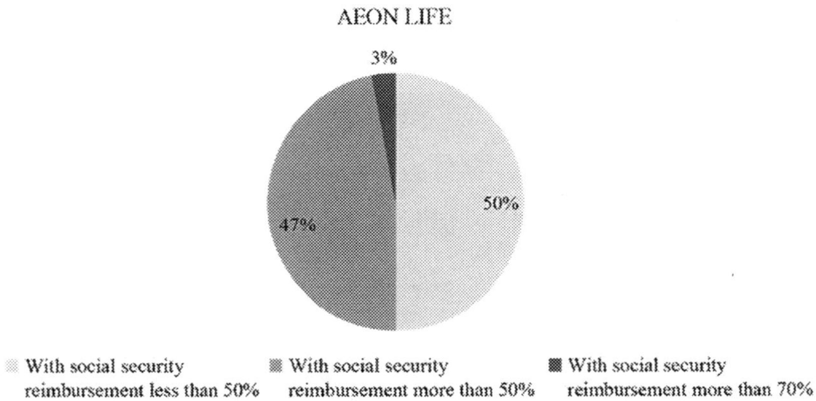

Figure 5.14 Reimbursement Rates of Social Insurance as Shown in 2018 Hospitalization Claim Statistics of Taikang Life and AEON LIFE

Source: 2018 annual claim reports of Taikang Life and AEON LIFE

According to statistics from New China Insurance, about 36% of medical costs incurred by its customers were within the scope of (social) medical insurance but were paid out of pocket, and another 13% were outside the scope of such insurance and paid out of pocket. China's basic medical insurance covers medical costs at a rate of about 50%. Clearly, social insurance is limited when it comes to covering the costs of hospital stays, and commercial health insurance can therefore play an enormous role in covering this need.

In comparing the settlement data on (social) medical insurance and (commercial) critical illness insurance, the per-incident average amount of reimbursement was substantially different. Social medical insurance areimbursed on average at a level of thousands, whereas critical illness insurance reimbursed at a level of tens of thousands (Table 5.9).

Although the overall amount of settlements paid for critical illness insurance is fairly high, the per-incident average amount is not. To take Taikang Life as an

Table 5.9 Claims for Medical Insurance and Critical Illness Insurance of Some Insurers

	Medical Insurance	*Critical Illness Insurance*
CPIC	CNY 3,810	CNY 43,900
Assicurazioni Generali (Individual insurance)	CNY 1,538.7	CNY 89,200
Aegon THTF	CNY 2,229.3	CNY 150,000
Taiping Life	CNY 3,900	CNY 100,000
AVIVA-COFCO Life Insurance Company Limited	CNY 934	/
Taikang Life	/	CNY 70,000
AEON LIFE	/	CNY 11

Source: 2018 annual claim reports of the listed insurers

Table 5.10 Percent of Coverage or Indemnities of Critical Illness Insurance by Some Insurers

	Assicurazioni Generali (Individual Insurance)	*Taiping Life*	*Aegon THTF*	*Greatwall Life*	*Taikang Life*	*Union Life*
<100,000 yuan	68.62%	60%	16%	65.75%	82%	68%
100,000–200,000 yuan	16.90%	27%	40%	26.4%	13%	23%
200,000–300,000 yuan	11.36%	8%	33%	7%		
300,000–500,000 yuan	2.96%	6%	7%	0.85%	5%	9%
>500,000 yuan	0.16%	/	4%			

Source: 2017 and 2018 annual claims reports of the listed insurers

example, in 2018, its per-incident reimbursement amount was just RMB 70,000, vastly below the RMB 100,000 to 500,000 that it costs to treat and recover from critical illness.[11] Looking at the entire market for critical illness in 2018, the amount that is covered under insurance policies is still quite a bit below what is needed to cover treatment costs. From published statistics of insurance companies, we see that the insured amount for critical illness is mainly below RMB 200,000 and average reimbursement for most companies is generally not above RMB 100,000. Table 5.10 shows that more than 60% of companies insuring critical illness were asked to insure people for less than RMB 100,000 (with the exception of Aegon THTF). Policies with an average coverage of more than RMB 300,000 accounted for less than 10% of the total. It is hard to effectively cover the actual expenses of patients with critical illness in this kind of situation.

It is difficult to figure out how much people actually spend on drugs. Insurance companies rarely keep track of an individual's spending on drugs when that

11 *2018 Annual Health Insurance Claim Report of Taikang Life, Dec. 30, 2018.* https://mp.weixin.qq.com/s/nsR7s9uWmMOoffFSMGpOgA.

individual presents claims for settlement, and detailed information on drugs is not separated out when settlement is made. The reason for this is that the quantity of data is vast, recording it is a nuisance, and people often hand over paper receipts or Xeroxed receipts when claims are being processed, which means that insurance companies have no electronic record of these costs. Looking at overall settlements and underwriting by commercial health insurance, however, the rate of reimbursement of individual claims is very high. (Commercial insurance) can therefore play a major role in covering the spending on medical costs in the future.

At the same time, it can be inferred that the degree of individual coverage of medical and drug costs for critical illness has room to grow. Going beyond social insurance, critical illness insurance provides those who need it with greater freedom to choose their medical services. With respect to medical-treatment insurance, the cost of basic drugs is mainly paid for by social insurance and the individual, as limited by the deductible. Most policies pay, on average, a few thousand RMB, which includes the cost of examinations, operations, the bed fee, and so on. We deduce the percentage that drugs occupy by using the figure of 35% that drugs constitute in total healthcare costs. Average reimbursed drug costs in (social) medical insurance therefore come to around several hundred RMB. In general, given a situation in which social insurance covers roughly one half of the costs of a hospital stay, using individual commercial health insurance can well be an effective way for people to improve their healthcare safeguards.

3.2.3 Types of group commercial health insurance

Commercial group health insurance primarily includes supplementary insurance and comprehensive medical insurance, both of which insure medical expenses, and then critical illness insurance. Generally these policies are invested in by privately operated enterprises or foreign-funded companies. As employers, the companies purchase the insurance on a group basis as a benefit for employees. By safeguarding the interests of their staff, they hope to draw in and retain personnel. Some group policies also have household policies as one component.

In designing group policies, insurance companies take into consideration such internal factors as the number of people being covered and where they live, the internal management system of the enterprise, the average age of personnel, gender percentages, history of using medical and commercial insurance, previous claims settlements, and so on. At the same time, they take into account such external factors as the pricing of competitors, the market environment of the district and municipality, support for re-insurance, and policies and regulations. Different products, scope of coverage, and rates are determined according to the actual circumstances of the policy holder. Since the policy holder is a group, it has greater negotiating ability than an individual might have in dealing with commercial insurance. Determining the rates of group health policies is more complex than it is for individuals. According to what people inside companies have indicated to us, prices may sometimes be adjusted depending on competitors' situations when bidding is underway. Group policies depend much more on negotiations than individual policies. Generally speaking, since group health insurance is voluntary and done for a purpose, a company will invest in insurance for its employees only when its business prospects look good.

The following uses a particular industry leader in providing group health insurance coverage (called Company A). The example is used to illustrate the role that group commercial health insurance plays in the payment of medical expenses and drug costs that are covered under four types of medical insurance.

3.2.3.1 SUPPLEMENTARY COMMERCIAL MEDICAL INSURANCE

In its early period, supplementary medical insurance was a product used by private enterprises and foreign-funded enterprises as a counterpoint to publicly funded medical care. It provided medical care benefits to employees of the company and at the same time was used to supplement social security. By now, the government of China is offering preferential tax treatment to companies that purchase supplementary health insurance for employees as a way to raise the overall level of their medical safeguards. More specifically, premium amounts that do not exceed 5% of an employee's salary can be deducted from taxable income when a company figures its taxes.

Commercial supplementary insurance is one type of commercial health insurance and is meant to reimburse costs. It generally does not impose a lower limit or upper limit on reimbursements, and the term of policies is generally one year (Table 5.11).

With respect to the scope of coverage, unlike individual medical insurance, supplementary medical insurance does cover the normal costs of outpatient visits. Like social health insurance, it refers to the reimbursable drug list in evaluating claims, and it pays an agreed upon supplementary amount for that portion of costs that are not yet covered by social insurance or that are covered but have not yet received payment from social insurance. Group health insurance often has supplementary provisions that will insure for unexpected medical expenses. This kind of insurance specifically supplements those drug costs that are incurred due to an unexpected medical event. Policy coverage can also include dental insurance, maternity insurance, and so on – the policy holder may choose to have this kind of coverage or not, depending on circumstances. The persons being covered under group health insurance generally include not just an employee (who must generally be under 65) but also the family of the employee (the percentage of reimbursed costs is lower for them than for the employee, and there are age limits on children, either 18 or 23). When an employee retires, he or she automatically ceases to be covered. The policy holder can opt for different items of coverage, depending on need, but in general this kind of product is used to supplement costs of medicine that are within the scope of the reimbursable list but that social security has not yet paid.

3.2.3.2 COMPREHENSIVE MEDICAL INSURANCE

Comprehensive medical insurance is mainly designed for and aimed at people who do not have social insurance. The principle behind its pricing and length of term are basically the same as those of commercial supplementary insurance. Scope of coverage uses the reimbursable drug list of social insurance as a reference. The

Table 5.11 Basic Information on Some Supplementary Group Medical Insurance

Insurer	*Assicurazioni Generali*	*PICC*	*China Life*
Product	Supplement Group medical insurance	Supplementary group medical Insurance (administrative)	Supplementary group medical Insurance (Type A)
Age of the insured	16–65 years old	18–60 years old	All employees and retirees who have participated in the medical insurance for urban employees can be insured
Associated insured	Spouses aged under 65 Children at 30 days old–18 years old		/
Term of insurance	1 year	3 years	1 year
Hospitalization	√	√	√
General outpatient (or emergency) service	Optional	√	√
Dental care	Optional		/
Fertility care	Optional		/
Public insurance benefits	Optional		Optional
Physical examination fee		√	/
Traffic accident medical insurance			√

insurance sets a deductible amount and percentages of reimbursement according to specific rules. This kind of insurance provides basic medical safeguards for those who do not have social insurance.

3.2.3.3 GROUP CRITICAL ILLNESS INSURANCE

Group critical illness insurance is a lump-sum payment-based insurance product that pays according to the occurrence of agreed-upon illnesses. The insurance company pays the policy holder an agreed-upon sum, but the premiums for this insurance are fairly high. This kind of group insurance differs from individual critical illness insurance when it comes to the terms regarding ongoing coverage. Generally, a group will be insured for one year, but the insurance company may adjust premiums in the following year depending on the extent to which the group has used insurance.

The basic situation of several kinds of group critical illness insurance in the market is as follows in Table 5.12.

Table 5.12 Basic Information on Several Forms of Critical Illness Insurance

Insurer		*Taikang Pension*	*Ping An Pension*	*Taiping Pension*	*Citic Prudential*	*Generali China*
Product		*Health Commitment 2018*	*Care for One's Whole Life (VIP Version)*	*Enjoy Health 2018*	*Xinfuwuyou (Happiness and Health Forever)*	*Happiness and Health for Life*
Age of the insured		0–70 years old	0–69 years old	0–70 years old	0–75 years old	0–60 years old
Renewal term		60 years old	65 years old	30 years	20 years	20 years
Critical illnesses	Kinds of critical illnesses	100 kinds	100 kinds	105 kinds	110 kinds	82 kinds, 12 kinds of special illnesses
	Indemnities for critical illnesses	CNY 500,000	CNY 500,000	CNY 500,000	CNY 500,000	CNY 500,000 CNY 650,000 (for special illnesses)
Small illnesses	Kinds of small illnesses	60 kinds	50 kinds	50 kinds	60 kinds	20 kinds
	Indemnities for small illnesses	CNY 100,000	CNY 100,000	CNY 100,000	CNY 100,000	CNY 150,000
	Number of claims	5 times	5 categories/5 times	6 times	5 times	once
Death	CNY 500,000	CNY 500,000	CNY 500,000	CNY 500,000	CNY 500,000	CNY 500,000
Premium	20 years of payment, coverage of CNY 500,000, lifelong					
	30 years old, male	CNY 10,800	CNY 10,700	CNY 10,700	CNY 10,770	CNY 11,000

In terms of the items covered, group and individual critical illness insurance are not that different from one another, but group insurance generally pays out just once. Persons inside the industry indicate that insurance companies may well formulate their customers' policies depending on the budget of the entity insured, the strength of demand, and so on. By adjusting the scope of provisions, the company will attempt to meet the different demands of different employers. The per person cost of premiums for this kind of group insurance are generally lower than the premiums for individual critical illness insurance, by between 100 to 1000 RMB.

3.2.3.4 EMPIRICAL ANALYSIS OF THE RESULTS OF CLAIMS SETTLEMENT IN GROUP COMMERCIAL HEALTH INSURANCE

The following uses the in-house data of the joint venture insurance company, Company A, as an example. It analyzes the role that payments from group health insurance policies can play in covering the costs of drugs.

3.2.3.4.1 Insurance to cover medical costs Company A primarily engages in the business of supplemental medical insurance. Enterprises are the primary holders of its policies. They cover a range of industries, so they are insuring employees in the fields of insurance, electronic equipment, textiles and garments, air transport, and the chemical industry, among others.

The financial amount of claims that supplemental insurance pays out annually is roughly two times that of comprehensive medical insurance, and its annual income from premiums is roughly 1.5 times that of comprehensive medical insurance. Clearly, the utilization rate of supplementary insurance is higher than that of comprehensive medical insurance.

Within total reimbursed amounts for medical costs that were made among all cases in the group insurance program of Company A, reimbursements made by the company represented 45%. This percentage is higher than the percentage of reimbursements made by (social) basic medical insurance, as shown in Figure 5.15. (A small portion of costs are not represented in the figure.) It is obvious therefore that, in the bigger picture, the percentage of reimbursements contributed by social insurance is limited. The great majority of medical costs are being borne by commercial health insurance.

Since the industries that take out group health insurance policies are quite different from one another, the payment percentages going to each are also bound to be different. A selection of industries illustrates this, as in Table 5.13.

Table 5.13 shows that commercial health insurance maintains roughly 40% to 50% of the share of total health insurance reimbursements made to different industries, while social health insurance stays between 20% and 30%. The type of industry is not a significant factor in terms of the percentage of medical costs that each of these covers. Commercial supplementary insurance and comprehensive medical insurance play a greater role in paying for medical and drug costs than China's basic medical insurance. However, in looking at premiums as a percentage of total compensation and reimbursements, service industries show a lower

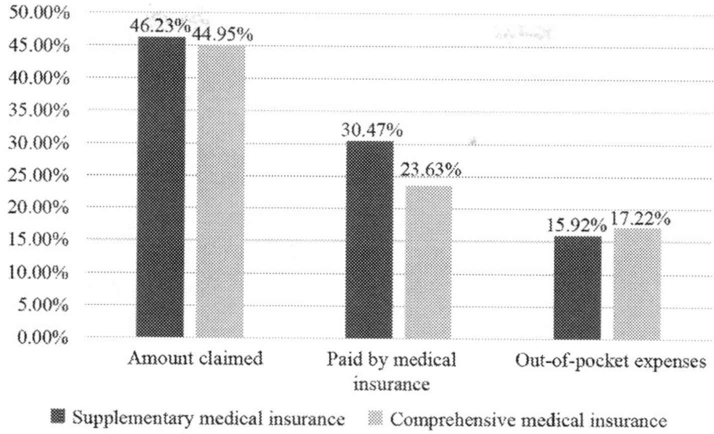

Figure 5.15 Comparison of Payment in Cases of Group Health Insurance

Table 5.13 Percent of Reimbursement of Medical Expenses in Different Industries

Industry	*Amount Claimed*	*Paid by Medical Insurance*	*Out-of-Pocket Expenses*	*Partial Self-Payment*	*Premiums/ Amount Claimed*
Social security industry	14.69%	60.09%	12.50%	5.61%	21.13%
Business services	33.51%	34.90%	24.02%	0.31%	31.25%
Retailing	39.06%	32.92%	16.86%	1.32%	41.36%
Computer service industry	43.83%	30.11%	18.37%	2.84%	54.06%
Insurance industry	48.75%	30.10%	14.15%	1.07%	63.02%
Banking industry	52.77%	24.17%	18.97%	0.37%	56.68%
Securities industry	36.26%	44.32%	12.07%	2.31%	67.52%
Real estate industry	49.89%	25.01%	18.16%	1.55%	75.94%
Chemical raw materials and chemical products manufacturing industry	48.77%	27.53%	16.83%	0.25%	88.57%
Oil and gas exploration industry	53.81%	24.40%	15.11%	0.10%	88.11%
Petroleum processing, coking, and nuclear fuel processing industry	49.93%	33.53%	10.23%	0.46%	84.90%

percentage than the financial industry. The percentage for the chemicals industry is higher than for either of these two. This may be because the occupational nature of the chemicals industry and also manufacturing industries leads to higher risk than service industries, and therefore premiums are higher. The degree to which safeguards are different among different industries is not substantial, even though

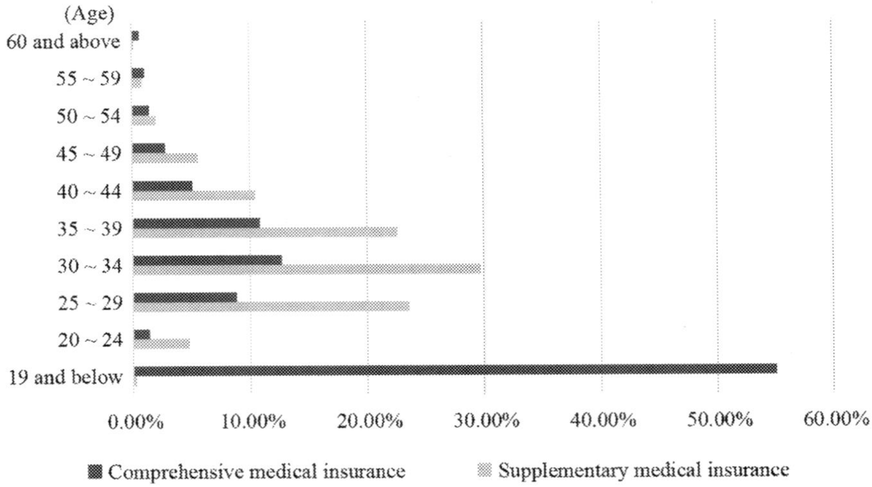

Figure 5.16 Comparison of Indemnity Payment Percentages by Age

the premiums taken in by group health insurance policies among different industries are different.

In terms of the age distribution of claims settlements, more than half of settlements of comprehensive medical insurance are concentrated in the age group below 19, which presumably relates to the medical costs of children of policy holders (Figure 5.16). In contrast, roughly 75% of claims for group health insurance were for the age group between 25 and 44. Since group health policies are taken out by employers, this figure is influenced by the age of their work force, which tends to be able-bodied adults.

3.2.3.4.2 Critical illness insurance Within group health insurance for critical illness, nearly 90% of claims related to malignant tumors. The most common cancers were thyroid cancer, breast cancer, lung cancer, cervical cancer, and stomach cancer. Other frequent critical illnesses included acute myocardial infarction, benign tumors, and cerebral apoplexy (stroke). The probability of occurrences of critical illness among group policies was similar to that of individual insurance policies. According to the statistics of Company A, companies and employers preferred to purchase medical policies rather than critical illness policies, so the number of critical illness policies was fairly low. Other statistics indicate that the petroleum and natural gas mining industries purchase more policies for critical illness, and reimbursements per incident average around RMB 102,000. Given inadequate statistics, analysis of other industries cannot be seen as sufficiently representative so is not discussed here.

Company A's statistics on claims reimbursement show that the overall payment ratio of commercial insurance is higher than it is for social insurance. Commercial insurance is able to compensate for expenses not paid by social insurance reimbursement to a greater extent. Moreover, since the holders of commercial insurance policies are mainly companies or employers, they can provide effective medical security to those who are insured. Reports are now indicating that at this point in time small and medium-sized enterprises are facing a shortage of qualified labor and it is hard for them to retain good people. The package of benefits that a company offers, therefore, has become a major consideration in holding onto people at a time of labor mobility.[12] It is second only to that of salary. Meanwhile, government policies are supportive of micro enterprises and health insurance is expanding – the market for group health insurance is expected to become a 'blue-sky' market in the future, which means that the role of group health insurance in covering medical and drug costs is going to be ever more important.

4 The international experience

4.1 United States

The medical insurance system in the United States is dominated by commercial health insurance, while social health insurance plays a supplementary role. Social health insurance (social security) is a mandatory program aimed mainly at older people and low-income groups and includes Medicare and Medicaid. Certain plans are targeted specifically at children and retired members of the military. At the end of 2017, 67.6% of the population in the United States was covered by some form of commercial health insurance,[13] and the great majority of the policies were employer-subsidized. That is, an employer took out policies on behalf of employees and also paid the greater part of the cost. This kind of policy covered more than half of the population. In order to motivate employers to purchase commercial health insurance for employees, the U.S. government has determined that pension expenses can be deducted from income as a tax-deductible expense. In terms of the types of safeguards, commercial health insurance in the United States is similar to that in China. It includes insurance for medical costs, loss of income due to disability, and long-term care insurance. In terms of the payment of claims, before medical costs occur, the insurance company pays an advance payment to the medical institution and this pre-payment covers roughly 35% of total medical costs (2016; see Figure 5.17).[14]

With specific regard to drug costs, in 2017, the total value of drug prescriptions in the United States was around USD 333 billion. The percentage of this that commercial health insurance covered, namely 42%, was higher than any other source of payment (Figure 5.18). Prescription drug costs accounted for 13% of all medical costs covered by commercial health insurance. This could not be considered very

12 *2018 Insight Report on China Enterprise Flexible Benefits Industry*, published by CBN date, https://max.book118.com/html/2018/1125/8057073100001134.shtm.

13 Iyiou.com, *Development of U.S. Health Insurance*, www.iyiou.com/pA13869.html.

14 As previous.

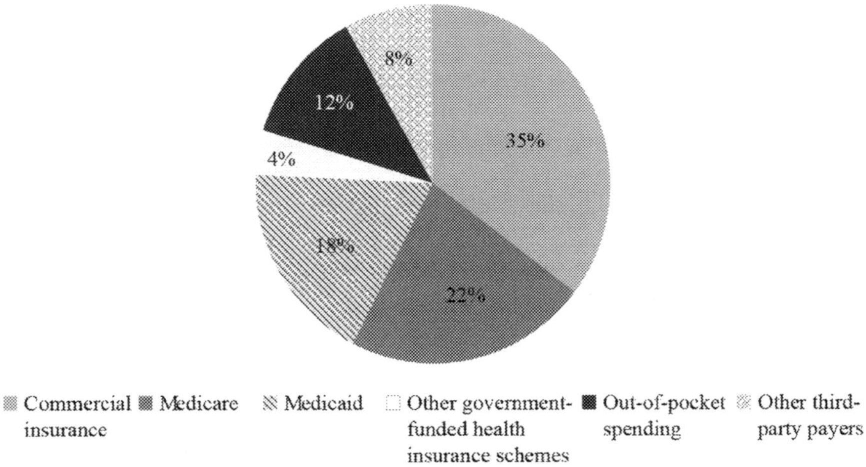

Figure 5.17 Composition of Medical Expenses in the U.S. in 2016

Source: Industrial Securities, collated by Sinohealth Industry Capital Research Center

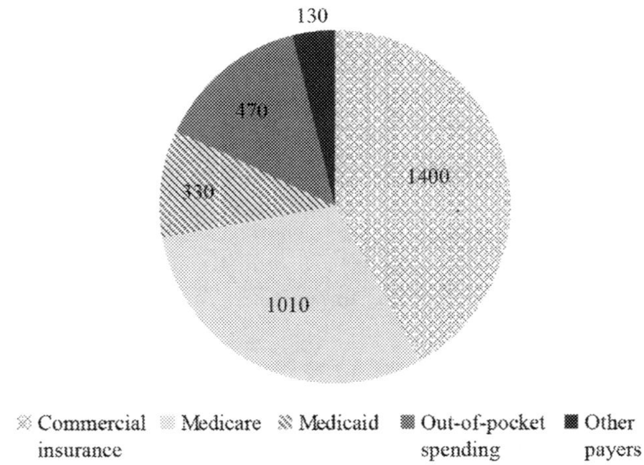

Figure 5.18 Composition of Prescription Drug Expenditures in the U.S. in 2017 (in USD 100 Million)

Source: KFF analysis of 2017 data from National Health Expenditures Accounts Get the data PNG

high, in relation to the various other medical costs such as diagnosis, examination, rehabilitation, and so on. Meanwhile, Medicare spending on drugs was 15% of total spending on drugs, and Medicaid spending was 6% of total spending (Table 5.14).[15]

15 Juliette Cubanski, Matthew Rae et al. *How does prescription drug spending and use compare across large employer plans, Medicare Part D, and Medicaid?*, published on May 20, 2019, www.healthsystemtracker.org/chart-collection.

Table 5.14 Composition of Medical Expenditures for Three U.S. Insurance Plans in 2017

	Prescription Drug Expenditures	*Other Medical Expenditures*
Commercial health insurance	13%	87%
Medicare	15%	85%
Medicaid	6%	94%

Source: KFF analysis of CMS National Health Expenditure data, 2017

The United States implements a system whereby drugs and 'medicine' are operated as separate businesses. Pharmacy Benefit Management companies play a pivotal role in helping control costs during the drug fulfillment process. They connect insurance companies, medical services providers, pharmaceutical suppliers, distributors, and, ultimately, patients. Pharmacy Benefit Managers designate specific pharmacies for policy holders, and these pharmacies thereby become the sales channel for drugs and at the same time pay the Pharmacy Benefit Managers a commission. Holders of insurance policies pay a specified amount of 'self-pay' and can then get their prescriptions fulfilled at pharmacies. In terms of controlling the costs of prescription drugs, once a doctor has made a diagnosis and written out a prescription, the pharmacy enters this information into an online system. The Pharmacy Benefit Manager reviews the prescription and the insurance policy of the patient, and provides feedback on both the drugs and their price while not compromising the aim to provide effective treatment. This helps control drug costs and furthers the goal of prescribing drugs in a rational manner.

There have been some problems along the way in how Pharmacy Benefit Managers operate in the United States, and the system has had to be improved over time, but it must be confirmed that these companies do in fact save on drug costs. Over 70% of the drug expenses in the administrative districts of the U.S. are paid for through Pharmacy Benefit Managers, and 45% of the entire U.S. population is covered in this way. Between 2001 and 2010, spending on prescription drugs went down by a total of RMB 1.39 trillion.[16] The American Nutrition and Health Association predicts that between 2012 and 2021, Pharmacy Benefit Managers will have saved patients and insurance companies some USD 2 trillion in drug costs.[17] By controlling claims and the cost of drugs, these companies are therefore of vital importance to American insurance companies.

In the United States, the system of Pharmacy Benefit Managers primarily uses market measures to manage drug costs, whereas in China, drug distribution and selling is mainly handled through medical institutions (Figure 5.19). In 2015, 68% of drug sales that went through insurance in China were sold out of hospitals as

16 Zhao W. Application of Pharmacy Benefit Management (PBM) in China's Medical Insurance and Commercial Health Insurance. Southwestern University of Finance and Economics, 2014.

17 Official WeChat Account "Investment Brainstorming", *"Feature Report on Medical Payment": PBM*, https://mp.weixin.qq.com/s/AHxhSX64U-vTOx8pikxJsA.

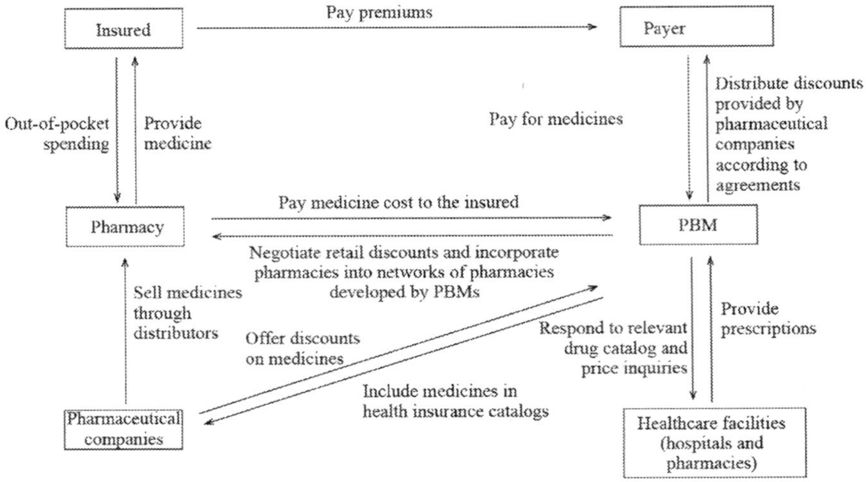

Figure 5.19 How Pharmacy Benefit Managers in the U.S. Serve the Function of Connecting with Various Parties

the end-point of sales. This is partly due to the long-standing habits of where people seek medical care, and partly due to the difference in types of drug available in hospitals as opposed to pharmacies. Drugs and hospitals cannot be completely separated in China; meanwhile, public hospitals dominate China's entire medical system. The 'basic medical insurance' system is China's main system of medical safeguards, but this system is limited by the level of IT in the country's medical system. This is very substantially different from the United States. Judged purely from market share, commercial health insurance in China currently has little ability to control medical costs or control health risks. One breakthrough that could change the situation, which is worth evaluating, is either reconfiguring and integrating the drug distribution system with commercial insurance, or setting up Pharmacy Benefit Managers departments within commercial insurance.

4.2 The U.K.

The U.K.'s system is a typical example of a national healthcare system in which publicly funded medical services serve the entire population, while commercial health insurance is supplementary and can satisfy the different levels of medical needs that people might have. The U.K.'s National Health Service (NHS) model is one that basically provides universal coverage. The NHS system is highly inefficient however, which has given privately operated medical services room to grow. In order to improve efficiency, the British government has begun to encourage this growth of private medicine and is even attempting to incorporate competition into the public model. Private medical services are highly efficient and provide a better environment for patients. Such patients tend to be high-income people who want individualized services and high-end treatment, so the costs of this treatment are correspondingly high. This provides commercial health insurance with a role to play – it can insure the private medical costs of policy holders. Meanwhile, the insurance companies in the U.K. and the country's privately operated medical facilities are not at all cut off from one another. Instead, insurance companies go through privately held medical facilities to provide their services to customers. This improves the efficiency of medical services as well as the efficiency of payments (reimbursements) and it allows insurance companies access to customer's health records which can be used as the basis for adjusting insurance plans.

In terms of positioning in the market, commercial health insurance in the U.K. is mainly targeted at high-income groups of people. Roughly 11% of the population has commercial health insurance policies. Among this segment of the population, more than 80% are enrolled in group policies; individual policies account for less than 20%.[18] The group policies are mainly set up by companies to provide benefits for their employees. Insurance companies sign policy contracts depending on the group's rate, policies are flexible, and safeguards can include items that basic medical insurance does not cover. Individual policies are fewer in number but the rates are higher, so this segment of the market makes a contribution to the premium income of commercial health insurance companies that is not insignificant.

In terms of paying for medical costs: in 2017, government spending on social insurance accounted for 79% of all medical insurance costs in the U.K. (Figure 5.20).[19] Non-government spending accounted for 21% (Table 5.15). This latter

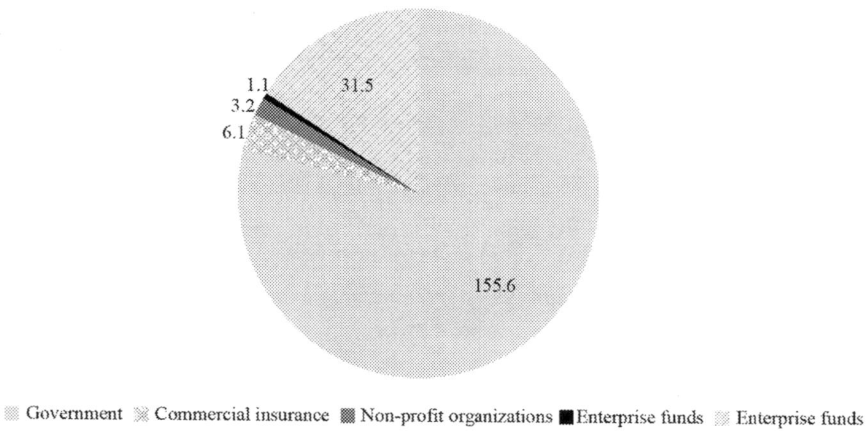

Figure 5.20 Medical Spending in the U.K. by Financing Method in 2017 (in GBP 1 Billion)

18 Iyiou.com, *Challenges of Developing Commercial Medical Insurance in Single-Payer Countries – A Case Study of the U.K.*, www.iyiou.com/p/61987.html.

19 Healthcare expenditure, UK Health Accounts: 2017 www.ons.gov.uk/peoplepopulationandcommunity/healthandsocialcare/healthcaresystem/bulletins/ukhealthaccounts/2017.

Table 5.15 Percent of Non-governmental Spending on Medical Costs in the U.K. (%)

	Non-profit Organizations	*Corporate Funds*	*Out-of-Pocket Expenditures*	*Commercial Insurance*
Treatment and rehabilitation	42	0	22	66
Long-term care	41	0	36	0
Medical materials	8	0	38	1
Preventive care	4	85	4	4
Supporting services	3	0	0	0
Financing and health management		0	0	26
Miscellaneous	0	15	0	3

Source: Office for National Statistics, LaingBuisson, Association of British Insurers

figure included commercial insurance, non-profit institutions serving households, corporate funding, and individuals paying for themselves. Within spending by non-government entities, commercial insurance mainly focused on covering medical costs and rehabilitation costs (66%) as well as health management and funding costs (26%). Non-profit organizations mainly focused on long-term care – 41% of non-profit spending went to this category. Corporate funds were predominantly used for preventive care, such as on providing occupational health services for employees.

With respect to spending for drugs: the National Health Service separates 'drugs' from 'medicine' (hospitals), so patients must go to a pharmacy that is independent from a hospital to purchase drugs. Those who are covered by an insurance plan pay extremely little out of their own pockets. Commercial insurance is mainly used for spending on diagnosis of the patient, procedures (operations), hospitalization, and nursing costs. If a person is diagnosed with a critical illness, a lump sum is paid after the diagnosis. With respect to drug coverage, commercial insurance will cover some drugs that are not included under basic medical insurance. Since commercial health insurance is not dominant in the country's medical security systems, however, the role that such insurance plays in paying for drugs is fairly limited.

4.3 Germany

Germany was the first country in the world to establish a mandatory social insurance system. Commercial health insurance plays a supplementary role to this system. In 2012, the premium income of commercial health insurance companies came to 19.2% of total premium income in the country,[20] and roughly 11% of the population chose to purchase separate commercial health insurance policies.[21]

20 Jiangsu Insurance Institute. Feng P.C., Liu Q. On German Commercial Health Insurance (Part I), published on Jun. 10, 2015.

21 *Just Landed Health insurance – How to cover your medical expenses in Germany*, www.justlanded.com/english/Germany/Germany-Guide/Health/Health-insurance.

In terms of how commercial health insurance operates, the risk that it covers is basically the possibility of critical illness – this is therefore quite different in nature from the risks that life insurance and property insurance cover. By law, commercial health insurance in Germany must be operated separately from other forms of insurance, that is, any company in the business of health insurance cannot also operate life insurance or property insurance businesses. This is to prevent the profits from different kinds of insurance from being commingled. With respect to underwriting, commercial health insurance companies must guarantee ongoing coverage according to German regulations. Once a company elects to underwrite someone, withdrawing from the policy can only be done by the person being insured.

With respect to product types and scope of coverage, Germany's commercial health insurance mainly can be divided into three categories. The first is commercial medical insurance, which represents more than 70% of all health insurance in Germany. Three types of people can take out this insurance. The first is high-income groups of people. According to statutory standards in Germany in 2019 (such standards are adjusted every year), if a person earns more than 59,400 euros in a year, or more than 4,950 euros in a month, then he or she must purchase commercial health insurance. The premiums are shared by the employer and the employee. The second type is government employees (civil servants). In this case, the government bears between 50% and 70% of the cost of premiums and the rest is paid by the individual. The third type is 'freelancers' or people who work for themselves. Since their income is generally fairly high, they too are required to purchase commercial medical insurance. This first category of commercial medical insurance covers such things as hospital stays, examination fees at clinics, treatment costs, the costs of procedures or operations, costs of diagnosis, and so on. Levels of coverage are not allowed to be lower than those of social medical insurance, and the patient may choose where to receive treatment. The second category of commercial health insurance is supplementary insurance. This mainly covers high-value medical services, such as single-room stays in hospitals, high-end dental costs (such as dental implants), the treatment of psychological problems, and so on. The third category is commercial nursing insurance. German regulations stipulate that anyone who purchases commercial health insurance must at the same time purchase commercial nursing insurance, to pay for long-term care costs.

In terms of the components of spending, in 2017, German spending on medical costs came to a total of EUR 374 billion (Figure 5.21). Of this, drugs accounted for 17%, including 10% from non-patented drugs and 7% from patented drugs.[22]

With respect to payments made by insurance, in 2016, total spending on medical costs in Germany came to EUR 357 billion. Spending by social insurance came to EUR 207 billion, while spending by private health insurance policies (commercial health insurance) came to EUR 31 billion, or 8.7%.[23] With respect to reimbursements for drug costs, a policy holder may submit bills

22 *Global Legal Insights Pricing & Reimbursement 2019 I Germany*.

23 *Assessment in Medicine Reimbursement of Medical Devices in Germany 2019*, www.aim-germany.com.

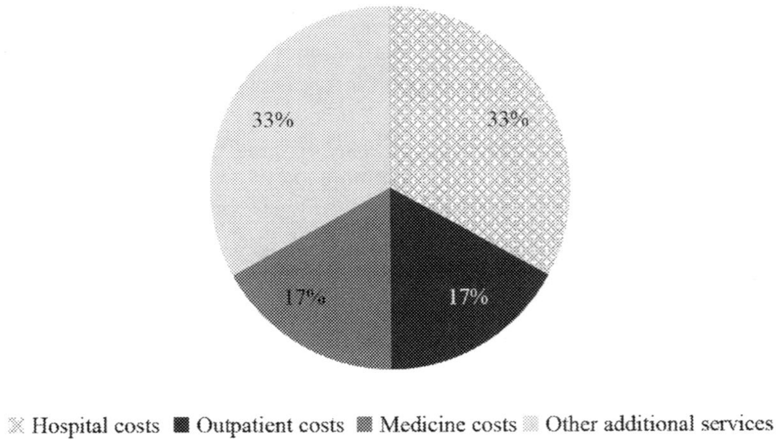

Figure 5.21 Composition of Medical Expenses in Germany in 2017

Source: Global Legal Insights

for prescription drugs directly to the insurance company for reimbursement. Non-prescription drugs (over-the-counter drugs) are generally not covered by commercial policies.

With respect to controlling spending on drugs and thereby controlling costs of drugs, Germany's health insurance industry has a high degree of autonomy. Commercial health insurance companies are all members of the health insurance association. Representatives of this industry association represent members in their price negotiations with medical facilities, pharmaceutical manufacturers, and other stakeholders. They help adjust prices and pricing standards for medical services, as well as discounts for drugs. This mechanism plays a crucial role in controlling drug costs that are paid for by commercial health insurance.

5 Discussion

5.1 The role that commercial health insurance plays in China's medical safeguards system

The role that commercial health insurance can play in a medical safeguards system, and how it plays that role, is intimately related to the social security system. The reason is that, theoretically at least, commercial insurance covers things that social security is not able to cover.

China's medical safeguards system is targeted at two groups of people and is composed of three different 'dimensions' of coverage. The two groups are 'urban and rural employees' and 'urban and rural residents.' The three dimensions are the social medical insurance system, which is the most basic, insurance for major illness, and finally commercial insurance as a supplement to social medical insurance.

Reimbursement of costs in China's basic medical insurance program has both a ceiling and a floor. Any costs under the threshold are borne by the person. Anything over the ceiling is either covered by major illness insurance or paid for by the person. In other countries, the situation is quite different. To take Germany as an example – in Germany, there is a ceiling on medical costs for which the person pays. That is, if medical costs go beyond a certain self-pay limit, they are paid for by medical insurance. Meanwhile, in China, percentages of reimbursement for those costs of social insurance that are indeed reimbursable can vary substantially, depending on the ranking of the hospital, the geographic location, and the social insurance plans of that location. Different parts of China have differing abilities to pool funding for social security. Not only is this due to different levels of economic development, but it also is due to different levels of government subsidies. Ultimately, the levels of security are different.

For example, in 2019, the pooled funding for social security in a certain part of Shandong Province came to RMB 910 per person. Of this amount, government subsidies came to RMB 520. In Beijing, pooled funding for social security came to RMB 1,610 per person, of which RMB 1,430 came from government subsidies. Meanwhile, reimbursement percentages also depend on the level of hospital – the higher the rank of the hospital, the lower the percentage of reimbursement. Statistics from 2018 show that, in addition, levels of funding and levels of treatment are vastly higher for the 'basic medical insurance program for urban employees' than they are for the same program for 'urban and rural residents' (Table 5.16). At the same time, with respect to payment of costs, costs incurred in one part of China will not be reimbursed in another part. As yet, there are either inadequate channels for reimbursement of out-of-region costs, or reimbursement rates are lower. In Japan, the situation is quite different – even out-of-country costs can be reimbursed at a rate of as high as 70%.

Meanwhile, less than 50% of the claims that are made by people who are insured under social insurance are actually reimbursed. This is according to claims settlement data of insurance companies. In contrast, commercial insurance can break through the restrictions that social insurance places on rank of hospital, out-of-region coverage, and so on. From this, we can realize that there should be enormous room for growth for commercial insurance, just by being able to reimburse actual costs.

The experience of countries like Germany indicates that commercial health insurance is targeted at high-income groups. Moreover, the cost of premiums is shared between employer and employee. In China, those who hold commercial insurance policies tend to be urban employees, but their basic medical insurance also gives them higher levels of protection. However, commercial insurance is for-profit by nature, and people's incomes are still low, which means that a large portion of urban residents cannot afford to purchase commercial health insurance or adequate protections under such insurance. Moreover, these people also have low levels of social security, making them even less able to withstand the risk of disease.

In other words, those who are greatest in need of a third-party entity to cover their risk of disease, especially major disease, are precisely those who can't afford

Table 5.16 Data on Per Capita Pooling of Basic Medical Insurance Funds in China, and Per Capita Spending out of those Funds in 2018

	Number of Participants (100 Million)	*Medical Insurance Income (CNY 100 Million)*	*Medical Insurance Expenditure (CNY 100 Million)*	*Current Fund Balance (CNY 100 Million)*	*Pooling Funds (CNY 100 Million)*	*Cumulative Fund Balance (CNY 100 Million)*	*Pooling Funds (CNY 100 Million)*
Basic medical insurance for urban employees	3.17	13,259.28	10,504.92	2,754.36	1,746.43	18,605.38	11,460.96
– Year-on-year growth	4.50%	8.70%	11.50%				
– Per capita premium (CNY)		4,182.74	3,313.86				
Basic medical insurance for urban residents	8.97	6,973.94	6,284.51	689.43	–	4,332.94	–
– Year-on-year growth	2.70%	27.10%	28.90%				
– Per capita premium (CNY)		777.47	700.61				
Basic medical insurance for rural residents	1.3	856.89	818.22	38.67	–	295.42	–
– Per capita premium (CNY)		659.15	629.4				

Source: National Healthcare Security Administration

sufficient safeguards. This intensifies the inequality in health safeguards due to differences in income. What these people need is a more universal-type health insurance plan that has real safeguards. With respect to reimbursement for drugs, a new drug-costs insurance has been under development in the past two years and is aimed at special anticancer drugs. The premiums are not expensive, a few RMB or ten or so RMB a month. This is a level that most households can afford, but in addition the insurance provides very strong benefits. This kind of product may well be a breakthrough point for commercial health insurance in the future.

5.2 The connection between commercial health insurance and the pharmaceuticals system

The experience of the United States, the U.K., and Germany indicates that each country's commercial health insurance has mechanisms by which to keep costs of drugs down and reimbursements for drugs under control. Commercial health insurance companies or related third parties participate in the various stages of the drug distribution system. Not only can they control spending on drugs through negotiated prices, but they also can benefit by the information channels that result.

In contrast, China's insurance companies are independent of both medical institutions and drug distribution entities. On the one hand, this pattern makes it hard for them to take the initiative in controlling reimbursement of claims. Other than carrying out health management during the underwriting process, all companies can do is passively wait for the bills once an insurable event occurs. On the other hand, it is hard for insurance companies in China to get hold of health information on policy holders. For all these reasons, it is extremely important that we upgrade the role that commercial health insurance can play in drug payment mechanisms. In this regard, we might consider making a start in the following two ways.

First, learn from the experience of the United States with respect to co-payments. Commercial health insurance participates in the payment of medical costs together with Medicare and Medicaid. Costs incurred from drugs that are included in the mandatory insurance plan list of drugs are shared by the commercial insurance company, the federal government, and the individual. To take Medicare as an example, the threshold for receiving any reimbursement is USD 360, so anything below that amount must be paid for by the individual. Over that amount, but within a ceiling, the individual co-pays 20% to 40%. For drug costs above the ceiling, the individual pays between 45% and 50%. The individual co-pays, but the insurance company bears a portion of the cost and the government provides subsidies. Although the standing of insurance companies in the medical systems of the U.S. and China is quite different, it would be very worth our while to look at connecting commercial insurance companies with the basic medical insurance system. Only when commercial health insurance systems, social security systems, and medical systems are on the same track will we truly be able to use the ability of commercial health insurance to underwrite and manage risk.

Second, integrate the industrial chain of drugs with the commercial health insurance industry. Commercial health insurance companies are the payer of drug costs;

they are essentially the buyer. They have the ability to use their advantage of scale to negotiate lower prices with pharmaceutical companies. This is especially true with regard to new drugs and special drugs whose extremely high prices place a particularly large economic burden on patients. Borrowing a lesson from Pharmacy Benefit Managers in the United States, commercial health insurance can connect pharmaceutical companies with the channels to reach larger sales targets in exchange for discounts on drug prices. Not only does this lighten the burden on patients, but it allows insurance companies to be proactive in controlling spending costs.

As the payer of medical costs, commercial health insurance companies should not be kept at a remove from the pharmaceutical and medical systems, and treated as just a teller who dispenses the money. Insurance companies have a technological advantage in terms of managing risk and can be more flexible in how they utilize funds. This advantage can only be fully realized when insurance is connected appropriately to China's basic medical insurance, its medical facilities, and its drug distribution companies.

5.3 A comprehensive development model: 'insurance + health'

All of the insurance companies we interviewed in the course of surveys for this study were keenly interested in the market for commercial health insurance. Under the encouragement of policies in recent years, they have begun to deploy resources in this segment of the industry. They are combining such things as their traditional commercial health insurance with health management, medical treatment, pensions, and so on to form a greater health industry chain.

Ping An of China has been taking full advantage of the Internet to build an online and offline comprehensive services system that can help build up its 'Greater Health' medical and healthcare lines. Taikang has set up a health management company and hopes to lower its probability of insurable events through the use of customer services. At the same time, this makes it easier for the company to draw in customers. From feedback within the company, setting up this health management business has indeed lowered the probably of insurable events, giving it two birds with one stone. On the 'care of the elderly' side of things, all of the companies are actively exploring what to do. Taikang is using a 'heavy-investment' method to invest in the actual building of nursing homes associated with hospitals, and has set up communities for the elderly that combine medicine with nursing care. It has already deployed this model in eight cities, including Beijing and Shanghai.[24] This has stimulated the sale of its long-term care insurance. At the same time, by holding the controlling percentage of shares in (private) hospitals, Taikang is directly investing in a hospital network. This then combines the claims settlement of insurance with the various links in hospital services. China Life has set up a

24 ChinaPension.com, *"Insurance + Health Management" Becomes an Important Field of Commercial Health Insurance*, http://invest.10jqka.com.cn/20171127/c601785377.shtml.

business that insures for unexpected injuries among older people. Ping An has used a 'light-investment' method to construct a health management platform and a medical services network. It is developing the 'Ping An Good Doctor' application to provide customers with real-time management and services. At the same time, it is connecting networks of offline physical checkup centers, hospitals, and pharmacies services in what it calls 'insurance + health.'

In the big picture, the way of the future appears to be that commercial health insurance companies will gradually take on the responsibility for national health management. At the current time, however, the space into which they might grow and be innovative is limited by such things as the unique nature of the institutional structures of China's medicine. This leads to only loose connections among commercial insurance and the services of hospitals and doctors, and makes it hard for commercial insurance to control risks as well as costs. Meanwhile, channels for sharing data among insurance companies and medical institutions are inadequate. For example, companies cannot receive claims settlements in electronic form, which makes it impossible for them to record and analyze claims in any detailed way. In the future, having information on the treatment procedures and drug costs of patients, in systematic form, will enable the insurance industry to use its own professional advantages to carry out more accurate risk evaluation, cost control, and management of health risks. We therefore recommend that the insurance, medical, and health security systems jointly set up a data platform in order to improve operational efficiency in the medical safeguards systems of the country.

5.4 *The impact of changes in the spectrum of diseases in China*

Chronic diseases have gradually become the most important cause of death in China, given economic development, improvement in medical technologies, and greater access to healthcare services (that deal with other causes of death). The incidence of chronic diseases has been going up rapidly in recent years due to industrialization, urbanization, and the aging of the population. In 2013, the prevalence of chronic disease among people over the age of 15 in China had already reached 33.1%. In 2012, the mortality rate from chronic disease was 86.6% of death from all diseases.[25] The incidence of malignant cancers, diabetes, psychoses, heart disease, and high blood pressure are rising at a particularly fast pace.[26] Such high incidences of these diseases signifies a very high cost burden of disease – indeed, these are already the primary cause of impoverishment or a return to poverty among the Chinese people. Statistics indicate that in 2010 the total sum of pooled funding that went into chronic disease prevention was already 3.2% of

25 National Health and Family Planning Commission of the PRC, *Report on Nutrition and Chronic Diseases of Chinese Residents (2015)*, June 2015.

26 Shen C.G. *The World's New Family Doctor Service System and the Development of a National Joint Health Security System*. China Book Publishing House, 2018.

GDP,[27] and 70% of the total cost burden of disease is related to chronic disease.[28] In 2015, the economic burden of just three chronic diseases came to RMB 3.8 trillion,[29] namely diabetes, stroke, and heart disease.

(Despite the need for it), China's basic medical insurance still provides inadequate compensation for the medical costs associated with the treatment of chronic diseases. On the one hand, this is due to the fact that chronic diseases require long-term treatment and repeated visits to outpatient clinics for checkups and medication. This puts a substantial cost burden on patients. In addition, as medical services change in China, some patients who would formerly have stayed in hospitals for treatment are now transitioning to treatment at outpatient clinics. What this means is that their expenses are no longer regarded as being within the scope of insurance coverage, since the coverage was originally defined in terms of coverage for other types of disease. Meanwhile, the reimbursement percentages under the rural insurance program called the 'new-style rural cooperative insurance' is lower for chronic diseases than it is for 'major diseases.' In addition, the surplus amounts in the 'individual accounts' (under the social security insurance system) are not enough to cover what is needed.

China's basic medical insurance does not allow for adequate reimbursement of clinic costs, which is where chronic diseases need to be addressed. Commercial health insurance, which already has a responsibility for covering reimbursement of routine clinic costs, will increasingly be a kind of supplementary insurance in this regard. However, generally speaking, commercial insurance has a deductible amount. If we intend to provide full coverage for the costs of treating chronic diseases among China's people, then, first, we need to expand the scope of what basic medical insurance will reimburse for, and we need to adjust the reimbursement percentages. Second, we should bestow advantageous policies on insurance companies and actively encourage them to institute the kind of policies that cover chronic disease. Given the high incidence of chronic disease, we may want to consider, in appropriate measure, relaxing the restrictions on health status of policy holders. We also may want to incline favorable policies in the direction of impoverished parts of the population. This requires joint efforts on the part of both companies and government, since it requires balancing the for-profit nature of insurance companies with the social responsibilities that insurance companies should bear, and it also requires taking market demand into account. Meanwhile, insurance companies may want to be proactive in testing markets for long-term care insurance by launching long-term drug insurance for chronic diseases and for covering the costs of long-term care.

27 Hao Y.D. *Measurement of Enterprise Labor Force Health Loss Caused by Chronic Diseases*. Air Force Medical University, 2017.

28 WJKF (2012) No. 34. *China's Chronic Disease Prevention and Control Work Plan (2012–2015)*, May 2012.

29 Hao Y.D. *Measurement of Enterprise Labor Force Health Loss Caused by Chronic Diseases*.

6 Conclusion

At present, commercial health insurance covers just a tiny portion of the claims made for medical and drug costs in China. Meanwhile, despite the fact that the country's basic medical insurance provides 'universal coverage,' the per capita amount of that coverage is rather limited. Costs that are not reimbursed by social insurance are a significant burden on those who are meant to be insured. In addition there are the inequities of unequal healthcare safeguards among people with different income levels and in different parts of China.

Nevertheless, it is virtually impossible for commercial health insurance to provide coverage for most groups that social insurance covers at a relatively low level. Right now, commercial insurance is mainly targeted at high-income groups in a way that could be called 'embroidering flowers on brocade.' It cannot 'provide coal in the midst of a snowstorm,' that is, to the great majority of urban and rural people who need it. In western countries, the most recent market positioning of commercial health insurance is aimed mostly at supplementary insurance for high-income groups – commercial health insurance cannot play a universal role. Even if it covers a broader spectrum of people, western-country premiums are still mainly shared between the employer and the employee.

It can be seen from this that commercial health insurance is not an option for the regular person in China. If health insurance aims to make breakthroughs in different groups of people, it must strengthen the way its policies provide real security. It must devise innovative product models and encourage health management, and it must rely on its technological advantages in controlling risk and controlling costs.

With respect to paying for drugs: costs of drugs for common diseases generally do not place an excessive economic burden on households, whether the costs are incurred through a hospital stay or at a clinic. China lacks adequate mechanisms, however, for covering costs relating to major diseases. Meanwhile, with respect to chronic illness: given the higher incidence of chronic disease and the aging of the population, insurance companies must pay more attention to building models that incorporate health management into insurance plans. As they do this, they should also adjust the structure of their insurance products, their service models, and the design of their reimbursable drug lists. Breakthrough points will come from insuring drugs that are outside the scope of the social insurance reimbursable drug list, and from policy clauses that cover drugs related to chronic diseases.

As the market for commercial health insurance expands, as people's material lives improve and they become more conscious of the need for insurance, the future of commercial health insurance is moving overall in a good direction. The government is adopting progressive policies that extend beneficial tax treatment to insurance companies that should help lower the burden of disease in an effective way on China's residents. It is also relaxing restrictive policies, which is mobilizing insurance companies to develop their health insurance businesses. In addition, (the government) is furthering the building up of information platforms. With the prerequisite that information must be kept secure, the sharing of information is generally more efficient than monopolizing information. Through the efforts of all sides, in government and in society at large, we should be able to lighten the cost burden that medicine currently places on the Chinese people.

Bibliography

[1] Jing T., Yang S., Status and Development Status of Commercial Health Insurance in Multi-level Medical Security System [J]. *China Health Insurance*, 2016 (6): 18–22.

[2] Qiu Y.L., Wang Z.Q., Comment and Analysis on the Integrated Development of Basic Medical Insurance System for Urban and Rural Residents [J] *China Health Insurance*, 2018 (02): 16–20.

[3] Dong Q.X., *Development Trend of Commercial Health Insurance [J]*. China Finance, published in 2015.

[4] Cui Z.M., *Research on Institutional Basis for the Development of Commercial Health Insurance under a Multi-level Medical Security System [D]*. Capital University of Economics and Business, published in 2018.

[5] Yu H.F., *Research on the Introduction of Market Mechanism Reform to China's Medical Security System [D]*. Postgraduate of Chinese Academy of Social Sciences, published in 2017.

[6] Liu Y.J., *Experience and Enlightenment of Commercial Insurance's Participation in Social Medical Insurance in Developed Countries [J]*. Reformation & Strategy, published in 2017.

[7] Wang M.Y., Yao Z.Y., Sharing the Disease Risk of Rural Chronic Disease Patients by New Rural Cooperative Medical System [J]. *Chinese Primary Health Care*, 2013, 27 (07): 15–17.

[8] Shen C.G., *The World's New Family Doctor Service System and the Development of a National Joint Health Security System [M]*. Beijing: China Book Publishing House, 2018.

[9] Hao Y.D., *Measurement of Enterprise Labor Force Health Loss Caused by Chronic Diseases [D]*. Air Force Medical University, 2017.

[10] Lin J., Overview of Outpatient Protection for Chronic Diseases in Medical Insurance [J]. *China Health Insurance*, 2015 (01): 40–43

[11] *Official WeChat Account: "Chadaoyanshu". Uncovering China's First Knowledge Map of Disease Insurance Industry*. https://mp.weixin.qq.com/s/OUkzvoqg2Vcehgdiku58Rg

[12] ChinaPension.com., *"Insurance + Health Management" Becomes an Important Field of Commercial Health Insurance*. http://invest.10jqka.com.cn/20171127/c601785377.shtml

[13] *2018 Industry Analysis Report on Commercial Health Insurance*. https://wenku.baidu.com/view70cb3fcdf162ded630b1c59eef8c7 5fbfc77d94f8.html

[14] Chinairn.com., *Average Exchange Rate of USD of 2015 against RMB: 6.4476 in December*. www.chinairn.com/news/20190211/145029974.shtml

[15] business.sohu.com., *In-Depth Report on Insurance Industry: Blue Ocean of Health Insurance*. www.sohu.com/a/225770521_620847.

[16] Lanjinger.com., *Insurance Association of China: Commercial Health Insurance Is in the Primary Stage of Development and the Market Size Will Exceed CNY 1 Trillion by 2020*. http://finance.ifeng.com/a/20180727/16410029_0.shtml

[17] Chinabgao.com., *Drug Costs in China Reached CNY 1,734.59 Billion and Represented 35.8% of the Total Health Expenditures in 2016*. 2018. http://data.chinabaogao.com/yiyao/2018/10253K1c2018.html.

[18] Juliette Cubanski, Matthew Rae et al., *How Does Prescription Drug Spending and Use Compare Across Large Employer Plans, Medicare Part D, and Medicaid?* 2019.5.20. www.healthsystemtracker.org/chart-collection

[19] Iyiou.com., *Challenges of Developing Commercial Medical Insurance in Single-Payer Countries – A Case Study of the U.K.* www.iyiou.com/pZ61987.html

[20] *Just Landed Health insurance-How to Cover Your Medical Expenses in Germany.* www.justlanded.com/english/Germany/Germany-Guide/Health/Health-insurance

[21] *Global Legal Insights Pricing & Reimbursement 2019 I Germany.* www.globallegalinsights.com/practice-areas/pricing-and-reimbursement-laws-and-regulations/germany

[22] *Healthcare Expenditure,UK Health Accounts:2017.* www.ons.gov.uk/peoplepopulationandcommunity/healthandsocialcare/healthcaresystem/bulletins/ukhealthaccounts/2017

[23] *Assessment in Medicine Reimbursement of Medical Devices in Germany 2019.* www.aim-germany.com.

[24] Ma X.Y., *Analysis of America's Pharmacy Benefit Management (PBM) and Its Enlightenment to China.*

[25] Deng L., Development Experience and Enlightenment of German Commercial Health Insurance [J]. *China Insurance*, 2015, (1): 47–49.

6 Research on drug-pricing mechanisms in other countries

Lü Lanting

1 Introduction

This chapter introduces the background to the subject of drug price-formation mechanisms. It covers concepts and theories related to drug pricing, and provides case studies of six major countries and regions that were included in the research.

1.1 Research background

Since its founding 70 years ago, the People's Republic of China has made substantial achievements in the sphere of healthcare. The overall level of health in the country has improved noticeably. With respect to medical insurance, China has realized universal coverage of its social insurance through the establishment of the country's 'medical insurance for urban employees' and the 'medical insurance for urban and rural residents.' With respect to medical services, the country has established a tiered system of diagnosis and treatment and has greatly enriched the extent of its medical resources. With respect to public health, major accomplishments have been made in preventing and controlling contagious diseases and in disease prevention in general. With respect to drugs, China has set up a 'national basic drugs system' and the country's pharmaceutical industry has grown tremendously. Moreover, by passing of a series of policies and measures, the country has begun to control drug prices, lowering the burden of health on patients.

China has already entered the new era that is being called 'Healthy China.' In October 2015, the Fifth Plenary Session of the 18th Central Committee of the Communist Party of China called for 'promoting the building up of a Healthy China.' In 2016, at the National Healthcare and Health Conference, General Secretary Xi Jinping pointed out that 'It will be impossible to have moderate prosperity in an inclusive way without having health for all, so we must give priority to the strategic position of health in the development of the country.' In addition, he noted, 'We must accelerate the building up of a Healthy China – all of our forces, at all cycles of planning, must safeguard the health of the people.'

This has therefore become the action plan and guideline for the health endeavor in the new era. In October 2016, the Central Committee of the Communist Party of China and the State Council issued the *Outline of the 2030 Healthy China Plan.*

DOI: 10.4324/9781003325345-6

In 2017, the 19th National Congress of the Communist Party of China issued its Report, calling for 'implementing the strategy of a Healthy China. We must improve policies that relate to the health of the people, and provide health services for the masses by mobilizing all of our forces at all times.' In July 2019, the State Council's Healthy China Initiative Promotion Committee issued the *Healthy China Initiative (2019–2030)*. The building up of a Healthy China has already entered the stage of actual implementation. This program marks a conceptual shift in thinking about improving health – that is, we have gone from a focus on treatment to a focus on health as the central concern.

Modernizing (our) governance of the healthcare sphere was called for at the national level. In October 2019, the Fourth Plenary Session of the 19th Central Committee of the Communist Party of China adopted a decision called the *Decision of the Central Committee of the CPC on several major issues to do with adhering to and improving the socialist system, pushing forward the governance system of the country, and modernizing our governance capacities*. This highlighted the need to 'Strengthen the systemic safeguards that improve people's levels of health. Improve national policies as they relate to the importance of the entire life cycle and the entire process of health.' The *Decision* called for full deployment of resources in modernizing governance capacities and governance levels in the sphere of public health and healthcare.

Reform of the institutional structures of medicine, pharmaceuticals, and healthcare is currently entering the 'deep-water zone.' A fairly large number of problems still need to be addressed. Reform of the systems that govern drug prices have become the breakthrough point in deepening reform of these institutional structures.

Right now, China's reform of the institutional structures of medicine, pharmaceuticals, and healthcare is facing the following problems. First, there has not yet been any fundamental resolution of the difficulties in accessing affordable medical care. The people are bearing the brunt of the substantial economic burden of paying for medicines and healthcare. Second, even as the scope of coverage of China's medical security funds is being broadened, the sustainability of these funds is facing quite serious challenges. Third, drug prices are still quite high. This affects the ability of patients to access and afford drugs, and the prices of patented drugs are a particular problem. The exorbitant prices of drugs and improper prescribing of drugs are one of the main reasons for the first two problems.

In 2018, China's total healthcare costs came to RMB 5799.83 billion, which represented 6.4% of GDP. Drug costs constituted 35.8% of total healthcare costs, which is much higher than the average level of OECD countries, which is 17%. Unreasonable spending on drugs is, beyond doubt, adding to the cost burden on patients and the burden on China's medical security funds.

Exorbitant drug prices have been a major and ongoing cause of the overly swift rise in China's healthcare costs and the relatively heavy cost burden that people have to bear. China's reform of the institutional structures that govern medicine, pharmaceuticals, and healthcare is aimed primarily at resolving this problem of inaccessible and unaffordable medical care. The 'unaffordable' part of the problem is mainly caused by exorbitant drug prices. The chain of distribution in the drug arena is not only long but involves the interests of quite a few stakeholders. At the same time, the existence of such structural factors as 'subsidizing medicine (hospitals) through (the sale of) drugs' has created a situation in which it is very hard to lower drug prices. The situation poses a relatively heavy economic burden on people and to a large extent is limiting the country's ability to deepen reform of the institutional structures of medicine. Therefore, exactly how to resolve this problem of ongoing exorbitant drug prices has become the main focus of drug-price-management policies.

The 13th Five-Year Plan will soon be coming to an end. We need to explore drug-pricing management models as we face the new reform situation in the 14th Five-Year Plan. In the Medical Reform Plan that was incorporated in the 13th Five-Year Plan, one of the 'five basic systems under construction' was 'building a safeguards system (social security) that ensures that drugs are supplied in an orderly and proper manner.' This makes it clear how important reform in the area of drugs is to the country's overall reform and integration of the institutional structures that relate to medicine. The Medical Reform Plan also highlighted the need to

> go further in improving the price-formation mechanisms for drugs, to strengthen the alignment of policies that relate to prices, medical insurance, and procurement, and to adhere to the management [of drugs] by category. Gradually, by implementing different forms of price management, [China should] set up a drug price-management system that conforms to the unique features of China's drug markets.

During the stage of the 13th Five-Year Plan, a number of reform policies had a major influence on generating mechanisms that helped formulate drug prices. Given that there must be constant improvement in the building up of the drug-supply safeguards system, these policies included pushing forward complete separation of 'medicine' and 'drugs,' establishing a National Healthcare Security Administration, carrying out pilot programs that link drug procurement to quantities, and applying the results of pharmaco-economic evaluations during negotiations for drug procurement. Under the new reform situation, with the 14th Five-Year Plan stage in mind, it is time to explore new models of managing drug prices.

The material that follows mainly presents a comparative study of the drug price-formation mechanisms of six countries and regions that typify certain approaches. The six are the U.S., the U.K., Germany, Japan, South Korea, and Taiwan, China. Through a deeper understanding of these advanced examples, we hope to be better prepared to resolve the difficulties that China currently faces in the realm of drug pricing. The aim in what follows is to look at how to improve China's own systems for managing drug prices and to propose relevant policy recommendations, so that the country can ensure that the demand of patients for affordable drugs is met, and so that policies also spur the healthy development of the pharmaceutical industry.

1.1.1 Economic background

In 2018, China's total population came to 1.39538 billion people. The country's gross domestic product (GDP) was RMB 8969.15 billion, and its per capita GDP was RMB 64,644. The efficiency of the country's healthcare services systems was fairly high. In 2018, total costs of healthcare were 6.4% of GDP, and per capita healthcare spending was RMB 4,148.1, which shows that the burden on people was fairly low. The allocation of healthcare resources was relatively reasonable – in 2017, there were an average of 2.4 doctors for every one thousand people, and there were an average of 6.03 beds per one thousand people. In 2018, the average life expectancy of the population was 77 years. The mortality rate of women in childbirth was 18.3 for every 100,000 people, while the infant mortality rate was 6.1%. Health levels of people were therefore fairly high.

1.1.2 Overall situation of China's medical and healthcare systems, and unique features

1.1.2.1 THE TIERED DESIGN OF THE SYSTEMS FOR MEDICINE AND HEALTHCARE

China's medical and healthcare systems are composed of three tiers, namely community healthcare institutions at the lower tier, then specialized hospitals, then high-level general hospitals. This structure and the management of the system has shifted and changed from a form suited to the planned economy to one suited to a market economy. The planned-economy system involved 'designated' diagnosis and treatment (i.e., medical care at designated locations), while the market-economy system involves 'guided' and 'tiered' diagnosis and treatment.

First stage: the embryonic period of a tiered diagnosis and treatment system (from the founding of New China until 1979) Once the country was established, it began to set up and improve upon systems involving medical services. Within urban areas, two tiers of municipal and district hospitals were established, as well as healthcare clinics at the local level, so that a three-tiered system of medical services took initial form. In rural areas, a three-tiered medical services network was established at the end of 1957, by measures that included rectifying all levels of government and setting up new healthcare organizations. Controls over medical care were quite stringent at this time. First, there were specific rules of all kinds, but added to that was the dual-mode economic structure that put strict limitations on mobility of the population between urban and rural areas. As a result, an embryonic form of medical care came about during the planned-economy period that was tiered, and that designated specific locations for where people went for medical care.

Second stage: disintegration of the tiered system of diagnosis and treatment (from the beginning of Reform and Opening Up to 2009) After Reform and Opening Up began, the system of designating where medical care was administered to specific populations went out of existence. This system had operated under the planned economy and was associated with tiers of medical care. The orderly pattern by which diagnosis and treatment was conducted in a tiered sequence also disintegrated. Starting in 1998, China began to reconstruct a 'basic medical insurance' system. This did not in fact have any noticeable effect on the rebuilding of a tiered pattern of medical care. The more acute the problem of unaffordable healthcare became, the more pronounced the lack of an orderly sequence became, and this could be seen particularly in the discrepancy between large and small hospitals. Large hospitals were overly full of patients while small hospitals had virtually none.

Third stage: rebuilding the tiered system of medical care and preliminary achievements (from 2009 to now) In 2009, China launched the New Medical Reform. Policy now emphasized the importance of establishing a tiered system of medical care as a major part of this reform. From this time on, China's tiered system has moved gradually in the direction of a 'guided' mode as opposed to a designated or mandated mode. In September 2015, the General Office of the State Council issued an opinion called *Guiding opinion on pushing forward the building up of a tiered system of diagnosis and treatment*. The national level of government asked each region to push forward the implementation of pilot programs for this endeavor in an orderly manner. The building of this system is currently underway and it is constantly being improved upon. The tiered pattern of medical care has basically been reconstructed.

1.1.2.2 OVERALL SITUATION AND UNIQUE FEATURES OF THE MEDICAL AND HEALTHCARE SYSTEMS

First, the way in which China's system has developed has been deeply impacted by the country's economic structures. Indeed, looking at the evolution of medical and healthcare systems, these structures have been massively influential. China has progressed from a planned-economy period to a period characterized as an 'early-stage socialist market economy' and then on to the current period of a 'mature socialist market economy.' Its medical and healthcare systems have been through corresponding changes – from a system of controls to chaotic management and now on to a system of governance.

Second, the definition of the functions at each level of today's systems is still 'chaotic,' however. Although China has by now set up a fairly mature and sound system of tiered medical care, the functions of the medical institutions at each level are still unclear. The division of labor is not adequately coordinated. Third-tier hospitals (the top level of hospitals) still effectively draw in high-caliber medical personnel and (most) patients. The phenomenon of too many patients at large hospitals and too few at small ones still prevails. Given this situation, the environment at third-tier hospitals is actually rather poor. Waiting rooms are crowded, people have to stand in line for a long time – these things are ubiquitous. Conflicts between doctors and patients are far more pronounced than they are in developed countries.

1.1.3 Medical safeguards systems

1.1.3.1 THE MEDICAL SAFEGUARDS SYSTEM OF CHINA HAS ALSO EVOLVED OVER TIME

Originally, only a person's 'unit' provided safeguards and coverage was therefore only extended to a minority of the population. This then moved in the direction of a social medical insurance system as the primary source of safeguards (i.e., reimbursement for medical costs), but with medical aid and supplementary commercial health insurance providing safeguards as well – that is, a multi-layered medical safeguards system. By now, an institutional system for universal coverage has been set up in China that has 'two verticals' and 'three horizontals.' The 'two verticals' refers to the 'basic medical insurance for urban employees' and the 'basic medical insurance for urban and rural residents,' and the 'three horizontals' refers to medical emergency relief, basic medical insurance, and commercial health insurance.

Under this pattern of a multi-layered medical safeguards system, the three layers have evolved separately yet have emerged with a certain degree of coordination, that is, aid assistance at the lowest level, the basic medical insurance level, and supplementary insurance at the highest level. Insuring the lowest level mainly implies medical relief and social philanthropy assistance. Basic medical insurance includes the 'basic medical insurance for urban employees' and the 'basic medical insurance for urban and rural residents' (this latter category includes two aspects, the 'basic medical insurance of urban residents' and the 'new-style rural cooperative medical insurance'). Finally, supplementary insurance is composed of a variety of things, including commercial health insurance but also critical illness insurance for residents.

1.1.3.2 THE BASIC SITUATION WITH RESPECT TO CHINA'S MEDICAL INSURANCE SYSTEM

1.1.3.2.1 The evolving nature of the institutions Within the multi-tiered system of medical safeguards, China's national system is the level called 'basic medical insurance.' This has gone through a long evolution since 1949. In the early period, after the country was established, medical insurance mainly provided coverage only to State-Owned Enterprises and collective enterprises. That is, it was a workers' compensation system for employees of 'units' (1951), and a system of publicly funded medical insurance for employees in public institutions and government 'organs' (1952). The extent of coverage was extremely limited.

By now, China has implemented a medical safeguards system that provides universal coverage. This system set up the 'basic medical insurance for urban employees' in 1998, the 'new-style rural cooperative medical insurance' in 2003, and the 'medical insurance for urban residents' in 2007. The system was therefore composed of three separate structures. Problems with this kind of divided system, and a separate administration for each, then became increasingly apparent, and the work of combining the systems was put on the agenda. On January 3, 2016, the State Council issued an opinion called *Opinion on restructuring and combining the systems of basic medical insurance for urban and rural residents*. This set forth the need to establish a unified system of basic medical insurance for residents in both urban and rural areas. In 2018, the National Health Security Administration was established, after which the official (formal) work of combining the two urban and rural systems was completed.

1.1.3.2.2 Operations of the system China's medical safeguards system is being run properly and has achieved fairly good results in terms of scope of coverage, funding policies, reimbursement benefits, administering of medical care, and funds management. By the end of 2017, the nationwide participation rate in the system of basic medical insurance overall came to more than 95% and has stayed stable at that figure for several years.

First, funding levels are constantly going up, and mechanisms for financing the system are also getting better. In 2017, the per capita contributions per employed worker under the employee's medical insurance system came to RMB 5,240. Per capita contributions for the residents' medical insurance came to RMB 605. Meanwhile, each level of government contributed RMB 439 in subsidies per capita from public finance. Second, initial attempts are being made to link incomes to contributions in a dynamic mechanism for the medical insurance of urban and rural residents. Some provinces have already been able to start pooling funds at the provincial level (that is, administering a province-wide system of health insurance). Third, the levels of benefits are being raised in a stable and reasonable manner. In 2017, 81.7% of the costs of a hospital stay were covered under the scope of medical insurance policies for employees' insurance, on average, and 66.2% were covered under the residents' insurance. Fourth, the scope of benefits is being expanded. At present, funding for the costs of clinics has already been generally established for the residents' medical insurance.

1.2 Concepts and theories that relate to the formation of drug prices

1.2.1 Defining the relevant concepts

1.2.1.1 DRUGS

As defined by the *Drug Administration Law of the People's Republic of China*, the term 'drugs' refers to substances that are used in preventing, treating, and diagnosing illnesses, that are used intentionally to regulate physiological functions, and for which regulations specify indications and functions for usage as well as dosages. Such substances include Chinese traditional medicine in a form to be infused in liquids and a plant-matter form, ready-made Chinese patented medicines, chemical-ingredient drugs and their derivatives, antibiotics, biochemical drugs, radioactive drugs, serum, vaccines, products made from blood, and diagnostic drugs.

Drugs can be classified according to various criteria

First, they can be prescription drugs or over-the-counter drugs. Prescription drugs can only be bought based on a doctor's prescription and taken in accordance with the guidance of a pharmacist. Prescription drugs are generally targeted at specific diseases. In contrast, over-the-counter drugs were originally also prescribed, but they became available to patients without a prescription as effectiveness and quality proved stable over time. Over-the-counter drugs are generally used for routine sicknesses that occur with some frequency. They can be further subdivided into Class A and Class B. Class A can only be purchased in retail pharmacies and require guidance on how to take them from a licensed pharmacist. Class B can be purchased in any store or other location, without the need of a pharmacist's guidance. The distinctions in this form of classification relate only to the use of a drug.

Second, drugs can also be classified according to their degree of innovation. This category includes innovative drugs, original-research drugs, and generic drugs or reproductions of the originals. 'Innovative drugs' mainly refers to newly developed drugs that are still under patent protection. 'Original-research drugs' refers to new drugs for which the patent term has expired. 'Generic drugs' refers to reproductions of original-research drugs that maintain the same quality and effectiveness as the originals. China's pharmaceutical registration system goes on to classify chemical (synthetic) drugs in more detailed fashion. When registering a chemical drug, it can fit into one of five categories. The first are innovative drugs that are already being sold on the market inside and outside China. The second are 'improved new drugs' that are already being sold inside and outside China. The third are drugs that are applying to be generics inside China and that are original-research drugs outside of China – however, the original-research drugs are not yet available within China (Reference Listed Drugs). The fourth are drugs that are applying to be generics inside China and the original-research counterparts are already being sold within China. The fifth are drugs that already available on the market outside China but are now being registered for sale within China. The distinctions with regard to degree of innovation primarily apply to the stage of registering the drug.

Third, drugs can be classified according to their degree of market competition and their clinical application. The first category includes mostly generic drugs. These are manufactured by many companies and are used in large quantities. The second category includes mostly innovative drugs and original-research drugs. These are manufactured either by a sole company or just a few companies. The third category includes those drugs which have relatively few clinical applications but are commonly used low-price drugs. They include emergency medicines, basic intravenous liquids, and non-patented drugs for women and children. The fourth category includes clinically necessary drugs which are used in small quantities and in short supply. The fifth category includes drugs provided at no charge (by the government), that are used in preventing infectious diseases and parasitic diseases. This category also includes narcotic/psychotropic drugs. This way of classifying drugs is mainly used in the course of procurement of drugs (by institutions).

1.2.1.2 DRUG PRICES

'Drug prices' generally refers to the prices at which consumers purchase drugs – the amount they actually pay, which is the sales price. This sales price is generally the end-point price at the end of the entire chain of distribution. In order to be more specific about the increase in prices due to various interests in the pricing chain, the price of each segment of the chain must be analyzed. The value chain of drug prices therefore includes the following aspects.

Ex factory price: this refers to the price that the manufacturer charges the wholesaler. The manufacturer's price includes the cost of raw materials, costs of manufacturing and processing plus associated management costs, and a legitimate amount of profit. After that, it also includes value-added taxes, which are as follows: the great majority of drugs pay a value-added tax of 13%. Some plant-based drugs pay a tax of 6%, while anticancer drugs and drugs for rare diseases pay 3%. Certain specific drugs pay no value-added tax.

Wholesale price: this price traditionally signifies the transaction price at the end of the distribution process. That is, it is the procurement price at which pharmacies, hospitals, and retail outlets procure drugs. It also refers to the settlement prices along the way, at each link in the chain of wholesale distribution – the settlement price at which distribution companies buy and sell drugs. As the number of wholesale links increases, the wholesale price goes up.

Bid-winning price: this is the price at which a transaction is completed between the manufacturer of a drug and the organization (a government department) that is conducting a bidding process for specific drugs. The winning bid results from specified bidding procedures and also agreed upon quantities that are to be procured.

Procurement price: this is the price at which hospitals purchase drugs from distribution companies once the drugs being purchased have won the bidding process. However, hospitals often undertake a second round of negotiations with drug suppliers, given their own cost considerations. This round of negotiations generally lowers the actual procurement price, so the procurement price is frequently lower than the bid-winning price of a given drug.

List/gross price and net price: in the price-formation systems of some countries, a second round of price negotiations is allowed in the course of procuring drugs, which provides for additional discounts. Such discounts are legitimized by specific laws.

For example, two prices are frequently mentioned in the drug-pricing system of the U.S., that is, the list/gross price and net price. The list/gross price is generally defined as an estimate in a list of prices. The net price is the real price, and it equals the wholesale price after taking off all discounts, rebates, and preferential treatment.

Selling price: this is the price at which medical institutions or retail pharmacies sell drugs to consumers. Prior to the separation between 'medicine' and 'drugs' in China, medical institutions could add a markup before selling drugs to consumers, and that markup was to be no more than 15%. After the reform, and the elimination of the drug markup, medical institutions now have to sell drugs at the bid-winning price.

Ceiling retail price: the National Development and Reform Commission and the relevant price authorities at the provincial level formulate and publicly announce a ceiling on the retail prices of drugs. No enterprise or individual is allowed to sell drugs at a price that is higher than this ceiling (in the process of distributing drugs).

Government-determined prices and government-guided prices: Both of these prices refer mainly to drugs that are being included in the list of drugs covered under China's basic health insurance. The terms are also applied to prices of drugs under monopoly-type production and monopoly-type operations that are not included in the reimbursable drug list.

1.2.1.3 DRUG-PRICING POLICIES

The term drug-pricing policies refers to policies that are specifically formulated with respect to drug prices, and they can be either direct or indirect. Direct pricing policies are aimed at the prices themselves. Policies include setting prices on drugs, rules and regulations on drug prices, price adjustment policies, and so on. Indirect pricing policies are aimed at key participants in the sphere of drugs, whose behavior is adjusted by the policies, whether on the supply side, the demand side, or the insurance side. Policies therefore have an indirect influence on prices. Examples would be adjustments to the medical insurance reimbursable list, procurement through bidding, the two-invoice system, and so on. The drug-pricing policies that this research deals with are both direct and indirect.

In addition, the characteristics of and market demand for different categories of drugs may vary considerably. At the same time we have to take into account the extent of demand for a drug, the degree to which the health insurance fund can afford to reimburse for it, and so on. Price policies can therefore differ, and the most common example of this is the way price policies are formulated according to amount of innovation. Specifically, price policies are different for non-patented drugs and for new drugs.

1.2.1.4 THE PRICE-FORMATION MECHANISMS THAT RELATE TO DRUGS

Price-formation mechanisms as they relate to drugs involve the process whereby the transaction and interaction of different entities in the drug market is combined with relevant adjustments of relevant drug-price policies to come up with a retail price that consumers actually pay. This research mainly looks at price-formation as it relates to the retail price of a drug. Specifically, it looks at market mechanisms and regulatory-adjustment mechanisms.

1.2.2 Analysis of the theory behind drug price-formation

1.2.2.1 THE MAIN PARTICIPANTS IN THE MARKET FOR DRUGS AND THEIR BEHAVIOR

There is a tremendous amount of unreasonable price distortion due to various interests in the realm of drugs, given the multitude of participants and the complexity of how their interests relate to one another. Not only is there competition among stakeholders, but there are alliances of interests among certain stakeholders. To shed more light on how prices of drugs are formed, therefore, it is necessary to clarify who the stakeholders are and what they want (Table 6.1).

Table 6.1 Major Stakeholder Groups and their Main Objectives

Stakeholder Groups	*Main Objectives*
R&D units	Reduce the costs, enhance the efficiency, and increase the output of research and development.
Producers	Reduce the production costs and related period expenses, enhance (or maintain) the *ex factory* prices, and increase the market share.
Distributors	Reduce distribution costs and related period expenses, enhance (or maintain) the distribution price, and increase the market share.
Medical institutions	Reduce the procurement and management costs, ensure safe and rational use, complete and meet the drug use-related performance indicators as provided by the competent authorities, and promote the application of drugs while markups are not canceled, so as to obtain greater profits.
Retail pharmacies	Reduce the procurement and management costs, enhance (or maintain) the retail prices, and increase the market share.
Consumers	Ensure safety, enhance the reimbursement ratio, and reduce the prices of drugs.
Drug administration authorities	Ensure the quality and safety of drugs in the entire process.
Health authorities	Promote the rational use of drugs in medical institutions (including the prescription by doctors – avoid extraordinary prescription, and the use of drugs in medical institutions – that is, regulate the drug ratio), cut down the acquisition prices of drugs (prior to the institutional reform), and crackdown on the tunneling between medical institutions/ personnel and drug makers.
Price authorities	Ensure rational drug prices.
Healthcare security authorities	Ensure fund safety and reduce the acquisition prices (after the institutional reform).
Information and industry authorities	Promote the development of the drug production industry.
Commerce authorities	Promote the development of the drug distribution industry.

The relevant parties in the sphere of drugs are as follows: production companies (including research and development units), distribution companies, medical institutions, retail pharmacies, consumers, and relevant government departments (these include drug regulatory departments, health departments, price departments, medical insurance departments, industry and information departments, and commerce departments).

Research and development departments: these are the main entities involved in developing drugs, and they include production companies and also the research institutes in academic organizations that participate in developing drugs. The R&D and production stages of drugs are generally closely tied in to one another.

Production companies: these companies make and produce drugs, and include companies producing the raw materials as well as the final products. Profits of these companies come mainly from the profits they derive by selling to wholesalers. The market positioning of these companies is determined by the technological content of their product. Producers of innovative drugs and original-research drugs (RLDs) are generally monopolies. They occupy a commanding position when negotiating with downstream entities, including distribution companies, medical institutions, and relevant government departments. They speak with considerable authority when it comes to determining prices and distribution channels. In contrast, generic drug producers are in a relatively weak position in negotiations, given the crowded market conditions and numerous substitute products.

Distribution companies: these are companies at the wholesale level who operate downstream from production companies. They buy in drugs and resell to the next level of wholesalers (prior to the implementation of the two-invoice system), or they resell to medical institutions and retail pharmacies. Their profit comes mainly from the margin they make in the course of reselling. The market standing of distribution companies depends mainly on their scale of operations. Those that are quite large can control numerous distribution channels and can thereby have a stronger say in determining price.

Medical institutions: these are mainly public medical institutions, which include public hospitals and the grassroots level of medical institutions (community healthcare service centers and health clinics at the township level). Medical institutions procure drugs at the bid-winning price (or at a price formed by secondary negotiations that are based on the bid-winning price). They sell to consumers at the bid-winning price (prior to the reform that separated out medicine and drugs, they sold to consumers after adding a 15% markup). Their profits come mainly by squeezing down the price they pay to production companies in the secondary negotiation or also from the markup. Medical institutions, including medical personnel, enjoy a double-monopoly position in the drug market due to their absolute advantage when it comes to information and technology. On the one hand, they enjoy a monopoly position by representing the consumer as the ultimate 'buyer' in the market, buying from producers and/or distributors. On the other hand, they enjoy a monopoly position by being the ultimate 'seller' in the market, selling drugs to patients. In China, moreover, they are the most important end-point of sales. Medical personnel in these institutions make the decisions for consumers.

Retail pharmacies: these are mainly retail operations that sell mostly non-prescription drugs but also some prescription drugs. They buy from wholesalers through a negotiated process. Based on the price they pay, they add a markup and then sell to consumers. The policies relating to procurement through bidding and the elimination of the markup do not apply to these retail pharmacies.

Consumers: consumers are the ones who have to bear the burden of the ultimate sales price. They are the final purchasers and users of drugs, yet they occupy the weakest position in the market for drugs. It is hard for them to have any influence whatsoever on pricing.

(Government) departments who administer and regulate drugs: these regulatory departments are the most important of all, since their responsibilities include the entire process to do with pharmaceuticals – research and development, registration, production, distribution, and prescribing. They are also responsible for regulatory supervision over drug quality throughout this entire process.

Healthcare departments: these departments are mainly responsible for regulatory supervision of the drug situation in public medical institutions. This includes drug usage, procurement, preparation, and prescribing by doctors.

Pricing departments: these departments mainly carry out regulatory supervision of drug pricing. Before China implemented the policy of allowing the market to adjust prices, they mainly formulated 'government-guided prices' and carried out government-pricing activities. After the great majority of drugs began to be priced by the market, these departments mainly became responsible for monitoring and supervising drug prices changes.

Medical insurance departments: the duties and responsibilities of these departments are twofold. First, they reimburse patients who have medical insurance for those drugs that are within the scope of the reimbursable drug list. They also deal with additions to or adjustments to the list. Second, they procure drugs – once the National Health Security Administration was established, the work of drug procurement was transferred from healthcare departments to these medical insurance departments.

Industry and information departments: these departments are responsible for the growth and development of the drug manufacturing industry.

Commercial departments: these departments are responsible for the growth and development of the drug distribution industry.

1.2.2.2 CHARACTERISTICS OF AND CLASSIFICATION OF THE DRUG MARKET

The drug market has the same basic features of normal commodity markets, but in addition it has certain distinct features, as follows.

First, it has quite high barriers to entry. The development of drugs requires high levels of technology and know-how, as well as large amounts of investment. Not only does the research and development process take a long time but the success rate is low. In addition, there are strict policy constraints on drugs which means that any drug maker must come prepared with very strong ability to carry out R&D. All of these make for high barriers to entry.

Second, the drug market is a classic example of an agented situation in which the transfer from supply to demand is indirect. The agent relationship in the drug market is manifested in the relationship between doctors and patients. Patients are unable to make accurate assessments of any information to do with drugs given the highly specialized nature of knowing how to prescribe drugs. They must rely on doctors to make choices for them. They 'authorize' doctors to be their 'agents.' In addition, their demand for drugs must go through doctors and hospitals as the suppliers of the drugs, who also decide on the types, quantities, and price at which drugs are supplied. This therefore creates an atypical supply-and-demand market.

Third, a great number of players participate in market transactions, which is highly controlled by government. Not only are there many participants in drug market transactions but there are a great variety of selling channels, leading to severe problems of non-transparent dealings and collusion of interests. Supply and demand cannot truly be balanced given a high degree of market inflexibility. In addition, due to the need to make sure drugs are absolutely safe and that access to them is fair and affordable, the government places very high controls over the market. Such controls extend to quality as well as price, through numerous policies that government has enacted.

Fourth, the market is highly segmented. Completely different niche markets are created by the differing amounts of innovation and technology content in drugs, as well as quality, efficacy, and market positioning. Each market segment then has its own market characteristics including pricing mechanisms and mode of selling. Moreover, in order to expand the market for a given drug, and increase profits, some drugs can be sold in different niche markets at the same time, using a variety of pricing systems and market behaviors.

Fifth, demand for drugs is highly rigid and there is little price elasticity of demand. Since drug consumption is of a mandatory nature, changes in price do not have a large impact on decisions about consumption. Consumers focus more on the quality and efficacy of a drug. Moreover, elasticity is reduced even further by the agent-relationship between doctors and patients together with the additional feature of having a third-party payer, namely medical insurance.

> Three different types of markets result from the characteristics listed previously, when combined with unique features of different categories of drugs.

A fully monopolistic market: this market results when there is only one manufacturer of a certain drug who monopolizes the market for that drug. This mainly happens in the case of innovative drugs. Once such a drug is successfully launched on the market it enjoys patent protection for a certain period of time, as per relevant regulations that protect international property rights. During this term, other companies are not permitted to sell either the same drug or copies of the drug. Manufacturers of innovative drugs will generally also construct an entire system of protections for their drug by applying for patent protection for any possible structural type and compositional pathway. During the term of the patent, therefore, they can be assured of a complete monopoly in the market for the drug.

A monopolistic competitive market: this occurs when there are only a few manufacturers of a particular category of drug who, together, occupy the dominant share of the market. Competition among these companies may be fierce, but at the same time they rely on one another and they often therefore form a price alliance that supports the market price of the product. A monopolistic competitive market forms when a drug comes out of patent protection and the maker of that drug and the first few makers of the generics for that drug form a market relationship. The original-research drug (in the U.S., the RLD or reference listed drug) enjoys an absolute advantage in market share due to its previous period of patent protection and its reputation in the market, since it has reliability. The initial generic for the drug receives preferential policy treatment. After coming to market, the maker of that drug may therefore decide on a pricing strategy whereby it lowers price dramatically in return for market share. The other leading generics for the drug follow the same logic. After a period of time in which there is market competition, a certain balance is formed in the market between the original drug, its first generic copy, and the several other generics on the market.

A fully competitive drug market: this indicates a situation in which a number of manufacturing companies produce a certain type of drug, and the impact on the market of each company is limited. Generally this happens in mature markets for generics. After a certain drug has been on the market for a long time, the technical obstacles to producing it are low and the original-research drug (RLD) has no clear advantage in terms of price or quality. A multitude of manufacturers then start producing the drug for the market, which means that there is intense competition at each level or stage of drug sales.

1.2.2.3 INITIAL PRICING IN THE DRUG MARKET

Price as determined by market supply and demand: in a market that is not completely competitive, the demand curve that each manufacturer faces is shown by line D in Figure 6.1. The corresponding marginal income is shown by line MR. Each manufacturer has its own average costs AC and marginal costs as shown in line MC. The strategy of manufacturers seeking to maximize profits must be when marginal costs are equal to marginal benefits, as determined by the equilibrium production quantity Q. The initial market price P is inevitably determined by the

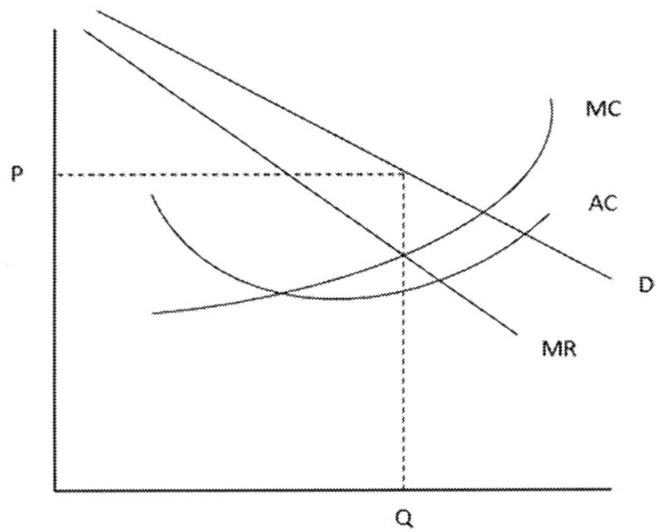

Figure 6.1 Drug Pricing in a Non-fully Competitive Market

demand curve. At this point, it is higher than the marginal costs and average costs of the manufacturer and the company is therefore able to receive excess profits.

Now consider a situation in which doctors and medical institutions 'induce demand.' Doctors are in fact able to push the demand curve outward, given that hospitals and doctors play an agent role on behalf of consumers. Depending on external constraints and economic incentives, doctors and hospitals can shift induced demand from D to D′, as shown in Figure 6.2. The new equilibrium in the market comes when the initial price Pe goes up to Pe′ and equilibrium production quantity does not change.

Generally speaking, when intervening in and regulating drug prices, government will take two factors under consideration. The first is the desire to control drug costs, and the second is the desire to maintain fairness and affordability. Intervention measures that are taken to correct market failures are done to improve the efficiency of monopolistic/competitive markets and thereby improve levels of social welfare. This requires that the government or the insurance payer control drug prices at reasonable levels and force them as close as possible to the average prices of drug producers. The problem with this is figuring out how to describe demand curves and average prices of producers in an accurate way, one that describes levels in reality, and that describes the new demand situation and degree of deviation when doctors induce demand. (In Figure 6.2, P′ is the price at which government controls prices, and the ideal situation is when this equals

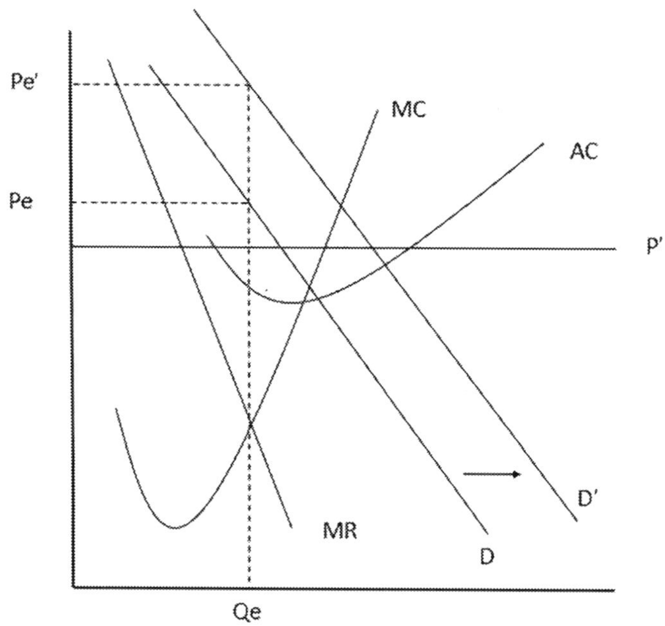

Figure 6.2 Changes in Drug Demand and Pricing under the Combined Monopolistic Competition and Induced Demand

the long-term average cost of drug makers.) What actually happens is that the two sides, the regulator and drug producers, begin a game of controlling and counter-controlling market information. This only adds to social costs. The ultimate result of intervention is determined by the balance of power between social costs of intervention and social benefits derived from regulatory controls.

1.2.2.4 TYPICAL REGULATORY POLICIES TO DO WITH DRUG PRICES

The initial price of a drug is generally affected by supply and demand factors in the market and by induced demand. In most cases, the ultimate selling price is formed by the *ex factory* price from drug manufacturers, the markups involved in the distribution process, and all kinds of policies aimed at moderating drug prices. The elements influencing price-formation mainly include the value of the drug itself, market supply and demand, and policy adjustments. Of these, policy adjustments play an extremely important role in price-formation. Countries around the world formulate regulatory policies to moderate drug prices, in order to overcome the possibility that market forces cease to work in the drug market (Table 6.2).

Regulatory policies with respect to drug prices have two main objectives. One is to control an excessively fast rise in overall costs associated with drugs. The second is to lower drug prices and improve the fairness of access as a result of affordability. Policies are mainly formulated with respect to the supply side and the demand side. Since medical institutions and doctors act as agents on behalf of patients, in this study they are included on the demand side of the equation.

If policies are classified according to their impact on the ultimate selling price of drugs, they can be divided into three groups, strong, moderate, and weak. Policies that have either a strong or a moderate influence on ultimate prices are generally aimed directly at the supply stage of the entire drug process. Those that are relatively weak are mainly aimed at the demand side. These attempt to change demand-side behavior by making purchasing decisions more price sensitive.

Direct government pricing: in this situation, the government directly determines prices at each stage of the drug process. It relies on specific rationales to do this, such as the cost of production for cost-based pricing. During the planned-economy period in China, all stages of the drug process, including production, distribution, and usage were priced directly by government. It is difficult for this kind of pricing to respond fast enough to changes in supply and demand, however, so the result is misallocation of resources and inefficient production. At the current time, essentially no countries adopt this kind of direct government pricing.

Placing restrictions on *ex factory* pricing: this kind of control mechanism is primarily used at the production stage of drugs, and is intended to prevent *ex factory* prices from deviating too far from the real cost of production. The main method adopted in this case is to set prices according to cost, that is, to use actual cost of production as the basis and then add on a certain amount of profit, in order to arrive at a price at which factories sell downstream to wholesalers. Production costs generally include costs of raw materials, R&D costs, and other costs occurred in the interim. In theory, this kind of pricing should accurately reflect the real value of

Table 6.2 Various Measures that are Taken to Regulate Drug Prices

Rigidity	*Regulatory Measures*	*Development/Influence Methods*	*Direct Regulate*	*Applicable Period*
High	Direct Government Pricing	– Direct pricing	Supplier: Producers and distributors Demander: Medical institutions	Production, circulation, and distribution
	Ex Factory Price Limiting	– Cost-based pricing	Supplier: Producers	Production
	Ceiling Price Limiting	– Internal reference pricing – International reference pricing – Market reference pricing – Value-based pricing	Supplier: Producers	Distribution and payment
Medium	Profit Margin Limiting	– Production profit margin limiting – Circulation markup rate limiting – Distribution markup rate limiting	Supplier: Producers and distributors Demander: Medical institutions	Production, circulation, and distribution
	Quantity and Price Agreement	Rebate, discount, and plus tax	Supplier: Producers	Payment
	Budgetary Constraints	Total budget of drug expenses	Supplier: Producers Demander: Medical institutions	Payment
Low	Drug Reimbursement List	– Positive list – Negative list	Supplier: Producers Demander: Patients	Payment
	Reimbursement Ratio Limiting	Providing different reimbursement ratios for drugs	Demander: Patients	Payment
	Reimbursement Threshold and Ceiling	Providing the reimbursement threshold and ceiling	Demander: Patients	Payment

a drug. In fact, however, arriving at a true cost of production is quite difficult due to asymmetry of information and the very specialized nature of pharmaceuticals. This kind of pricing is generally applied to pricing generic drugs. In certain OECD countries, such as Slovakia, the prices of generic drugs produced in the country are controlled by placing limits on production-cost prices.

Ceiling price limits: this kind of pricing places a ceiling on the top price of a drug, and is generally aimed at the selling stage of the drug cycle, which includes the payment stage (when insurance reimburses for drug purchases). Drugs can be sold at prices under this ceiling. With regard to 'the payment stage,' this form of pricing refers to formulating the payment standards at which medical insurance pays out reimbursements. Although such payment standards are not the true ceiling on a sales price, they take on the function of limiting what medical insurance will pay out, so this study uses such payment standard limits as one category of price ceilings.

Ceiling prices include four categories: formulating an internal reference price, an international reference price, a market reference price, and a price based on value. *Internal reference price*: this mostly involves comparing a certain drug with another of the same type, and placing a higher price on the one that has higher quality. For example, if the same type of drug has three versions, the original-research version (RLD or reference listed drug), the initial generic form, and generics that were later put on the market, then pricing will go down in a sequence of steps, starting from the original-research version. *International reference price*: this mostly involves pricing the domestic version of a drug by reference to the same type produced in another country or region. The domestic price takes China's actual circumstances into account. This kind of pricing is generally applied to innovative and patented imported drugs. *Market reference price*: this kind of pricing is generally applied to generic drugs for which there is considerable market competition. First, drugs are classified or grouped according to certain principles. Reference prices are formulated based on the market price of the group. *Price based on value*: the basis for formulating this kind of price is the usage value or the results that patients derive from using the drug. The most important methodology used in this form of pricing is the pharmaco-economic evaluation. Such an evaluation is generally carried out on innovative drugs when the drug is going to be put on the market, requiring a price negotiation.

Controls on profit rate and markup rate: this kind of pricing policy sets upper limits on the profit rate or markup rate at different stages and is to prevent excessive profits at each stage. Limits on profit rates are mainly aimed at drug transactions in the distribution process and include placing limits on the profit rates of drug manufacturers. (In this case, one kind of restriction limits the profit on the prices at which a manufacturer sells to wholesalers, and a second kind limits the overall profit rate of the manufacturer.) In the distribution process, this kind of limitation puts restrictions on the profit rate at which wholesalers sell to retailers. At the usage stage, limits are put on the markup rate at which retailers sell to patients. For example, prior to 2014, the National Health Service system in the U.K. limited the annual profit rate of drug companies to no more than 21%. In Spain, wholesalers' profit rates are limited to 10% to 12%. In China, at one point the price differential of a distributor could not exceed 15%. At the usage (prescribing) stage, China also limited the markup rate at which hospitals can sell to patients to no more than 15%.

Quantity and price agreements: in this kind of situation, a drug manufacturer and relevant authorities determine the corresponding relationship between price and quantity to be sold before a drug is put on the market. If the quantity sold turns out to exceed what was agreed upon, then the manufacturer must lower the price of the drug in one way or another, such as by offering greater discounts, returning profits (to the government), paying a value-added tax, and so on. This form of pricing is generally applied to price negotiations with medical insurance, and is generally used to control the risk of innovative drugs after they go on the market. France and Australia, among other countries, have implemented the practice. In China, the thinking behind the current policy of linking quantity to price, for health insurance reimbursement purposes, is similar. 'Determine market share in advance, and then exchange (lower) price in return for (higher) quantity.'

Budget limitations: this is when a country or a region sets aside a fixed percentage of its budget for drug costs – this money is to be used to supplement the potential increase in use of a drug when its price goes down. Such a pricing policy can force medical institutions and doctors to improve their cost consciousness, and can force them to prescribe drugs in a more rational way. Prior to 2003, Germany used a base of reference prices,[1] but on top of that, the country implemented a total-cost budget for drugs. To a certain degree, in China, the control over the percentage of a hospital's income that comes from its pharmacy also belongs to this category of budget limitations.

Drug reimbursement list: China's medical insurance fund establishes a reimbursable drug list, including both positive and negative lists. The question of whether or not a drug can be included in this list massively affects the public's price sensitivity for a given drug and therefore the list has a large impact on the market share that the drug enjoys. In order to gain access to the list, therefore, manufacturers may choose to lower drug prices to a degree.

Establishing reimbursement percentages: this refers to the way China sets different reimbursement percentages on different categories of drugs. For example, the drug reimbursement list has category A and category B, and reimbursement percentages for these are different. By affecting the price sensitivity of patients, this too will affect market share to a degree.

Reimbursement threshold and ceiling: China sets different limits on the lowest amount and the highest amounts that will be reimbursed for different drugs.

1.3 Case studies of six countries and regions

This study presents examples of price-formation mechanisms in six other places, the United States, the U.K., Germany, Japan, Korea, and China's Taiwan region. It uses structuralized comparative analysis to do this, looking at the process,

1 Chang Feng. *A Study on Drug Price Regulation Policies in China: Drug Pricing and Compensation Mechanism* [D]. Southeast University, 2010.

methodology, and mechanisms used in price-formation in each place. The hope is that it can serve as a reference and provide information for the policy recommendation section that forms the primary objective of this report.

Each of the six countries and regions has its own unique features when it comes to price-formation mechanisms.

1 The United States: The U.S. uses a pluralistic model for medical insurance, in which three types of insurance co-exist, namely public medical insurance, private non-profit insurance, and private for-profit insurance. Drug price-formation is influenced by centralized procurement and by payment standards under the public medical insurance system (Medicare).
2 The U.K.: The National Health Service model uses a combination of public hospitals and private general practitioners. Pricing is done by controlling the overall profit at the level of drug manufacturing.
3 Germany: This country uses a long-standing social medical insurance model. It uses drug reference prices (payment standards) for medical insurance as well as value-based pricing (AMNOG). (See later for acronyms.)
4 Japan: Uses the model of social medical insurance. The pricing system for drugs is completely government administered and uses examination reviews and price adjustments. Pricing basically relies on audits and the newest health technology assessment tools.
5 Korea: Uses the model of social medical insurance. The government sets prices on prescription drugs. Imported drugs in Korea are priced with reference to prices in seven other countries. In order to encourage domestic production, Korea's government prices domestic medicines and preparations that are made from domestically manufactured materials at the same price as (imported) original-research drugs (RLDs, reference listed drugs).
6 Taiwan China: Uses a model of social medical insurance + comprehensive private medical services. Decisions on reimbursement and pricing are made at the Conference for Drugs and Reimbursement Standards. Generally this is attended by personnel from the healthcare and drug regulatory departments, by specialists in the field, by people in the medical insurance business, by doctors, pharmacists, and so on.

The case studies of these places are presented next in sections two through seven.

1 Case study of the United States

1.1 Overview of the U.S. medical system

1.1.1 Background to the economic system

The full name of the U.S. (*meiguo* in Chinese) is the United States of America. Located in the central part of the North American continent, it covers 93,700 square kilometers and is composed of 50 states, the special district of Washington, D.C., and a number of overseas territories. In 2018, it had a total population of 327 million. It is a federated constitutional republic. It is the largest economic entity in the world, with a 2018 GDP of 2.06 trillion and per capita GDP of USD 62,853. Spending on healthcare is relatively high. (See Figure 6.3.)

The country operates through a capitalist market-economy system with a relatively low level of government intervention. Although the government influences economic functioning through the use of macro-economic adjustments, in overall terms it could be said that the free market is the primary force behind the growth of the U.S. economy, and that economic structures revolve around private companies and market systems.

2 Features of medical systems

FIRST, the American healthcare system is clearly market-oriented, with limited intervention by government.

Private institutions are the main providers of healthcare services. American medical institutions can be divided into public hospitals, private hospitals, and grassroots clinics (such clinics are primarily operated by individual doctors and most are for-profit entities). Private hospitals can be further subdivided into for-profit and not-for-profit hospitals. In 2017, there were a total of 6,210 hospitals in the country, of which roughly 79% were private hospitals. Public hospitals are in a minority and mainly serve low-income groups of people or special groups such as psychologically disturbed people, retired military, and so on. Each state has the authority to decide whether or not to establish public hospitals.

The costs of medical insurance are borne by both government and the market, and the role of commercial health insurance should not be overlooked in the

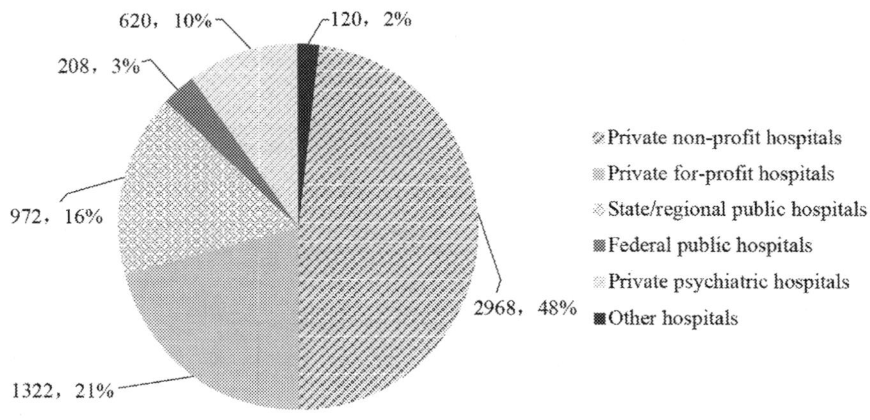

Figure 6.3 Numbers and Percentages of Various Types of Medical Institutions in the U.S. in 2017

Source: American Hospital Association (AHA)

process. In 1920, the U.S. Congress began to use market-based measures to deal with problems of medical insurance. However, due to failures of the market, it was hard for vulnerable groups of people to get insurance – such people included the elderly, low-income groups, and people with disabilities. In 1965, therefore, Congress passed the Social Security Act with an amendment that set up Medicare and Medicaid. Other government-led programs to do with health insurance include the Children Health Insurance Plan (CHIP), the Civilian Health and Medical Program of the Uniformed Services (CHAMPUS), and so on. In 2017, commercial health insurance plans covered 42% of total U.S. healthcare costs (Figure 6.4).

Government intervention is less than in other countries. On pricing, the U.S. allows pharmaceutical companies to set their own list prices. Such things as rebates and net prices are arrived at through negotiations with such commercial entities as Pharmacy Benefit Management organizations, and intermediary organizations that provide services to the payer side, such as Group Purchasing Organizations and Pharmacy Services Administration Organizations. This is in contrast to other countries, which may require the use of reference prices and healthcare technology evaluations and which therefore place restrictions on pricing at the government level.

SECOND, relationships among stakeholders in the U.S. healthcare system are complex. The role of the market in the system is pronounced, which means that each party relies on price negotiations to satisfy its own interests. This spawns all kinds of intermediary organizations and the formation of complex contractual and financial flows. In the process of price-formation, Pharmacy Benefit Managers are the primary intermediaries and they in turn interact with medical insurance, pharmacies, drug manufacturers, and Pharmacy Services Administrative Organizations and take in information and funds from a variety of sources. Net prices are finally formed after a complicated process of multiple negotiations to determine the extent of rebates.

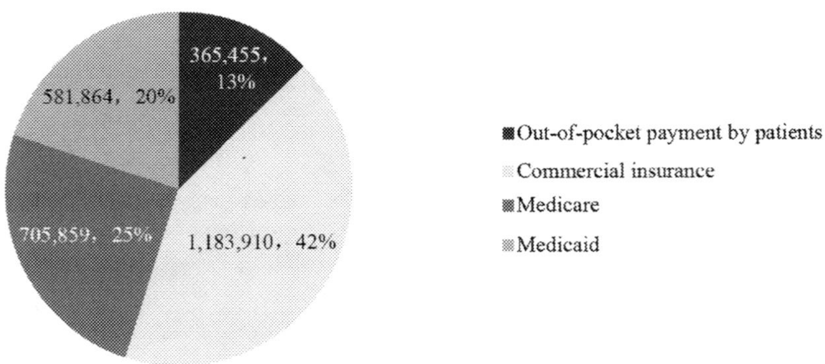

Figure 6.4 Percentages of Total Healthcare Expenses in the U.S. that are Covered by Various Types of Insurance, 2017

Source: American Hospital Association (AHA)

THIRD, the U.S. has made remarkable achievements in the field of pharmaceutical innovation. According to a study by the Information Technology and Innovation Foundation, the U.S. ranks first in the world in such innovation. Critical factors include a high degree of intellectual property protection and a willingness to spend on research and development. The U.S. contributes around 20% to global GDP, but it contributes around 40% to world spending on medical and healthcare R&D. Meanwhile, the U.S. market for drugs is around 40% of the world market (Table 6.3).

FINALLY, medical services and products in the U.S. are particularly expensive, while performance of healthcare on an overall basis is lower than might be expected. According to the World Health Organization, healthcare results in the country rank lower than average. The U.S. has not set up universal healthcare insurance, which is quite rare among the world's developed countries. At the same time, healthcare costs are high. In 2017, they came to USD 3,492.1 trillion, or 17.9% of GDP (Figure 6.5). Not only does this rank second in the world, but it is higher than the average level of high-income countries as prescribed by the World Bank (12.6%). In 2017, the U.S. had an average of 2.61 doctors per one thousand people, and 2.77 hospital beds per one thousand people. Its average lifespan for women was 81.1 years, and 76.1 for men, and its infant mortality rate was 5.8%.

With respect to spending on drugs (Figure 6.6), although the percentage of total healthcare spending that goes toward drugs has not changed substantially over the past 15 years, spending on prescriptions fulfilled at outpatient clinics have consistently stayed at around 10% of total healthcare spending, while spending on prescription drugs in hospitals has stayed at around 4% to 5% (of total healthcare spending).[2] In 2017, spending on prescriptions at clinics came to 9.5% of total drug spending (this is the most recent year for which we have data), while the peak

Table 6.3 National Origins of Newly Established Chemical Enterprises, 1971–2010

Country	*1971–1980*		*1981–1990*		*1991–2000*		*2001–2010*	
	NCEs	*%total*	*NCEs*	*%total*	*NCEs*	*%total*	*NCEs*	*%total*
U.S.	157	31	145	32	75	42	111	57
France	98	19	37	8	10	6	11	6
Germany	96	20	67	15	24	13	12	6
Japan	75	15	130	29	16	9	18	9
Switzerland	53	10	48	11	26	14	26	13
U.K.	29	6	29	6	29	16	16	8
Total NCEs	508	456	180	194				

Source: Arthur Daemmrich, "Where is the Pharmacy to the World? International Variation and Pharmaceutical Industry Location," Harvard Business School Working Paper, 2009 Milken Institute.

2 As pharmacy is separated from medicine in the U.S., outpatient prescription drugs excluded from hospitals are available in retailers, e-distributors, long-term healthcare facilities, and specialty pharmacies. Specialty pharmacies sell the so-called specialty drugs directly to patients, which mainly include biological products and other expensive innovative drugs.

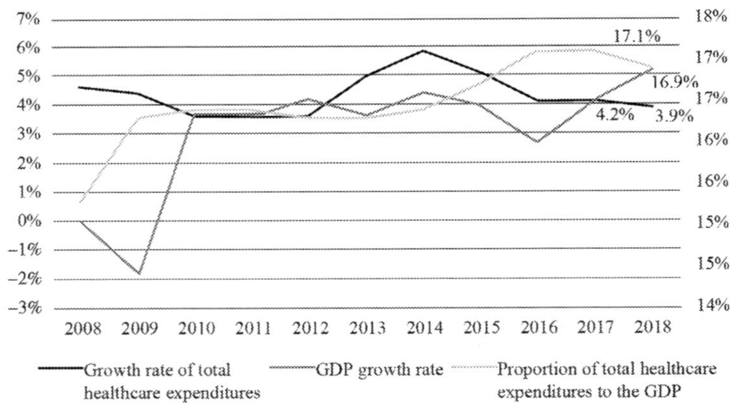

Figure 6.5 Growth Rate of Total Health Care Expenditure, GDP Growth Rate, and Health Expenditure as Percentage of GDP in the U.S. (2008–2018)

Source: World Bank Database and OECD Database

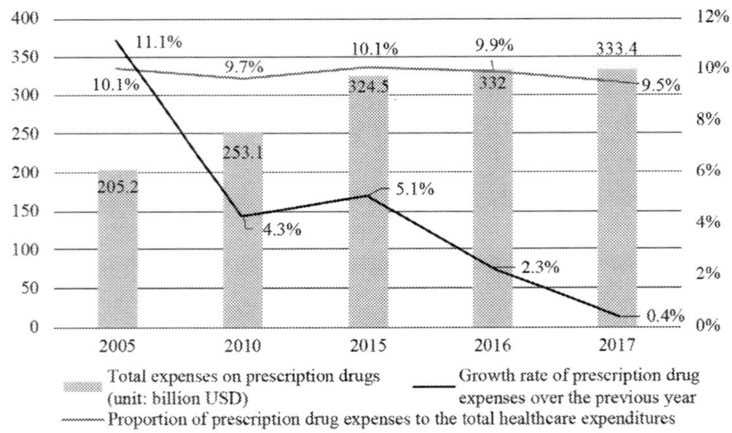

Figure 6.6 Spending on Prescription Drugs in the U.S. in 2005–2017

Source: Centers for Disease Control and Prevention and the U.S. Health Data Center

of this spending came in 2006 (the year the Medicare D plan was launched),[3] and was 10.4%. However, the out-of-pocket costs of patients have been going up every year (as seen in Figure 6.7), and elderly people in the U.S. are spending more and

3 Medicare is a medical insurance system provided by the U.S. government for the elderly over 65 years old since 1966. Medicare A mainly covers inpatient services; Medicare B covers outpatient and physician services; initiated in 2006, Medicare D is a prescription drug reimbursement plan undertaken by commercial insurance agencies; and the latest Medicare C is an 'advanced version' that combines Medicare A, B, and D.

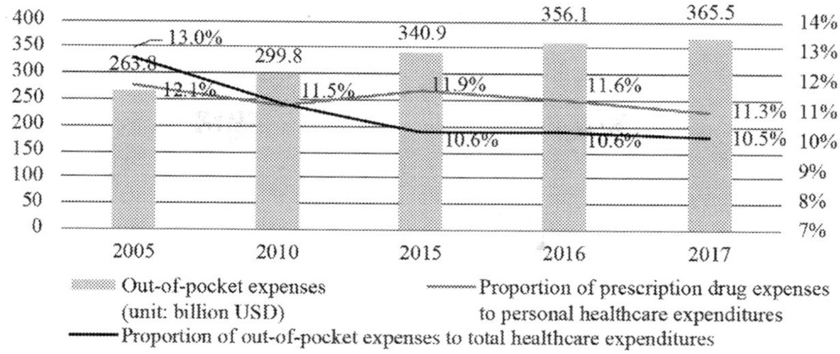

Figure 6.7 Spending on Prescription Drugs, Out-of-Pocket Healthcare Spending and Out-of-Pocket Healthcare Spending as Percentage of Total Health Expenditure in the U.S. (2005–2017)

Source: CDC Database

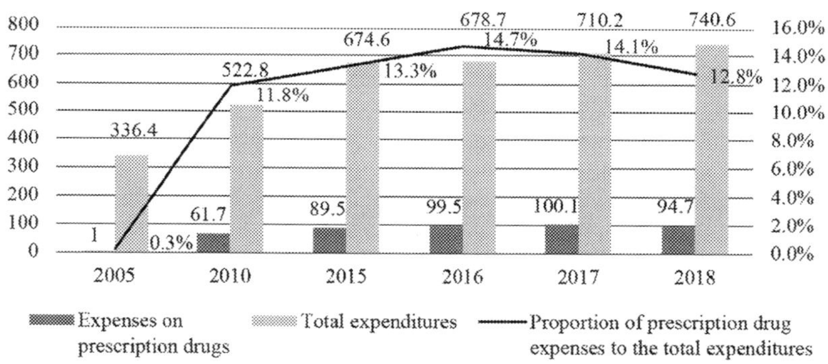

Figure 6.8 Data on Total Medicare Spending and Medicare Spending on Prescription Drugs in the U.S., 2005–2017 (Unit: Billion USD)

Source: The US National Health Data Center of the US Center for Disease Control and Prevention

more on drugs (as seen in Figure 6.8). Not only is the absolute volume of spending increasing, but the percentage of total spending on drugs is also increasing every year. Moreover, in 2017 this percentage came to roughly 14.3%, which is far higher than percentage of drug spending in the U.S. to total healthcare spending (9.5%).

Drug prices in the U.S. have three distinct characteristics. First, prices of some drugs are undeniably higher than in other developed countries (Table 6.4). Second, the differential between net prices[4] and list prices[5] is noticeably increasing, as shown by Figure 6.9. Third, drug prices are dramatically different when purchased

4 Net price refers to the actual selling price that equals the nominal selling price minus various discounts and rebates.

5 List price refers to the publicly announced price.

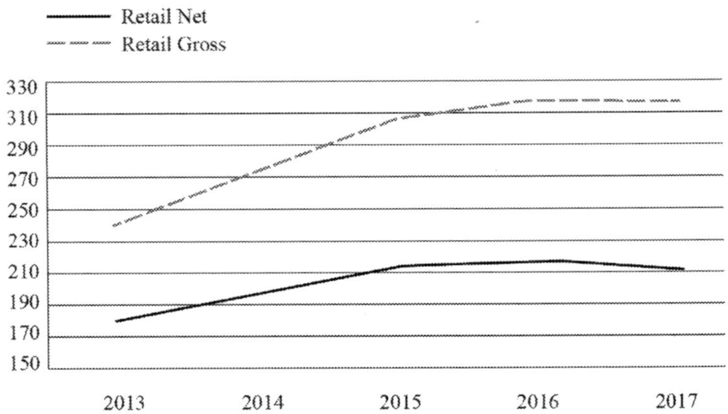

Figure 6.9 Sales Volume of Drugs in the U.S., 2013–2017: List Price vs Net Price (Unit: Billion USD)

Source: Report on Drug Use and Expenditures in the U.S.: A Review of 2017 and Outlook for 2022

through different types of insurance, at different pharmacies, and in different parts of the country (Table 6.5). As noted, the percentage of spending on prescription drugs at pharmacies as a percent of total spending on healthcare has stayed at around 10% over the past 15 years. This figure is arrived at by using the net price of drugs.

3 Features of the medical insurance system in the U.S.

With respect to medical insurance: commercial health insurance in the U.S. plays a key role in the medical insurance system of the country.

Spending that covered personal healthcare costs in 2017 was as follows: 35.1% came from spending by commercial health insurance, next was Medicare at 22.3%, and finally Medicaid at 17.6%. In recent years, out-of-pocket costs that individuals spend on their healthcare have been going down as a percent of total costs. In 2005, the figure was 15.6%. By 2017, it had gone down to 12.3%.

Commercial insurance still covers the largest portion of spending on prescription drugs – in 2017, this spending came to 30.3% of medical costs. In recent years, however, spending by Medicare on prescription drugs has gone up noticeably – from 1.9% in 2005 to 30.3% in 2017. Out-of-pocket spending has gradually gone down as a percentage of total medical costs, going from 25% in 2005 to 14% in 2017 (Figure 6.11).

2 Drug-pricing mechanisms in the U.S.

1 The drug system

Table 6.4 A Comparison of the Prices of Some Drugs in Different Countries in the Second Quarter of 2017

Drugs				*Price per Dose*					*Potential Savings for the U.S.*			
Name	*Specifications*	*Origin*	*Manufacturer*	*U.S.*	*Canada*	*U.K./ Australia/ New Zealand*	*India*	*Turkey*	*Canada*	*U.K./ Australia/ New Zealand*	*India*	*Turkey*
Abilify (psychosis, depression)	5 mg	Japan	Otsuka	$34.51	$4.65	$6.23	N/A	$2.25	87%	82%	N/A	93%
Advair Diskus (asthma) [1]	250 mcg/ 50 mcg	U.K.	GSK: Glaxo operations	$1,277.00	$377.62	$217.41	$84.99	$102.00	70%	83%	93%	92%
Bystolic (high blood pressure)	10 mg	U.S.	Forrest Pharmaceuticals	$4.71	$2.36	N/A	N/A	N/A	50%	N/A	N/A	N/A
Celebrex (pain, inflammation)	200 mg	Singapore	Pfizer	$13.72	$1.91	$1.05	N/A	N/A	86%	92%	N/A	N/A
Cialis (erectile dysfunction)	5 mg	U.S. (Puerto Rico)	Lily	$12.13	$4.44	$4.36	N/A	$3.52	63%	64%	N/A	71%
Crestor (cholesterol)	10 mg	Germany	CordenPharma GmbH	$11.37	$2.04	$1.82	$0.39	$0.40	82%	84%	97%	96%
Flovent HFA (asthma) [1]	110 mcg	U.K.	GSK	$781.00	$173.27	$152.40	N/A	$65.99	78%	80%	N/A	92%
Januvia (diabetes)	100 mg	U.K.	MSD	$14.88	$4.35	$3.04	$2.00	$1.17	71%	80%	87%	92%
Lantus Solostar (diabetes) [2]	3 ml	Germany	Sanofi	$1,160.39	$447.00	N/A	N/A	N/A	61%	N/A	N/A	N/A
Namenda (dementia)	10 mg	U.S.	Forrest Pharmaceuticals	$5.78	$3.56	$1.50	N/A	$1.38	38%	74%	N/A	76%
Nasonex (nasal allergies) [1]	50 mcg	Singapore	MSD	$648.00	$132.53	$113.92	$50.00	$43.97	80%	82%	92%	93%

(*Continued*)

Table 6.4 (Continued)

Drugs				*Price per Dose*					*Potential Savings for the U.S.*			
Name	*Specifications*	*Origin*	*Manufacturer*	*U.S.*	*Canada*	*U.K./ Australia/ New Zealand*	*India*	*Turkey*	*Canada*	*U.K./ Australia/ New Zealand*	*India*	*Turkey*
Nexium (acid reflux)	40 mg	Sweden	Astra Zeneca AB	$7.78	$3.37	$2.21	$0.35	$0.36	57%	72%	96%	95%
Spiriva Handihaler (bronchitis) [1]	18 mcg	Germany	Boehringer-Ingelheim	$1,303.00	$234.90	N/A	$90.00	$269.00	82%	N/A	93%	79%
Symbicort (asthma) [3]	160 mcg/ 4.5 mcg	France	AstraZeneca Dunkerque Production	$1,446.00	N/A	$319.11	$73.01	$227.00	N/A	78%	95%	84%
Synthroid (thyroid)	100 mcg	U.S.	Abbot Laboratories	$1.69	$0.30	$0.66	$0.36	N/A	82%	61%	79%	N/A
Tamiflu (influenza) [4]	75 mg	U.S.	Genentech	$473.91	$175.65	N/A	N/A	N/A	63%	N/A	N/A	N/A
Ventolin HFA (bronchial conditions) [1]	18 g of 90 mcg	U.K.	GSK (Glaxo Operations)	$206.00	$95.16	$83.31	$37.50	N/A	54%	60%	82%	N/A
Viagra (erectile dysfunction)	100 mg	Ireland	Pfizer	$58.72	$10.77	$8.31	$4.44	$9.27	82%	86%	92%	84%
Xarelto (clots and stroke)	20 mg	Germany or Puerto Rico	Janssen or Bayer	$15.38	$6.19	$6.22	$3.83	N/A	60%	60%	75%	N/A
Zetia (Cholesterol)	10 mg	U.S.	MSD	$10.17	$2.19	$2.13	N/A	$2.68	78%	79%	N/A	74%
Average Saved Amount									70%	76%	89%	86%

Table 6.5 Price Comparison of Top Ten Drugs of Three Pharmaceutical Manufacturers in 2016

Brand name (generic name)	*Sales*[a]	*WAC*[b]	*FSS*[b]	*VA price*[b]
Eli Lilly				
Humalog (insulin lispro)	2.8	25.33	4.72	4.72
Cialis (tadalafil)	2.5	54.76	32.81	26.02
Alimta (pemetrexed)	2.3	3203.10	3033.48	2238.28
Forteo (teriparatide)	1.5	1125.46	477.39	477.39
Humulin (insulin human regular)	1.4	13.71	1.25	1.25
Cymbalta (duloxetine)	0.9	10.47	7.27	5.44
Trulicity (dulaglutide)	0.9	310.96	124.49	93.17
Strattera (atomoxetine)	0.9	14.32	6.89	6.34
Zyprexa (olanzapine)	0.7	26.55	13.80	13.80
Erbitux (cetuximab)	0.7	11.47	10.81	7.97
Johnson & Johnson				
Remicade (infliximab)	6.0	1110.60	656.46	582.10
Stelara (ustekinumab)	3.2	17570.10	9693.19	9693.19
Invega (paliperidone)	2.2	1456.67	1198.75	932.18
Zytiga (abiraterone)	2.2	71.33	45.24	45.24
Xarelto (rivaroxaban)	2.2	11.91	7.42	7.15
Prezista (darunavir)	1.8	22.48	20.74	14.51
Simponi (golimumab)	1.7	7561.99	1716.81	1761.81
Invokana (canagliflozin)	1.4	12.95	8.91	7.78
Imbruvica (ibrutinib)	1.3	123.37	69.56	69.56
Velcade (bortezomib)	1.2	1612.62	1498.68	1200.70
Merck				
Januvia (sitagliptin)	3.9	12.70	9.01	7.98
Zetia (ezetimibe)	2.5	10.46	8.65	4.92
Janumet XR (metformin/sitagliptin)	2.2	6.35	5.36	4.00
Gardasil (human papillomavirus vaccine)	2.1	1601.68	1409.88	961.29
ProQuad (MMRV vaccine)	1.6	1906.18	1613.73	1067.62
Keytruda (pembrolizumab)	1.4	1111.63	1100.26	813.49
Isentress (raltegravir)	1.4	23.16	19.45	13.92
Remicade (infliximab)	1.3	1110.60	656.46	582.10
Vytorin (ezetimibe/simvastatin)	1.6	10.36	8.57	4.88
Cubicin (daptomycin)	1.1	445.49	317.44	289.94

Source: Mattingly, T.J., Levy, J.F., Slejko, J.F. et al. Estimating Drug Costs: How Do Manufacturer Net Prices Compare with Other Common US Price References?. Pharmaco Economics 36, 1093–1099 (2018) doi:10.1007/s40273-018-0667-9

WAC wholesale acquisition cost, *FSS* federal Supply Schedule, *VA* Veterans Affairs, *XR* extended release, *MMVR* measles, mumps, rubella, and varicella

a In billion

b Per unit cost in U.S. dollars

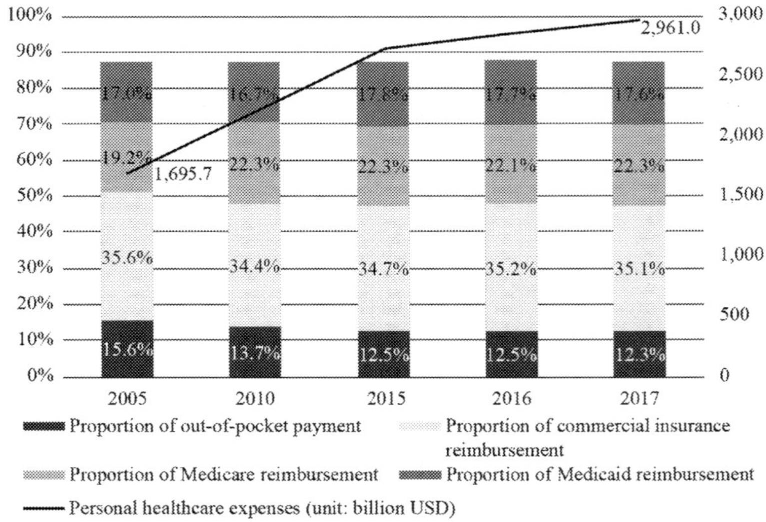

Figure 6.10 Trends in Personal Healthcare Expenditures Borne by Different Payers in the U.S., 2005–2017

Source: Centers for Disease Control and Prevention and the U.S. Health Data Center

Note: Personal healthcare expenditures include all expenses on healthcare except government administrative expenses, net medical insurance expenses (the difference between medical insurance premiums and the insured amount, invested in non-medical services, e.g., management costs, taxes, and profits), and expenditures on public health activities, public health research, and public medical devices.

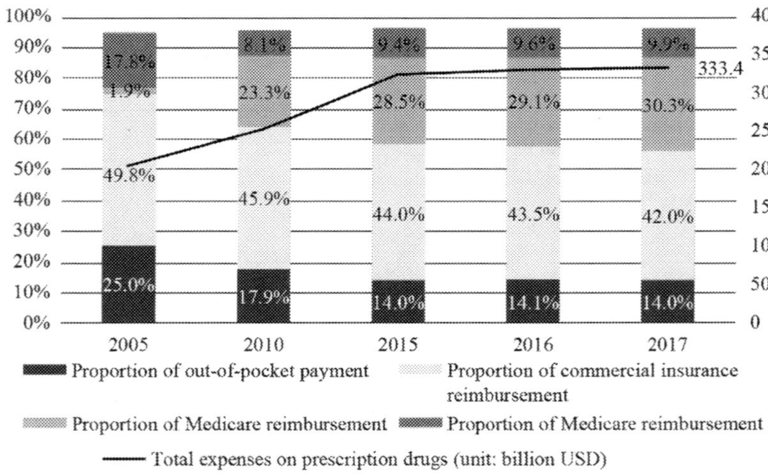

Figure 6.11 Trends in Personal Healthcare Expenditures Borne by Different Payers in the U.S., 2005–2017

Source: Centers for Disease Control and Prevention and the U.S. Health Data Center

1 History of the systems pertaining to pharmaceuticals in the U.S.

In 1820, 11 doctors set up the *U.S. Pharmacopeia* and recorded the first list of standard drugs.

In 1848, Congress passed the *Drug Importation Act*, which required the U.S. Customs Administration to carry out strict inspection of foreign drugs in order to avoid the importation of contaminated low-quality drugs from overseas.

In 1883, the American Medical Association began to implement independent auditing of drugs, which continued up until 1995. Drug manufacturers now needed to provide evidence that their drugs were as effective as advertised, and only then could these drugs be advertised in the journal of the AMA and its other publications.

In 1906, the Congress passed and Roosevelt signed the *Food and Drug Act*, prohibiting states from conducting business in mislabeled and contaminated food, drinks, and drugs. A regulatory agency which was the predecessor of Food and Drug Administration was established.

In 1912, Congress passed the *Sherley Amendment*, which prohibited drugs from being labeled in a deceptive manner.

In 1933, the Food and Drug Administration (FDA) passed a resolution calling for a complete rewrite of the outdated 1906 *Food and Drug Act*.

In 1938, the Congress passed the *Federal Food, Drug, and Cosmetic Act*, which required that newly developed drugs be guaranteed for safety before they could be distributed. This served to launch a new drug regulatory system, under which the FDA was authorized to regulate medical products. The legislation also set limits on quantities of any unavoidable toxic substances and it allowed for inspection of factories.

The Federal Trade Commission was authorized to oversee the advertising of all FDA-regulated products except prescription drugs.

The FDA stressed that sulfanilamide and other dangerous drugs must be used under the guidance of medical experts, which was considered the prelude to regulation of prescription drugs (see the *Durham Humphrey Amendment* of 1951).

In 1941, the irrational use of sulfathiazole tablets caused the deaths or injuries of nearly 300 people. In response, the FDA made radical adjustments to the production and quality regulation system, which significantly promoted the development of good manufacturing practices (GMPs).

In 1944, the *Public Health Service Act* ruled that the scope of regulatory supervision over biological products should be expanded.

In 1948, the Supreme Court ruled that the jurisdiction of the FDA should be extended to retailers, under the case of the *U.S. v. Sullivan*. The authority of the FDA was thereby extended to allow it to stop pharmacies from illegally selling such drugs as barbiturates and amphetamines.

In 1950, the U.S. Court of Appeals ruled that the instructions for use on labels must indicate the purpose of the drug.

In 1951, the Congress passed the *Durham Humphrey Amendment*, which defined the drugs that could only be used safely if they had passed regulatory supervision. It also stipulated that such drugs could only be used when prescribed by medical professionals, while all other drugs did not require a prescription.

In 1952, a nationwide FDA survey showed that the antibiotic chloramphenicol caused nearly 180 people to suffer from fatal blood diseases. Two years later, the FDA, the American Society of Hospital Pharmacists, the American Society of Medical Record Administrators, and the American Medical Association volunteered to participate in the drug response reporting program.

In 1953, the *Factory Inspection Amendment* required that the FDA provide a written report to manufacturers, providing the results of the conditions discovered during investigations as well as results of sampling of factory products.

In 1962, Congress passed the *Kefauver-Harris Drug Amendments*, which for the first time required drug manufacturers to prove that their drugs were effective before the FDA would grant approval for distribution.

The First Conference of the Advisory Committee on Investigational Drugs made policy recommendations to the FDA on product examination and approval.

In 1938–1962, safety evaluations were carried out on 4,000 drugs on the market under a contract entered by and between the FDA and the National Academy of Sciences/National Research Council.

In 1966, the *Fair Packaging and Labeling Act* required that the packaging of all consumer products in interstate trade should provide accurate information and also sufficient information about the products.

In 1968, the FDA established the Drug Efficacy Study Implementation, DESI which was expected to implement the recommendations that the National Academy of Sciences made as a result of its survey on the efficacy of drugs put on market from 1938 to 1962.

In 1970, the FDA for the first time called for inserts to be put in drug packaging that described the risks and benefits of the drugs for patients.

In 1972, the U.S. increased efforts to inspect over-the-counter drugs for safety and efficacy. It also began to look into the reasonableness of over-the-counter drug labeling.

In 1973, the Supreme Court authorized the FDA to regulate all classes of products.

In 1983, Congress passed the *Federal Anti-Tampering Act*, which criminalized tampering with the packaging of consumer goods.

Congress passed the *Orphan Drug Act*, under which the FDA was asked to encourage research and sale of drugs for rare diseases.

The FDA temporarily stopped direct advertising of prescription drugs to consumers. This prohibition was lifted in 1985.

In 1984, the *Drug Price Competition and Patent Term Restoration Act* (also known as the *Hatch-Waxman Act*) ruled that the FDA could approve the applications for generic copies of branded drugs, provided it was unnecessary to resubmit research on the safety and efficacy of the branded drug that was being reproduced. This thereby resulted in an increased supply of low-priced generic drugs. This Act also allowed the makers of branded drugs to extend patent protection for as long as five years for newly developed drugs, in order to make up for loss of sales during the time the drug application was being processed.

In 1987, drug-related laws and regulations were studied and revised, which effectively improved the availability of experimental drugs for patients with severe diseases that had no alternative therapies.

In 1988, The *Food and Drug Administration Act* formally put the FDA under the direct jurisdiction of the Department of Health and Human Services. It confirmed that the Commissioner of Food and Drugs should be appointed by the president with the recommendation and consent of the Senate, and it broadly defined the duties of the secretary and the commissioners of research, enforcement, education, and information.

The *Prescription Drug Marketing Act* prohibited prescription drugs from being sold through illegal channels, in order to prevent the mislabeling, adulteration, and counterfeiting caused by illegal selling. The Act made it obligatory for drug wholesalers to obtain permits from state governments, so as to restrict the re-import of drugs from other countries and to prohibit the marketing, trading, or procurement of drug samples, as well as the distribution or forgery of exchange-able drug coupons.

In 1989, the FDA issued a guideline under which drug manufacturers should determine whether or not a drug would be effective for the elderly, and to include the elderly in research if they were in fact using the drug.

In 1991, more than a dozen federal agencies adopted rules to protect participants in research studies that used humans in clinical trials. This ruling had already been issued by the FDA and was known as 'the Common Rule.'

In 1992, the *Prescription Drug User Fee Act* allowed the FDA to collect fees from the makers of drugs and biological products to pay for costs associated with product applications. It went on to require that the FDA use these funds to hire more personnel to expedite applications for products.

In 1993, the FDA launched Med Watch, a system designed to collect reports from medical professionals on drugs and issues related to other medical products.

The FDA issued guidelines for measuring gender-specific differences in responses to drugs. These also encouraged pharmaceutical manufacturers to include both male and female patients in their research, and to study the influence of gender on results.

In 1994, the *Uruguay Round Agreements Act* extended the patent protection of U.S. drugs from 17 to 20 years.

In 1998, the FDA introduced the Adverse Event Reporting System to store and study the safety reports on drugs already available on the market.

The Pediatric Rule required manufacturers of specific newly developed drugs and already existing drugs to study their safety and effectiveness with regard to children.

In 1999, Drug Facts Label (DFL) was applied to non-prescription drugs (over-the-counter drugs). Laws now required the labeling of such drugs to conform to standard formats with certain required information.

Clinicaltrials.gov was established, to provide the public with up-to-date information on the registration of federally and privately supported clinical studies, so as to encourage the participation of patients in promising medical studies.

The FDA issued guidelines on e-submission that provided for accepting and filing e-applications for the registration of newly developed drugs without accompanying paper copies.

In 2002, the *Best Pharmaceuticals for Children Act* was promulgated, under which drug manufacturers might be entitled to exclusive marketing within six months, provided that they carried out research on the drugs for children.

In 2003, the *Pediatric Research Equity Act* ruled that the FDA may require drug manufacturers to study the effectiveness of newly developed drugs with respect to children.

The *Medicare Prescription Drug Improvement and Modernization Act* required that research be done into how to use new technologies to provide basic information on prescription drugs to the blind and the visually impaired.

In 2004, the FDA stipulated that OTC drugs must use barcodes to prevent patients from receiving the wrong drugs.

In 2005, the Drug Safety Board was established. Its committee is composed of FDA officials and representatives of the National Institutes of Health and the Veterans Administration. It advises the director of the Drug Evaluation and Research Center of the FDA, and it cooperates with that organization. It communicates information on drug safety to health professionals and patients. At the same time, three guidelines were published with a view to honoring the commitment to risk management performance goals as part of the 2002 Prescription Drug User Fee Act (PDUFA). These were the *Risk Assessment Prior to Drug Marketing, Development and Implementation of the Risk Minimization Action Plan*, and *Good Pharmaco-vigilance Practices and Pharmaco-epidemiologic Assessments*.

In 2006, the *Requirements on Content and Format of Labeling for Human Prescription Drug and Biological Products* were approved. These stipulated that the labels of medical products should make it easier for healthcare professionals to derive and use information on the labels.

In 2012, the *Food and Drug Administration Safety and Innovation Act* expanded the authorities of the FDA. It allowed the FDA to charge fees within the industry, in order to support the review of innovative drugs, medical devices, generic drugs and bio-generic drugs; to promote drug innovation, help patients buy safe and effective products; and to encourage stakeholders to participate in FDA-regulated processes so as to improve the safety of the drug supply chain.

In 2013, the *Drug Quality Safety and Security Law* outlined the procedures for identifying and tracking certain prescription drugs via electronic and interoperable systems.

In 2017, the user payment plan for drugs, medical devices, generic drugs, and bio-generic drugs was revised and expanded under the *U.S. Food and Drug Administration Reauthorization Act* (FDARA).

2 Features of the U.S. drug system

The parts of the U.S. legal system that have to do with the pharmaceutical industry mainly involve patent protection, free-pricing, drug substitution, and medical insurance reimbursement. Price-formation of drugs in the U.S. is somewhat hard to understand, and is dominated by a combination of drug manufacturers, wholesalers, Group Purchasing Organizations, and Pharmacy Benefit Managers. Nobody can say with any accuracy what the prices of all drugs are.

2 Introduction to the main entities involved in drug price-formation in the U.S.

1 Pharmacy Benefit Management companies

Pharmacy Benefit Management companies serve as intermediaries among drug manufacturers, pharmacies, and third-party payers. They organize and also pay for the drug costs of patients. The drug costs that are paid for by third-party payers and relevant rebates are all transmitted through Pharmacy Benefit Managers. These entities are also authorized by third-parties to negotiate rebate amounts with drug manufacturers, using the drug formularies and drug tiers that they manage as a negotiating tool. They assist third-party payers in determining the scope of reimbursements under insurance plans, and the portion of costs that are to be paid out-of-pocket by patients. In addition, Pharmacy Benefit Managers negotiate with pharmacies on the pricing of drugs, and they establish networks of pharmacies which makes it more convenient for patients to obtain drugs.

All pharmacies throughout the U.S. have contracted with at least one Pharmacy Benefit Manager, and more than 80% of the U.S. population is serviced by Pharmacy Benefit Managers when they purchase drugs. These entities can be divided into three main categories. The first are independent organizations. The second are affiliates of medical insurance companies and handle the consolidating and managing of drug benefits on behalf of the insurance company. The third category works with employers through either cooperation agreements or alliances. Prior to 2018, there were more than 30 Pharmacy Benefit Managers in the U.S., among which the top six handled 95% of payments for prescription drugs in the country. By 2018, five of the top six had already been purchased by insurance companies. This means that 95% of the payment for prescription drugs in all of the U.S. is now handled by just two Pharmacy Benefits Managers. Moreover, the parent companies of these two not only provide medical insurance but they also provide specialized pharmacy services. In 2018, between 23% and 30% of the income of Pharmacy Benefit Managers came from drug manufacturing companies.

2 Third-party payers

Third-party payers and medical insurance are composed of commercial insurance and government-sponsored insurance. The most important components of the government-sponsored insurance are Medicare and Medicaid.

Medicare is made up of four parts, A, B, C, and D. Part A is hospital insurance, and its coverage includes care while hospitalized, nursing care from professional nursing institutions, end-of-life care, and family health maintenance. Part B is medical insurance, and its coverage includes services provided by doctors and other health-maintenance providers. It also covers outpatient healthcare at clinics, family health maintenance, durable medical equipment (such as wheelchairs, walkers, medical beds, and other equipment), and a number of preventive services (such as examinations, vaccinations, and injections). Part D covers prescription drug costs (including a number of recommended injections and vaccines). Responsibility for covering Part D falls to private insurance companies according to rules formulated by the medical insurance industry.

Patients can be included under Medicare coverage via two methods. One is to join a traditional medical insurance plan, which includes Medicare Part A and Part B. Part D is an optional choice in this case. If patients want medical insurance to pay for the portion of costs that they originally would have to pay out of pocket, then they may purchase supplementary insurance. (The original out-of-pocket amount, for example, might be 20%.) Patients who elect traditional coverage plans may receive reimbursement of costs at any hospital that supports such medical insurance and any clinic run by a licensed medical practitioner. The second method is to join directly in a preferred medical insurance plan, that is, the Part C plan. This is an integrated plan that substitutes for and includes Part A, Part B, and often also Part D. Once a patient opts for Part C coverage, his or her out-of-pocket costs may be lower than traditional plans, but this plan generally supports only doctors who are within a given network. In the great majority of cases, Part C provides benefits that go beyond the traditional medical insurance plans, for instance, vision, dental, and hearing insurance.

In 1992, the federal government launched the 340B plan which all hospitals, clinics, pharmacies, and convalescent homes could join. This plan required a drug manufacturer (or supplier) to grant a large discount for drugs being reimbursed through Medicare Part B to these institutions, if the supplier wanted to sell them drugs. In 2016, drugs sold through the preferred sales plan of 340B reached a volume of USD 1.6 billion.

Medicaid was founded in 1965, and is a public health insurance plan that is sponsored by the federal government and by state governments. It primarily provides medical insurance to low-income groups, who can include children, parents, infants, elderly people, and disabled people. Funding for Medicaid comes jointly from the federal government and state governments. Each state makes its own specific arrangements, under the guidance of federal programs. The federal 'guidance' is in the nature of 'orientation,' while each state has considerable leeway in terms of design and management of programs. There may be and often is a considerable difference among states between the qualifications required for assistance and the benefits. Moreover, not all medical institutions support Medicaid. According to the Medicaid Report of August 2019, at present 65,200,000 people are covered by Medicaid.

Medicare and Medicaid are at times confused with one another. Medicare is a health insurance plan that is managed by the federal government, with federal assistance that targets people who are over 65 as well as disabled people. It is not restricted to people with low incomes or modest resources. Around 10 million low-income elderly people and disabled people are covered simultaneously by both Medicare and Medicaid.

3 Group Purchasing Organizations

Group Purchasing Organizations of pharmacies (GPOs) are organizations that represent independent pharmacies in negotiations over drugs. Their core objective is to obtain somewhat lower wholesale prices from suppliers by lowering transaction costs. By improving the quality of services that their members (pharmacies) provide, they also aim to lower pharmacies' operating costs. Each GPO generally sets up long-term contractual relations with either one or more wholesalers. At present, there are roughly 16 GPOs in the United States. Each one represents from 250 to 5,000 pharmacies. Every pharmacy in the country has signed a contractual relationship with at least one GPO, but each pharmacy may have contractual relations with more than one GPO.

4 Pharmacy Services Administrative Organizations

Pharmacy Services Administrative Organizations represent independent pharmacies in their negotiations with Pharmacy Benefit Managers. They assist independent pharmacies in developing contractual relationships with Pharmacy Benefit Managers and in gaining additional reimbursement for drugs. They also provide other services, for example, some large-scale PSAOs may also provide Group Purchasing Organization services. The great majority of independent pharmacies will have a relationship with one PSAO, but in some cases, pharmacies may develop relationships with more than one. As authorized by small pharmacies, PSAOs negotiate payment plans with Pharmacy Benefit Manager enterprises. Most PSAOs are affiliated with (i.e., under the purview of) drug wholesalers. The rest are affiliated with chain drugstore groups.

5 Pharmacies

Pharmacies in the U.S. can be divided into independent entities and those that are part of chains, but they also can be divided into traditional pharmacies and specialty pharmacies. These distinctions are not clear cut, but in general it is understood that the drugs that specialty pharmacies sell are completely or in large part specialty drugs, while traditional pharmacies sell non-specialty drugs.

Traditional drugs are non-biodrugs (or biologics). Traditional drugs include mineral or plant extracts, antibiotics, and hormone products. Specialty drugs are used as part of the comprehensive treatment of chronic diseases and complex diseases. Drugs used for cancer, rheumatoid arthritis, AIDS, and multiple sclerosis all belong to the category of specialty drugs. These drugs are distributed through private pharmacies but also through hospital channels. Since many of the treatments for chronic diseases and complex diseases rely on the services of medical institutions, some specialty drugs are prescribed in hospitals and at the clinics of licensed medical practitioners. However, Pharmacy Benefit Managers themselves have opened specialty-medicine pharmacies, and have licensed practitioners. Hospitals are therefore in competition with pharmacies when it comes to the distribution of specialty drugs. Pharmacy Benefit Managers will generally limit the scope of drugs which can be reimbursed through various channels, so specialty drugs are sold through a minority of channels.

6 Patients

Patients can go through pharmacies to get drugs, or they can get the drugs directly from within a hospital. When they get the drugs themselves, they must buy them from a prescription pharmacy that meets regulatory requirements, and such drugs include oral medications and injection drugs. Reimbursement depends on the pharmacy benefit part of their insurance plan. When institutions provide drugs for a patient, this mainly involves medications used in the process of diagnosis and treatment. The patient does not go to a pharmacy to buy the drugs. Reimbursement depends on the medical benefit part of a patient's insurance plan, and such drugs may include those used in inpatient medical services, X-ray filming, diagnostic services, follow-up services, outpatient transfusions, and so on.

A patient may get some drugs through a pharmacy and others through a medical institution. For example, 76% of the injection drugs used for multiple sclerosis are reimbursable under pharmacy benefit insurance plans, another 5% under medical benefits, and 19% under both. However, the percentages of reimbursement are different for these two options, so the choices patients make will affect the reimbursement price.

3 The process of price-formation of drugs in the U.S.

In the U.S., the *ex factory* price of a drug is determined by the manufacturer of the drug, and this company and the wholesaler then negotiate on the wholesale procurement price. Generally speaking, the retail price is determined through negotiations between Group Procurement Organizations that have been authorized to act on behalf of pharmacies, and the wholesalers. In contrast, the final selling price depends on discounts and rebates between Pharmacy Benefit Managers, as authorized by third-party payers, or PSAOs as authorized by drug manufacturers and either large pharmacy chains or independent small-scale pharmacies, and the resulting reimbursement price.

Figure 6.12 describes the flow of contractual relationships, funds, and medical materials that lead to price-formation of drugs in the U.S.

Once the manufacturer of a drug determines price, the distribution of that drug, as one key task of the process of price-formation, proceeds separately from reimbursement, as another key task.

1 Price-formation in the course of distribution

In retail channels, first the wholesaler buys drugs from the manufacturer at the procurement price. After that, either a pharmacy or a Group Purchasing Organization that the pharmacy authorizes to act on its behalf will negotiate a retail price for the drugs with the wholesalers. Large pharmacy chains will often use their enormous purchasing quantity as a bargaining chip to negotiate directly with wholesalers, while small pharmacies will go through Group Purchasing Organizations to try to get more advantageous prices. If the drug being purchased is a

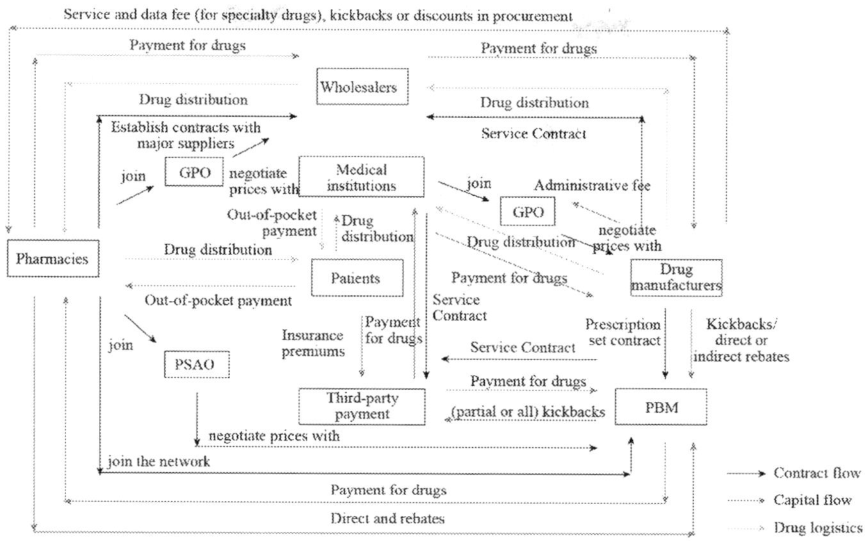

Figure 6.12 Inter-relationship among Different Drug Price-Formation Entities in the U.S.

newly patented drug, then the manufacturer may require the Group Purchasing Organization to purchase a certain quantity. When a patient purchases this drug from a pharmacy, they first pay out a self-pay (out-of-pocket) portion. This portion is generally determined by the conditions set forth in the health insurance plan, and those conditions are in fact the result of negotiations between Pharmacy Benefit Managers, drug producers, and third-party payers.

Certain special costs may be generated by the process of distributing or allocating drugs. For example, for specialty drugs, pharmacies may provide services for drug manufacturers that include targeted guidance on usage, advice on following the doctor's orders in continuing use of the drug, and so on, and the manufacturer may in this case pay service charges and data fees to the pharmacy.

Within hospital channels (for drug distribution), group purchasing is the common practice, which is covered more specifically in 'Four. Centralized drug procurement in the United States' later. Since the great majority of drugs in the U.S. are distributed through retail pharmacies, the following focuses on price-formation and profit allocation in the pharmacy channels.

2 Price-formation in the course of payment (or reimbursement)

First, the third-party payer goes through Pharmacy Benefit Managers to reimburse pharmacies for the cost of drugs that a patient has purchased. The reimbursement price is composed of two parts. The first is the Estimated Acquisition Cost, which is the cost of the drug. The second is the cost of services associated with providing the drug. Each prescription has a fixed service fee but small-scale pharmacies will sometimes ask their PSAO to seek an extra fee from the Pharmacy Benefit Manager for handling drug reimbursements, since one possibility is that the payment they get from third-party payers is lower than the actual retail selling price. In this case, the PSAO will represent small pharmacies in getting an extra reimbursement fee from Pharmacy Benefit Managers. One of the large Pharmacy Benefit Managers, called the Elevate Provider Network, notes that each week Pharmacy Benefit Managers receive some 500 such applications but only around 25% are successful.

Next, drug manufacturers pay rebates to Pharmacy Benefit Managers. These then return back either all or some of the rebate to third-party payers. This generally applies to branded drugs. Once the retail transaction is complete, the rebate goes directly to either the third-party payer or the Pharmacy Benefit Manager, without going through the wholesaler or pharmacy. The amount of rebate is determined before the contract with health insurance becomes effective, and is the result of negotiations between the Pharmacy Benefit Manager, as authorized by the third-party payer, and the drug manufacturer.

Finally, upon completion of the retail process, the pharmacy may also make a concession on the payment price that goes to Medicare D. This can be thought of as a rebate paid by the pharmacy. It is a similar operating procedure to that used by the manufacturer in its rebate toward third-party payers.

4 The allocation of profits (or benefits) in the course of drug distribution and payment

Our study group has not been able to obtain extremely accurate data on how much of the pie different stakeholders in the U.S. drug market get when the pie is split up (in fact, the figures are obscure to everyone). We therefore use a sampling method to estimate roughly how much in the way of benefits each entity receives in the course of distributing prescription drugs. In this example (Table 6.6), we assume that the list price of the drug is USD 450. Since there is no data to support the extent of rebates for PSAOs, Group Purchasing Organizations, and pharmacies, those are not included in the following example.

1 Drug manufacturers

The profit derived by drug manufacturers in the course of drug distribution is the actual procurement price less the rebates provided to Pharmacy Benefit Managers and any service fees. (This is after subtracting the costs of manufacturing the drug.) The list price of the drug is determined by the manufacturer, but the actual selling price is negotiated between the manufacturer and downstream buyers. It is based on the list price but is generally lower and is generally not disclosed to the public. Given indeterminate figures, the third-party payer generally refers to this actual selling price as the Estimated Acquisition Cost when it makes payment.

Table 6.6 An Example: Distribution of Profits in the Course of Distributing a Prescription Drug in the U.S.

Stakeholders	*Capital Flow*	*Item*	*Amount (USD)*	*Profit (USD)*	*Profit Margin*
Drug Manufacturer	In-going	Price actually paid by wholesalers	450*94%=423	423-180-18=225	53.2%
	Out-going	Rebate paid to the PBM	450*40%=180		
	Out-going	Service fee paid to the PBM	450*4%=18		
Wholesaler	In-going	Wholesale price actually paid by pharmacies	450*96%=432	432-423=9	2.1%
	In-going	Price actually paid to drug manufacturers	450*94%=423		
Pharmacy	In-going	Price paid by the third party for drugs	450*99.1%=446.6	446.6+1-432=15.1	3.5%
	In-going	Prescription fee paid by a third party	1		
	Out-going	Price actually paid to wholesalers	450*96%=432		
PBM	In-going	Service fee paid by a third party	450*0.5%=2.25	2.25+180+18-1-171-9=19.25	9.6%
	In-going	Rebate paid by drug manufacturers	450*40%=180		
	In-going	Service fee paid by drug manufacturers	450*4%=18		
	Out-going	Prescription fee paid to pharmacies	1		
	Out-going	Rebate paid to a third party	180*95%=171		
	Out-going	Service fee paid to third-party drug manufacturers	18*50%=9		
Third-party Payer	In-going	Rebate paid by drug manufacturers minus the part retained by the PBM	180*95%=171	171+33+9-445.9-1-2.25=-236.15	-
	In-going	Out-of-pocket payment by patients	33		
	In-going	Service fee paid by drug manufacturers minus the part retained by the PBM	18*50%=9		
	Out-going	Price paid to pharmacies	450*99.1%=445.95		
	Out-going	Prescription fee paid to pharmacies	1		
	Out-going	Service fee paid to the PBM	450*0.5%=2.25		

Source: Drug Channels

Notes:

1. This describes only the overall capital circulation process of each market entity in the drug distribution process. It does not cover the manufacturer's costs for research and development and production of drugs, the insurance premiums collected by third parties from beneficiaries, etc.
2. Intermediary prices are mainly expressed as a percentage of list prices, and list prices are mainly set by the manufacturer. Percentages have been estimated based on market surveys conducted by researchers and from Drug Channels.

2 Wholesalers

The profit derived by wholesalers is the differential between the retail price of the drug and the actual procurement price of the drug. The actual procurement price is generally lower than the list price but higher than the wholesale price. According to estimates of 'Drug Channels,' the three largest wholesalers of the drugs in the U.S. had a combined turnover of USD 453.7 billion in 2018, which represented a 6.8% increase over the previous year.

3 Pharmacies

The profit derived by pharmacies is mainly the drug price and prescription fees that third-party payers pay less the wholesale price of the drugs. According to surveys done by Drug Channels, the amount of third-party payment is based on the Estimated Acquisition Cost system, and comes to roughly 99.1% times the list price.

In this example, the profit of the pharmacy is 3.5%. More complete survey data indicates, however, that the average gross profit rate of pharmacies has been stable over a long period at 20%–25%. (The gross profit rate[6] is gross profit as a percentage of turnover.) This (higher) rate reflects both the gross profit rate on new drugs (3%–6%) and that on generic drugs (40%–50%). The profits of large chain pharmacies are higher than those of small independent pharmacies. The gross profit rate has not been changing much, but the turnover of pharmacies has been going up every year, which means that the gross profits of pharmacies have also increased.

4 Pharmacy Benefit Managers

The profits derived by Pharmacy Benefit Managers equal the sum of service fees from third-party payers and payment of rebates and service fees from manufacturers, less the sum of prescription fees paid to pharmacies and a portion of the rebates and service fees that third-party payers pay to manufacturers. Pharmacy Benefit Managers are intermediaries in the payment process for drugs, so capital flows are the most complex in this segment of the whole process. Rebates are the primary source of their profits. Since these organizations control the right to negotiate prices, the profits they derive from rebates can be around 40% of the list price of a drug. Over ten years, the price of rebates has almost tripled. Pharmacy Benefit Managers can return all or a portion of rebates to third-party payers, and in fact the portion that they retain for themselves is declining. However, it cannot be denied that Pharmacy Benefits Managers earn massive profits from rebates (Figures 6.13, 6.14).

6 Gross profit equals the turnover minus operating costs.

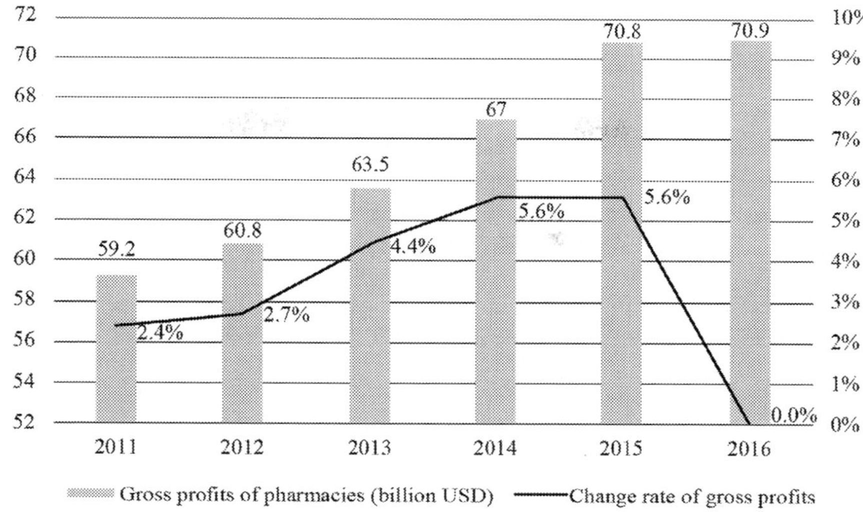

Figure 6.13 Changes in the Gross Profits of Pharmacies in the U.S., 2011–2016

Source: 2016 Annual Retail Trade Report, U.S. Census Bureau 2018.

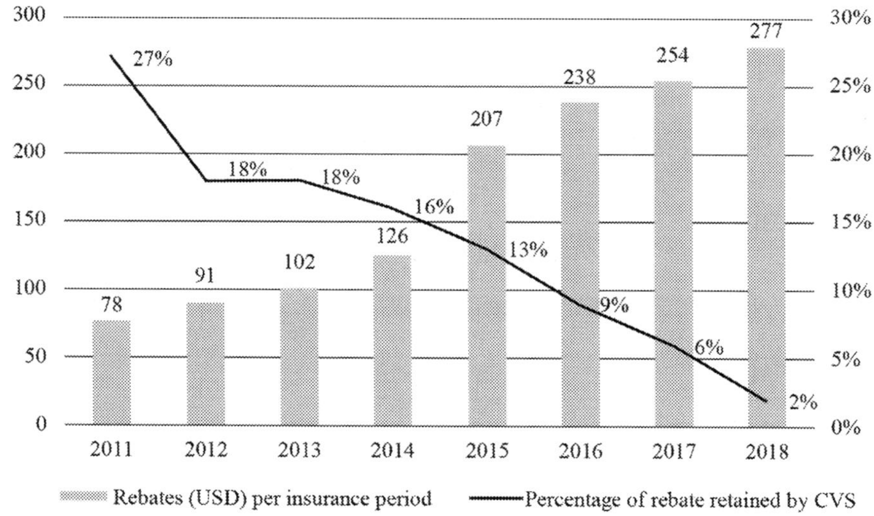

Figure 6.14 Rebates and Retention that CVS Received from Drug Manufacturers, 2011–2018

Source: Drug Channels

5 Third-party payers

The profits derived by third-party payers are the sum of all or a portion of the manufacturer's rebates and service fees plus the self-pay portion that patients pay, less the amount that third-party payers pay out in reimbursement, the prescription fees they pay to pharmacies, and the service fees they pay to Pharmacy Benefit Managers. According to the (former) head of the Health and Human Services Department in the U.S., Secretary Azar, drug manufacturers pay as much as USD 150 billion every year in rebates. Rebates just for Medicare Part D come to the high figure of USD 29 billion. Given the ubiquitous use of rebates, the real price that third-party payers pay for drugs is actually far lower than the list price of drugs. Patients, however, do not derive any benefits from the rebate system in terms of lowering their out-of-pocket amounts. This is one of the reasons that out-of-pocket costs are high.

5 Price-formation of drugs – in microcosm

1 Fees that third-party payers pay to pharmacies

Third-party payers generally do not know the acquisition prices of drugs, so they need to use Estimated Acquisition Costs in order price drug costs. (There are different ways to do that.)

1 Estimates may be made through reference to list prices: by referencing public data on average wholesale prices and also public data on wholesalers, third-party payers can estimate prices. This method is generally used for brand-name drugs and specialty drugs.
2 Method of pricing by using fixed prices: this method is generally used for generic drugs and it mainly puts limits on prices, for example, ceilings on costs.
3 Method of pricing by acquisition price: fixed prices are set according to the acquisition price of pharmacies. This method is mainly used for Medicaid services. Pharmacies that are participants in these plans have terms in their contracts with Medicaid that require that they report drug prices directly to Medicaid.
4 Method of pricing by the producers' price: this type of pricing is set according to the average sales price as derived from surveys of drug producers. This kind of pricing is mainly used for drugs that are physician-administered.

When third-party payers reimburse for drugs, the pricing methods that commercial insurers use are not publicly known. Drug Channels estimates that the service fee for each commercially reimbursed prescription is less than one U.S. dollar. With respect to Medicare D payments, however, the *Services Center of Medicare and Medicaid* requires that payers pay pharmacists a 'specialty-drug service fee.' This fee is much higher than what payers pay for commercial insurance plans, and the methods for determining it can be different in different states.

1 A fixed fee for services: 28 states use this method, and the average value of the fee is USD 10.53.
2 Fees for prescription services that are different for every pharmacy, depending on a number of factors: 14 states use this method, and the average value of the fee is USD 12.

The profits derived by pharmacies come primarily from the differential between the reimbursement for the Estimated Acquisition Price and the actual acquisition price. The service fee is not a major part of their profits.

2 Rebates that drug manufacturers pay

With respect to commercial insurance and Medicare Part D: rebates are determined by negotiations between drug manufacturers and Pharmacy Benefit Managers. Tools that Pharmacy Benefit Managers can make use of include the ability to administer consolidated prescriptions and different levels of drugs.

With respect to Medicaid and medical plans administered under the Defense Department, such plans enjoy a partial rebate as prescribed by law and they also receive extra rebates through negotiations with Pharmacy Benefit Managers.

By the requirements of the Medicaid Drug Rebate Program of 1991, drug manufacturers must enter into rebate agreements with CMS and must pay the rebates on a quarterly basis. Medicaid will provide coverage for the drugs of those manufacturers who sign such contractual agreements. The drug manufacturer reports the Average Manufacturer's Price to CMS (the drug price that wholesalers pay), as well as the lowest price of each drug (which includes rebates, discounts). Based on the Average Manufacturer's Price, CMS calculates the legally prescribed rebate per unit:

1 The rebate equals the Average Manufacturer's Price less the lowest price
2 The rebate equals the Average Manufacturer's Price times a given percentage
3 An extra rebate must be offered when the increase in the Average Manufacturer's Price is greater than a given indicator of inflation

In addition, Pharmacy Benefit Managers may receive an extra rebate through negotiations with drug manufacturers. The reason manufacturers may offer such rebates is to increase their competitiveness and to be included in the preferred drug list.

3 Recent administrative issues to do with the pricing of drugs

1 America-First Healthcare Plan

The Blueprint for this (Trump administration) initiative holds that four main reasons are causing drug manufacturers to set overly high prices on drugs. 1) Drug manufacturers set overly high prices on drugs. 2) Government programs and the elderly are paying excessive costs given a lack of the newest negotiating tools. 3) The self-pay portion of drugs costs is constantly increasing. 4) Foreign governments are taking advantage of the results of U.S. investment in drug innovation.

1 The list price of manufacturers is too high.
2 The elderly and government programs pay excessive costs due to a lack of the newest negotiating tools.
3 The self-pay portion that patients pay for drugs is not only high but constantly increasing.
4 Foreign governments are jumping on the bandwagon and enjoying the results of U.S. investment in innovation.
5 Drug manufacturers are facing pressures that lower their income, including international price restrictions, rebates for Pharmacy Benefit Managers, and increasing amounts of taxes and duties, including those imposed by the Affordable Care Act. They therefore raise prices.
6 Current Medicare regulations limit the ability to carry out effective price negotiations on high prices (especially the Part D drug plan).
7 More patients are paying higher deductibles as a percentage of their health insurance plans. Together with the increases in the price of drugs, this is leading to an increase in the amount of out-of-pocket they pay.
8 Drug manufacturers are developing more innovative drugs for which there is no substitute. This means that more and more drugs are highly priced. Only 1% of patients reap the benefits of such drugs, but they increase overall healthcare spending by as much as 35% to 40%.

Four strategies for lowering the prices of drugs, as proposed by this Blueprint, are: increasing competition, improving negotiating ability, providing incentives to lower list prices, and lowering the self-pay costs of patients. Specific measures for these four strategies are detailed next. They include some that the Trump administration felt could be implemented immediately as well as others that are still under discussion.

To increase competition, measures that can be taken immediately are: prohibit manufacturers from using regulatory procedures to hinder competition (such as risk evaluation and mitigation strategies REMS); promote measures that speed up the development of biologics. Measures still under discussion include: consider how to encourage the greater dissemination of original-drug samples (reference listed drug samples) in order to encourage more generics; encourage other measures to make use of biosimilars.

To improve bargaining capability, measures that can be taken immediately are: attempt value-based procurement within the framework of the federal medical insurance plan; address the problem of rising prices of generics that come from a single source by expanding the scope of drugs covered under Medicare Part D;

continue reforming Medicare Part D by giving more negotiating authority to insurance providers (that is, government health insurance) in their negotiations with manufacturers; report to the president on whether or not the drugs under Medicare Part B can be shifted to Part D for price negotiation; launch a competitive procurement plan for drugs under Part B; mobilize all administrative departments to evaluate the problem of foreign companies taking advantage of U.S. innovation. Future measures that might be pursued would include: consider launching value-based procurement under the framework of the federal insurance plan, including indications-based pricing, given the need to take long-term funding of health insurance into account; eliminate obstacles to value-based procurement under government health insurance programs; make prices of drugs that are available through different channels more consistent with each other; evaluate the accuracy and validity of statistics on government spending on drugs.

To provide incentives to lower list prices, actions that can be taken immediately are: under FDA monitoring, require drug manufacturers to state prices of drugs on advertising; make competition between generics and other drugs and the rise in prices of drugs more transparent by updating the federal health insurance drug spending dashboards. Actions that might be pursued in the future are: adopt measures to limit kickbacks, including revisiting the safe-harbor provisions under the Anti-Kickback Statute; undertake other reforms to do with the whole rebate system; provide incentives to prevent drug manufacturers from raising prices of drugs under Part B and Part D; evaluate the authorizations that Pharmacy Benefit Managers are allowed; reform the rebate plans for drugs covered under Medicaid; reform the rebate plans for drugs covered under 340B; revise the regulations put out by the Health and Human Services Department on drug discount coupons for co-pays.

To lower self-pay (out-of-pocket) costs, actions that can be taken immediately are: prohibit pharmacists from using Part D provisions as an excuse not to inform patients that they could reduce their cash outlays by not going through medical insurance for some drugs; improve the benefits statement of Part D to add in information on drug price increases and potential substitutions. Measures that could be taken in the future are: inform beneficiaries of Medicare Part B and Part D of lower-cost alternatives; provide more frequent information on prices under Part D, or provide better information on an annual basis.

Once the Blueprint was released, the Trump administration adopted various measures to lower drug prices, including encouraging greater competition in biosimilars, providing greater negotiation authority to government health insurance programs, using an international price-index to formulate drug prices, cracking down on kickbacks, and making an attempt to import less expensive drugs from other countries.

2 Other follow-on actions

June 2018: the FDA approved a generic form of opioid as a supplementary form of treatment.

July 2018: the FDA passed new guidelines that opened up new channels for patients to obtain over-the-counter drugs.

July 2018: the FDA launched a Biosimilar Action Plan, intended to promote competition in the biosimilar pharmaceutical market.

July 19, 2018: Secretary Azar asked the FDA to set up a Working Group to research how to import low-cost drugs from other countries whose patent protection had expired.

August 7, 2018: a new bargaining tool was developed for Medicare Part B so that it could have the same negotiating power as commercial insurance companies.

Early October 2018: Trump signed an injunction that broke through previous restrictions on pharmacists that prevented them from advising patients of cheaper alternative drugs.

October 15, 2018: Secretary Azar announced that further steps would be taken to increase transparency of drug pricing.

October 15, 2018: Secretary Azar declared that drug manufacturers would now be required to state prices in television advertisements that advertised their drugs, which went a step further in making prices transparent.

October 25, 2018: The U.S. announced it intended to use an International Pricing Index model to control prices of drugs used in medical institutions (such as drugs for transfusions). Secretary Azar declared that the main point of this was to control the high prices that Medicare was paying for drugs, but that it was also to lower drug prices in general and to reduce the phenomenon of having foreign countries take advantage of the situation. The Centers for Medicare and Medicaid declared that the plan was to launch a test run of using the IPI model in the spring of 2020, and to use it for five years, until 2025. Requests for opinions were to come in prior to December 31, 2018. The original intent was to start in the spring of 2019, but as of January 10, 2020, there has been no further guidance.

November 26, 2018: Medicare and Medicaid Services recommended adjusting Medicare Part D to increase its negotiating ability and thereby lower drug prices.

January 31, 2019: the Trump administration declared that it intended to rein in the system of rebates that drug manufacturers provide to intermediaries, and instead to have such rebates provided directly to patients.

May 2019: Medicare and Medicaid Services finally approved the proposal that drug manufacturers should declare their prices in television advertisements. This applies to drugs that cost more than USD 35 for a one-month supply or one course of treatment.

June 24, 2019: In an Executive Order, Donald Trump again stressed the need to improve transparency in drug pricing.

July 2019: Under pressure from Trump, the Department of Health and Human Services and the FDA passed the 'Safe Drug Importation Plan,' which allows for the import of low-priced drugs from Canada and other countries.

November 27, 2019: the Federal Register made public final regulations on making drug prices more transparent – this relates to newly introduced drugs in hospitals that are in the outpatient pre-payment system. Another regulation regarding the public disclosure of drug prices is still under consideration (as of January 10,

2019). Both of these are expected to improve the transparency of drug pricing in the U.S.

December 13, 2019: in a vote of 230 to 192, with votes divided along party lines, the U.S. House of Representatives passed bill HR3, on new drug pricing. This bill holds three major provisions that are aimed at controlling the constant increase in prescription drug prices. First, it holds the self-pay portion of health insurance for the elderly to within the limit of USD 2,000. Second, it requires drugs whose prices have exceeded the inflation rate since 2016 either to lower prices or to hand over the sales amount that exceeds inflation to the Treasury. Third, it allows the Department of Health participate in setting prices on at least 50 drugs but at most 250 drugs. Speaker of the House Pelosi noted that the third provision was key, and that drug prices of six advanced countries would be used as price indicators for determination of U.S. prices. If this bill passes (the Senate), over the next ten years, the U.S. is expected to save USD 456 billion in spending. However, since this will also lower investment in R&D, the bill may also result in keeping at most one hundred types of new drugs from coming to market. Naturally, the chances that this bill will become law are essentially zero, since the Republic Party controls the Senate. President Trump also declared that he opposed it. The Republican Party in the House has recently put forth a more moderate bill on price reduction called HR 19, and the Senate also has a similar proposal. Both of these recommend limiting self-pay to USD 3,100, but neither has mandatory price limits nor do they allow the Department of Health to cut prices. Although both the House and Senate proposals are more moderate, they are still a threat to the drug industry, since any restriction at all will have a direct impact on investment in new drug R&D. Not only will the quantity of new drugs that are produced go down, but outstanding products that have the highest risk and greatest degree of innovation will be affected. Looking at the way things have worked in the past, worldwide, the most innovative products come from markets that provide the greatest return.

4 Centralized drug procurement in the United States

Centralized procurement happens in both the channels that supply drugs to commercial pharmacies and the channels that supply medical institutions. Such procurement is mainly carried out by Group Purchasing Organizations.

1 Centralized procurement of drugs that go through commercial (retail) pharmacies

Small, independent pharmacies generally go through Group Purchasing Organizations for centralized purchasing operations in order to derive either discounts or rebates from the suppliers of the drugs. Virtually all independent pharmacies cooperate with at least one GPO, and each GPO has ties with either one or many wholesalers. Pharmacies that enter into relationships with a GPO mainly procure drugs from the wholesaler that the GPO has chosen, but there are situations in which a pharmacy carries out procurement apart from a GPO. In such a case, the wholesaler may provide the pharmacy with more favorable prices than it has negotiated with the GPO. The price-formation of preferential prices comes about when the wholesaler provides the pharmacy directly with either discounts or rebates that it pays on an annual or a quarterly basis.

2 Centralized procurement of drugs that go through medical institutions

Some medical institutions go through GPOs to carry out procurement. GPOs are organizations that help medical institutions (such as hospitals, clinics, nursing homes, and home-health organizations) gain discounts through combined (larger) purchasing quantities and through negotiations with wholesalers. GPOs themselves do not buy drugs. They are responsible for negotiating contracts with wholesalers and with drug manufacturers. Once they have achieved a successful negotiation for group procurement, each hospital still retains the right to make final decisions on specific drug purchasing. The great majority of medical institutions will have a committee that deals with drug procurement matters, and it is generally made up of doctors, nurses, clinical practitioners, and professionals in the field of medical insurance. This contributes to making sure procurement decisions are rational. Some GPOs provide electronic procurement systems and other services. In 2018, the United States had more than 600 GPOs, around 30 of which were quite large.

The history of GPOs can be traced back to 1909, when the authority responsible for overseeing New York's hospitals thought of setting up a centralized procurement organization to handle laundry services. In 1920, the very first GPO in New York was launched, in New York City's Department of Hospitals. In the latter half of the 20th century, the importance of GPOs became more apparent with increased aging of the population and tighter finances in both the public and private sectors. The number of GPOs in the early period had increased only slowly, with just ten in existence in 1962. The beginning of Medicare and Medicaid spurred greater growth, however, so that there were 40 in existence by 1974. Between 1974 and 1977, this number tripled. By 2007, there were several hundred GPOs throughout the United States, as well as subsidiary organizations and cooperatives; 96% of comprehensive hospitals and 98% of community clinics were now members of at least one GPO. One important point is that 97% of the not-for-profit private hospitals participated in group procurement, and 72% of hospital procurement in general went through contracts with GPOs.

GPOs vary widely in size, ownership, and services. Some are owned by hospitals while others exist independently. Some only provide specialized services to such institutions as non-profits and nursing homes, while others provide services to all kinds of institutions. There are also those who provide only medicines of a particular kind.

The operations of GPOs depend in part on administrative fees from drug suppliers. These are generally calculated according to the price of the medicines that the medical institution, with which the GPO has a contract, purchases. The GPO informs the medical institution of these administrative fees, and that institution then informs Medicare.

5 Price-formation of drug payments (reimbursement)

The actual payment price of drugs in the United States is the price that insurance pays when drugs are consumed, less a rebate. This price is mainly estimated by medical insurance (since actual purchasing prices are not disclosed under most circumstances). The rebate is mainly determined by negotiations between medical insurance and the authorized Pharmacy Benefit Manager.

6 Brief summary of drug price-formation mechanisms in the United States

Drug pricing in the U.S. mainly relies on negotiation, and the payer generally seeks to strengthen its bargaining power via two approaches. One approach is to gain a bargaining advantage by going through organizations that process a larger amount of drugs in the distribution process. At the retail end of the process, independent retailers therefore enter into agreements with Group Purchasing Organizations to carry out negotiations on their behalf, and they take advantage of the power of PSAOs to improve their negotiating capacity when it comes to payment. In negotiating rebates from manufacturers, all forms of insurance use the powerful intermediary role of Pharmacy Benefit Managers to gain higher rebates.

The second approach is for insurance to use its influence on patients and their purchasing intentions to create a bargaining advantage. This is generally seen when Pharmacy Benefit Managers seek to gain higher rebates for medical insurance through the use of formularies and drug hierarchies.

7 Lessons for China in how drug pricing works in the U.S.

1 Increase the transparency of drug pricing

In overall terms, prices of drugs in the U.S. are too high, and one main reason is that pricing is not transparent. The profits at each stage of sales and payment are essentially unknown, which provides the perfect opportunity to raise selling prices. This then indirectly causes the payment price at which insurance reimburses for drugs to rise to exorbitant heights. On the one hand, figures on drug rebates are not transparent, which leads to net prices being non-transparent. Net prices are equivalent to list prices less all kinds of rebates and discounts. Since the rebates that drug manufacturers pay out do not go through distributors or pharmacies, only third parties or pharmacy benefit managers know, so the net price of drugs are not available. Meanwhile, the markup at each stage of the process is very likely high. In addition, procurement prices of drugs are not transparent, which means that insurance payments, or reimbursements, must essentially be based on estimates.

Third parties (insurance companies) have no way of knowing the true price at which pharmacies are buying in drugs – all they can do is make estimates of drug costs through various ways in order to pay reimbursements. (In China), improving the transparency of drug pricing will therefore provide insurance with a better basis on which to price payments. It will help control medical costs and force the prices of drugs to fall in the course of distribution.

2 Put limits on drug rebates

In the United States, drug prices are basically not determined by doctors – the behavior of doctors is disengaged from pricing. Nevertheless, a tremendous amount of all kinds of rebates, preferential treatment, and kickbacks still exist and the total quantity is moving upwards at a fierce rate. The main reason patients pay such high out-of-pocket costs is that list prices for drugs are high and they are high due to rebates. Drug rebates are the means by which drug manufacturers expand the size of their markets. They provide Pharmacy Benefit Managers and insurance payers with profits. They also, however, lead to exorbitant list prices of drugs. Since patients pay out-of-pocket costs based on the percentage of a list price, their self-pay portion is also exorbitantly high. Therefore, (in China), prohibiting rebates on drugs may well be an effective way to hold down the increasing amount of self-pay that patients have to pay.

3 Raise bargaining capabilities of payers by promoting bargaining mechanisms

Pharmacy Benefit Managers are massive intermediary organizations – by managing drug formularies and drug tiers, they have effectively raised the bargaining power of medical insurance payers in the United States. In China, the establishment of the National Health Security Administration and its successful negotiations indicate that the country has already realized the key role that medical insurance, as payer, can play in lowering drug prices.

Abbreviations and acronyms

AMP: Average Manufacturer Price
CHAMPUS: Civilian Health and Medical Program of the Uniformed Services
CHIP: Children Health Insurance Plan
CMS: Center of Medicare and Medicaid Service
EAC: Estimated Acquisition Cost
FDA: Food and Drug Authorities
GPO: Group Purchasing Organization
HHS: The U.S. Department of Health and Human Services
IPI: International Pricing Index model
PBM: Pharmacy Benefit Management
PSAO: Pharmacy Services Administrative Organization
REMS: Risk Evaluation and Mitigation Strategies

2 Case study of the United Kingdom

2.1 Introduction to relevant conditions in the U.K.

2.1.1 Economic background

The full name of the U.K. is The United Kingdom of Great Britain and Northern Ireland. It is located in western Europe, has a land mass of 244,100 square kilometers, and in 2017 its population was 66.05 million. As the world's sixth largest economic entity, it has an advanced economy, and in 2018 its Gross Domestic Product totaled 2.03 trillion British pounds, or USD 2.4563 trillion. Per capita GDP in 2018 was 30,750 British pounds, or USD 37,207.5. The country's healthcare services system operates with high efficiency. Total medical and healthcare costs in 2018 came to 9.8% of GDP, or a per capita spending on healthcare of 451.1 British pounds. The burden of healthcare costs in the U.K. is lower than it is in the great majority of developed countries. The allocation of healthcare resources in the country is fairly reasonable – in 2018, there were 2.85 doctors per one thousand people, and in 2013, there were 28 hospital beds per one thousand people. In 2017, the average life expectancy of women was 83.1, and that of men, 79.5. The infant mortality rate in that year was 3.9%. In overall terms, the health status of people is quite high.

2.1.2 Medical services system

There is a clear-cut division of labor in the medical system of the U.K., with different levels of services. There are a total of 5,534 medical institutions in the country, which can be divided into two types or three levels. The two types are primary healthcare services, and emergency and hospital services. The three levels are community basic care institutions, regional hospitals, and training hospitals. Primary healthcare facilities provide routine clinic services and basic medical and public-health services to patients, and they are manned by general practitioners. The emergency and hospital services are provided by specialist physicians. Their services cover only those patients who have been referred from general practitioners or those who have emergency symptoms and need immediate treatment.

The U.K. has set up a mature and sound system of two-way referrals and hierarchical medical care (diagnosis and treatment):

First, the hierarchical system of medical care is based on high-quality general practitioners. The country puts great emphasis on the training of general practitioners – all must be certified and licensed by the Royal College of General Practitioners. Once they are employed, general practitioners must continue to further their professional development for the rest of their careers, which ensures that they have the ability to provide quality medical and healthcare services. Moreover, the U.K. makes sure that salaries are set at levels that provide incentives. Salaries of general practitioners are roughly three to four times general salary levels in the country, and they are even higher than salaries of specialists. In 2016, salaries of general practitioners were about 116,000 pounds per year (USD 140,360). Salaries of specialists were roughly 106,000 pounds per year (USD 128,260). The pay of general practitioners in the U.K. is the highest of any in Europe. It is far greater than salaries in Australia and Canada, and can even be more than twice the average income of other doctors. In addition, the U.K. has provided incentives for doctors through reform of payment methods. The main tool in this regard is the Quality and Outcomes Framework (QOF). The index system and scoring system of the QOF are quite specific – not only is the system easy to operate, but it is highly transparent and its fairness can be verified. At the same time, it recognizes the value of medical services. All of these things guide the professional behavior of general practitioners in the country, and motivate them to work in the interests of a patient's good health. Not only are they unwilling but they are also unable to do unethical things in order to receive 'gray' income.

Second, the two-way referral system in the U.K. has as its bedrock a very strict gatekeeper system. From birth, all residents of the U.K. must enter into contracts and the rate of agreeing to these contracts is essentially 100%. Other than emergency situations, when a British resident has a health problem, they first must be seen by the general practitioner from whom they have contracted to receive healthcare services (the gatekeeper). Treatment is then determined by the results of this first diagnostic visit. Once patients have been referred up to further, more specialized, medical care, and received such care, they are then again referred down to the general practitioner for rehabilitation and health maintenance. Statistics indicate that general practitioners cost the NHS just 10% of total spending but resolve nearly 95% of medical problems. Given the system, the people of England have become accustomed to waiting in orderly fashion to see a doctor – this has become a social custom, or one could even say a cultural atmosphere. It is rare that patients and doctors are in conflict with one another due to waiting. From time to time, however, unfortunate incidents are reported in which a patient's condition has deteriorated over the waiting time, to the extent that the patient has died.

2.1.3 Provision of healthcare resources

The provision of healthcare resources and their management are handled on a flat (as opposed to hierarchical) basis in the U.K. Management of all matters to do with health is concentrated in the Department of Health. This unified control extends to managing the National Health Service, the collection and allocation of funds for healthcare, and administering the provision and quality of medical services. The organization called NHS England determines the pricing of medical and healthcare services at the national level, and the scope of payment (reimbursement). It has jurisdiction over the Clinical Commissioning Group (CCG) of general practitioners. Specialty medical services and primary healthcare services in the country are purchased by the National Commissioning Board via the National Health Service, and this takes up around 40% of the budget of the NHS. The other 60% is taken up by community healthcare services, emergency medical care, mental health services, and so on, which are purchased through the CCG.

The Clinical Commissioning Group officially went online on April 1, 2013, after a period of trial operations that started in October 2010. By the time trial implementation was completed, CCG services covered essentially all of the U.K. At this time, local general practitioners unions are authorized to provide specific services and payment in all parts of the country, under the guidance of Clinical Commissioning Groups, which have the authority to set prices and adjust prices of services at the local level. When the NHS provides budgets to the CCG to carry out purchasing of medical services, the main method of allocating costs is called a 'weighted capital formula,' that is, weighted by per capita demand. When local CCGs purchase services for the local population, types of services may be different and methods of payment are therefore also different. Primary healthcare services are mainly paid for through payment in advance per capita. Community healthcare services are mainly paid for through payments by lump sum (block budgets) in advance, while payments for hospital services are mainly paid for according to results. Meanwhile, different standards for measuring performance correspond to different methods of payment, in order to ensure the quality of healthcare.

The NHS Monitor is the independent regulatory body of the National Health Service. It is responsible for regulatory supervision of all matters to do with medical and healthcare services, and it also holds certain authority with respect to pricing medical services. That is, it reviews and authorizes the CCG to announce price adjustments.

With specific regard to the subject of drugs, the U.K.'s public hospitals implement a 'separation of drugs and medicine' policy. That is, patients are provided with drugs only when they are actually hospitalized. Hospitals do not prescribe drugs for outpatient use. As a result, drug use in public hospitals only accounts for 20% to 30% of NHS spending on drugs, while private pharmacies are responsible for providing the rest (70% to 80%). Patients must pay a portion of the cost of drugs when they pick up prescription drugs at a pharmacy in all parts of England, with the exception of drugs for children under the age of 16, students over the age of 19, elderly people over the age of 60, people suffering from chronic diseases, and people who earn a low income. In Scotland, Northern Ireland, and Wales, drugs are entirely free.

2.1.4 Characteristics of the medical insurance system

The U.K. passed the Beveridge Report in 1942, which had a National Health Service as its central pillar. Based on this, the country formally proposed a 'national healthcare services act' in 1944; four years later the law was promulgated that set up the country's national health services system. The NHS is a key component of the country's welfare (benefits) system. It emphasizes the fairness of medical and healthcare services.

Medical and healthcare costs in the U.K. are mainly covered by general tax revenues and premiums from social (non-commercial) insurance. Around 11% of NHS funds come from national health insurance premiums, and around 81% come from the state budget. The very small remaining portion comes from non-free medical income and contributions from various philanthropic organizations. With a strong focus on the obligations of the state to provide healthcare benefits, the U.K. was the first country in the world to provide benefits 'from the cradle to the grave.' When the NHS was first set up, personal medical spending in the U.K. approached 2%, a figure which then began to rise. Since the early 1990s, however, the percentage of personal medical spending has gone from over 4% to the current slightly over 1%. This level is even less than it was 60 years ago. It can be seen from this that the level of medical and healthcare services provided by the NHS has improved notably over more than 60 years, and the safeguards that are provided to the country's citizens have also improved.

Each of the four regions of the U.K. manages its own health services independently (England, Scotland, Northern Ireland, and Wales). Although the Department of Health of the U.K. is responsible for healthcare matters of the entire country, the Department of Health only directly administers specific matters to do with England. The systems governing healthcare of citizens in the other three regions are handled by their own governments.

Starting in the 1990s, the NHS has undergone two major changes. One was the 'market-oriented reforms' that began in 1991, and the other was an intentional weakening of the internal market that began in 1997, when efforts were made to increase cooperation. The market-oriented reforms were required by the loss of vitality in healthcare markets due to the way the country's medical services were provided. Efficiency was very low. A plan was drawn up in 1985 called the *Green Paper on Social Security Reform*, and in 1989 a *White Paper on Reform of the Medical System* came out. Guided by these two documents, the main reform approach involved separating the purchasing of services from the provision of services. Reforms to weaken the internal market began after the Labor Party took power. Under the slogan 'New U.K., New Economy,' and using the Blair administration's White Paper on a new national health service, this mainly aimed to improve the asymmetry in information between patients and doctors, it bestowed greater autonomy on hospitals in order to incentivize them, and it started paying (reimbursing) on the basis of health results. These measures were aimed at two objectives: controlling the costs of medical insurance, and improving the results of services.

2.2 Drug price-formation mechanisms in the U.K.

In 2018, total sales of drugs in the U.K. came to USD 29.201 billion, or a per capita amount of USD 411.60. The country clearly displays the attributes of a 'welfare state' when it comes to the drug market. For example, in 2017, government purchases constituted 66% of all spending on retail drugs, which is higher than the OECD average of 58%, and individual co-pays (out-of-pocket costs) were 34%, which is lower than the OECD average of 39%. The market for generics in the U.K. has developed fairly well – in a ranking of generics to all drugs in the market, the U.K. ranked first among OECD countries (this includes ranking by share of value as well as share of quantity). Generics were 36% of all drugs in terms of value, which was higher than the OECD average of 25%, and they were 85% of all drugs in terms of quantity, which was far higher than the OECD average of 52%. Meanwhile, the number of professional (licensed) pharmacists in the U.K. is also increasing. In 2000, there were 60 pharmacists for every 100,000 people (close to the same figure as the OECD average), but this had increased to 88 in 2017 (higher than the average of 83 for OECD countries).

2.2.1 The drug system of the U.K.

The sphere of 'drugs' is quite broad and involves the various aspects of production and distribution, price determination and control, wholesale and retail and so on. The U.K. was quite early in formulating laws and systems pertaining to this whole subject, and it also modified its approaches from time to time as the situation changed.

First, with regard to drug production. In 1968, the U.K. promulgated the 'Drug Act,' which stipulated that any activity to do with drugs (production, supply, importing and exporting, and so on) must have the corresponding license and any other necessary credentials (including exemptions). There are four main licenses to do with drugs in the U.K.: a product license enabling the product to be sold on the market, a manufacturers' license, the wholesalers' license, and a license that enables clinical trials. In order to avoid conflict between drug production companies and drug marketing, the U.K. separates the permits that allow for the two activities. The specific organization that handles such permits is the MHRA: Medicines and Healthcare Products Regulatory Agency. The MHRA places certain requirements on manufacturers of drugs – their factories, equipment, and employees must meet qualifications and permits are granted for only five-year periods. Permits for selling drugs on the market are determined by such things as safety, effectiveness, and quality. Permits are granted only after both internal reviews and external reviews by specialists.

The pharmaceutical industry in the U.K. has developed quite well under the system outlined here. In 2012, the U.K. had a total of 387 drug manufacturers, and 17 of these ranked among the top 20 pharmaceutical companies in the world. These 17 companies employed 59% of all employees in the industry in the U.K.; their gross revenues totaled 68% of the industry total in the U.K. The U.K. has a large share of the global market – GlaxoSmithKline and AstraZeneca are two of the largest ten pharmaceutical companies on earth. From the late 1990s up to now, R&D spending by U.K. drug companies has consistently held a higher percentage of total R&D spending than any other country. The U.K.'s pharmaceutical industry is of major significance to the country's economy. According to 2012 statistics, drugs made a larger contribution to the balance of trade than any of eight other major industrial sectors.

Second, with regard to wholesale and retail trade in drugs: four relevant laws and acts set forth regulations to do with drug licensing and advertising (the 1968 Drug Act), drug storage and recording (the 1971 Drug Management Regulations), pharmacy professionals (the 1999 Health Act), and drug wholesale licenses (the

2005 Medicine for Human Use Regulations). Licenses (permits) for wholesalers are valid for five years.

Third, with regard to drug pricing and controls: in the U.K., companies may set their own prices for branded drugs. Price regulation mainly relies on the PPRS – the Pharmaceutical Price Regulation Scheme. This operates on the basis of voluntary participation and is non-contractual. Its objective is to ensure that the country's healthcare services sector can use and promote innovative drugs as quickly as possible that are safe, effective, have good clinical results, and are cost-effective. The idea is to guarantee the common interests of all sides as much as possible. The first edition of the PPRS came out in 1993, as determined through negotiations between the Department of Health and British Pharmaceutical Industry Association (ABPI). The PPRS is adjusted every five years. The 2014 version proposed the idea of a Patient Access Scheme which pharmaceutical companies should submit to NHS England. The Pharmaceutical Access Scheme is a pricing agreement, created by pharmaceutical companies, the purpose of which is to enable people who are sick to receive drugs they need that have a high cost basis. These plans, including new pricing agreements, are intended to further the ability of patients to get cost-effective drugs and other technologies. The 2014 PPRS came into effect when the 2009 PPRS expired and when the 2009 version expired, in January 2019, it was replaced with the VPA: the Voluntary Scheme for Branded Medicines Pricing and Access. The two are quite similar and have the same goal. The National Health Service and ABPI are participants in the VPA, as well as the U.K.'s Department of Health and Social Care. In a certain sense, the VPA is a new version of the PPRS. It also is valid for five years, from January 1, 2019, to 2023.

2.2.2 Subjects related to price-formation of drugs in the U.K.

Price-formation of drugs is a highly complex process that necessarily involves a number of entities (Figure 6.15). In overall terms, these include government, drug manufacturers, wholesalers, retailers, pharmacists, and patients.

First, with regard to officially authorized organizations such as the U.K. government. The Department of Health is responsible for formulating national policy on drugs. It holds negotiations with companies that make patented drugs, and it promotes the PPRS (Pharmaceutical Price Regulation Scheme), and it also is responsible for centralized procurement through a bidding process of generic drugs for hospitals within NHS England. The MHRA, or the Medicines and Healthcare Products Regulatory Agency, is responsible for reviewing and giving approval to drugs and medical equipment for selling on the market, as well as regulatory supervision. Under it are the Committee of Safety of Medicines, and the Chemistry, Pharmacy, and Standards Sub-committee, which assist in carrying out drug evaluations. The Licensing Authority is responsible for issuing licenses. The Prescription Pricing Authority of the U.K. has the authority to make decisions on pricing, which includes formulating prices for prescription drugs but also deciding on the reimbursable drug list.

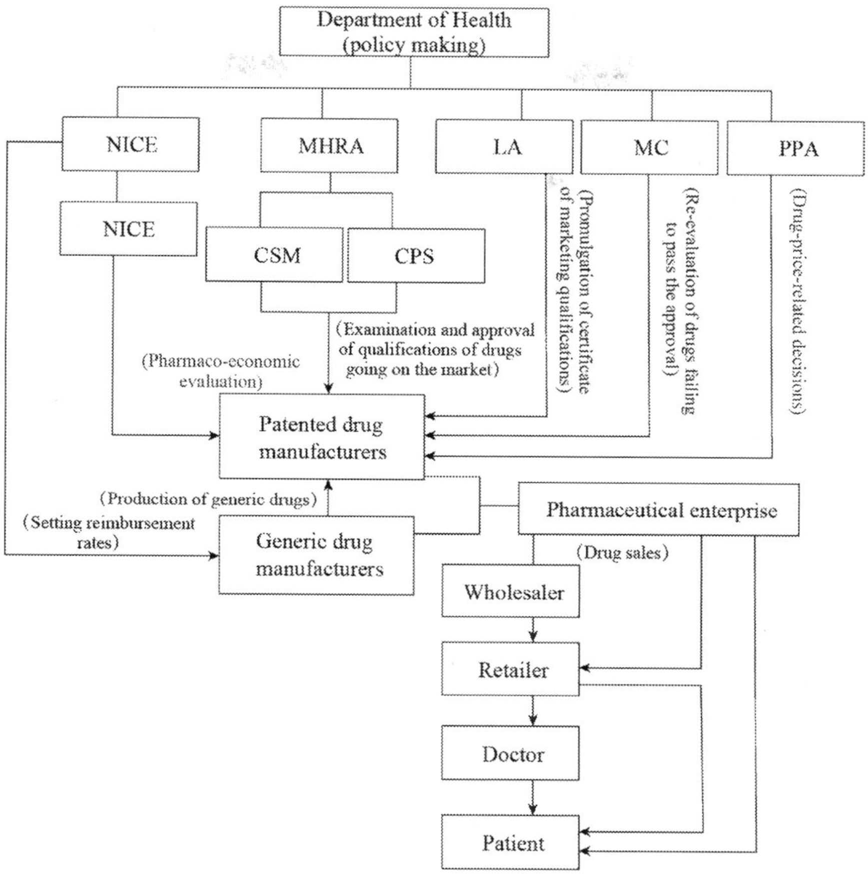

Figure 6.15 Relationship among the Primary Price-Formation Entities in the U.K.

The National Institute for Health and Care Excellence (NICE) is an organization that is financed by the NHS and that carries out pharmaco-economic evaluations. It presents its policy recommendations directly to the NHS and is supremely influential. At present, it has authorized nine evaluation centers in the country, including at the Royal Medical College, universities, and other places, in which nearly 2,000 clinical professionals, evidence-based medical experts, economists, clinical epidemiologists, and so on come together in teams to carry out health technology assessments and to formulate guidelines. This organization's activities cover four main areas. First, NICE assesses the cost-effectiveness of new drugs, medical equipment, and diagnostic and treatment procedures. The results of assessments directly determine whether or not a drug can be entered into the national reimbursable drug list. Second, it compiles guidance manuals on drugs that have already been put on the list, for the use of practicing physicians. Doctors use these as reference in making decisions on treatment methods. Third, it tests and evaluates the safety and effectiveness of drugs and medical technologies. Fourth, it composes guidance manuals on public safety at the individual patient level and community health level, covering such things as the standards for usage of needles, and health education. Except for subjects that impinge upon commercial confidentiality, the evaluations produced by NICE, and the procedures it undertakes in putting out its manuals are transparent and publicly available. The standards by which it decides whether or not to recommend a drug or a medical technology are not only the result of economic assessments, but also take into consideration the major impact such things as chronic diseases are having on a large range of people. Because of this, NICE does not set fixed requirements on the medical costs involved in decisions. NICE also does not take into consideration whether or not its recommendations will result in an added burden on public finance (the National Health Service). Its recommendations are based solely on evaluation standards. If the National Health Service determines it will be difficult to pay for something NICE has recommended, then it can refuse to adopt the recommendation. This situation has not yet occurred, however.

Second, with regard to drug manufacturers, wholesalers, and retailers: drug manufacturers include those who make innovative drugs and those who make generics. Innovative drug makers develop new drugs that, after review and approval, are placed on the market and enjoy patent protection for a specific period of time. Generic drug makers reproduce the ingredients in innovative drugs in order to make drugs that can be put on the market once patent protection of the original has expired. The efficacy of the generic is essentially the same as that of the original. The aims and requirements of the U.K. with respect to wholesalers are that drug supply should be uninterrupted and that it proceed through market competition in order to ensure efficiency in distribution. The drug wholesalers in the U.K. can be divided into two main categories. One type is a 'full-line' wholesaler that provides the majority of drugs on the market, and there are three of these. The second type is a 'short-line' wholesaler that only provides certain specialty drugs. This type is highly specialized and there are 50 of these. The full-line wholesalers occupy over 70% of the total value of the market. The gross profit that wholesalers can make from selling patented drugs is considerable, but these profits are subject to controls. What's more, some profits are lost due to discounts. The profits they can make from selling generics are not subject to controls. In the retail arena, community pharmacies are particularly important. There are three main sources of income for such pharmacies. They derive fees from their services in fulfilling prescriptions, their operations are subsidized when they provide health-related services, and they make profits off selling drugs. Right now, community pharmacies are expanding the types and range of services they provide. They are, for example, offering counseling on drugs and testing of patients who take drugs over a long period, and they are launching public-health related activities and disease-prevention activities.

Third, with regard to doctors and patients. Doctors decide what drugs patients should take and in what quantity, while patients are the ultimate consumers of drugs. How doctors prescribe drugs and how patients have a need (demand) for drugs are, to a large extent, what determine the price of drugs.

The role that doctors in the U.K. play in price-formation can be seen at all stages of the process. At the front end, when it comes to allowing access to the market and formulating clinical guides, the very powerful doctors' association influences market entry as well as list price, together with a small number of individuals. At the end-stage of the process, the prescribing of drugs basically follows the advice of user guides. If there are individual cases of specialized needs that do not fit into the guides, or if new drugs come to market that are urgently needed by patients, then special applications can be drawn up and submitted to the Department of Health, National Health Service, and NICE – these can request a revision of the guides or they can request an assessment of the new drug.

The citizens of the U.K. play a role in the pricing of drugs mainly through their participation in a group called the Citizens' Council. This consists of 30 members of the public who to the greatest extent can reflect the demographic characteristics of the population. Members of the council are recruited by independent organizations for a maximum term of three years. Each year, the Citizens' Council holds a two-day meeting that is open to the public. At this meeting, members solicit differing opinions of experts on a given subject, so that they can examine the issues in details and carry on thorough discussion based on their own points of view. Independent reporters collect the conclusions of members' discussions and opinions. Prior to finalizing the draft report, they circulate copies to members, solicit their advice, and then make revisions based on the results. Once the conference is over, the report is made public in order to solicit the opinions of the public at large. The summary of the opinions as well as the report are then passed on to the Board of Directors of NICE for further discussion. The Citizens' Council provides NICE with a public perspective on the primary moral and ethical issues that NICE must take into account in considering a given issue. The Citizens' Council safeguards the right of the public to participate in decision-making, but it is even more useful in facilitating public acceptance of and implementation of policies.

2.3 The process of and methods of drug price-formation in the U.K.

In the U.K., the methods of pricing patented drugs are different from those of generic drugs.

2.3.1 Price-formation for patented drugs

Only after a drug has been reviewed and approved can it be sold on the market as a patented drug (Figure 6.16). The U.K.'s Medicines and Healthcare Products Regulatory Agency (MHRA) was established in 2003. Once this Agency receives an application, it has two Committees within the Agency conduct assessments. These are the Committee of Safety of Medicines (CSM) and the Sub-committee of Chemistry, Pharmacy, and Standards (CPS). If the drug passes examination, the

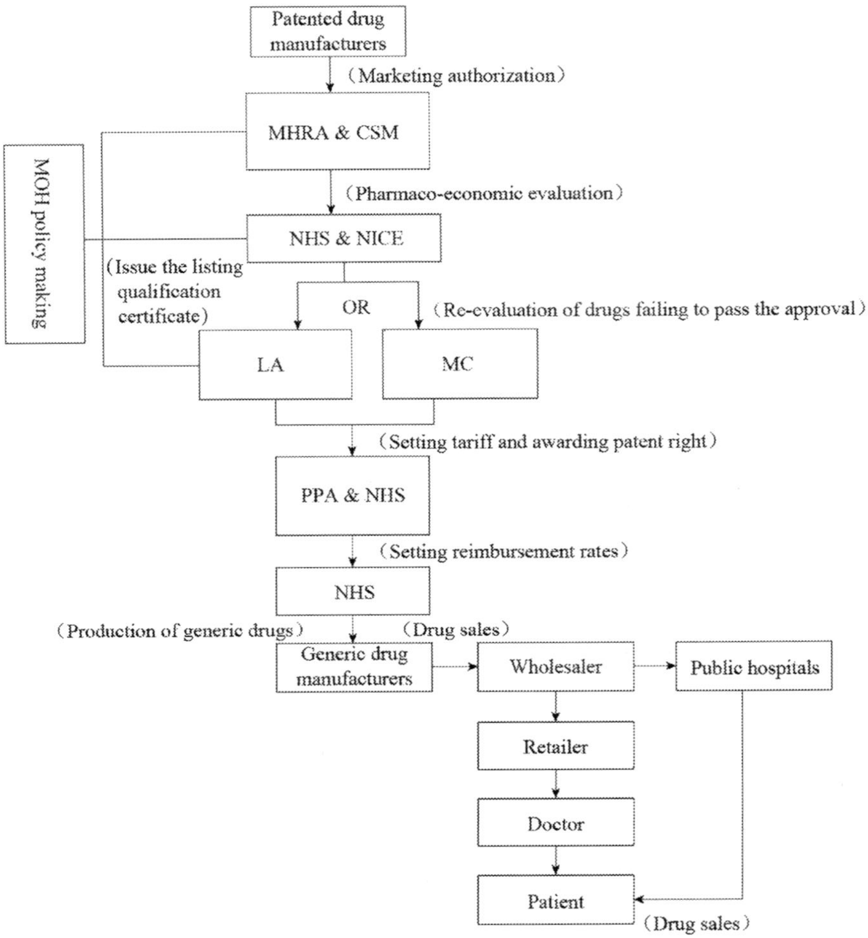

Figure 6.16 Flow Chart of Patented Drugs in the U.K.

Licensing Authority then issues a license to the company. If it does not pass, then the company can appeal and the Medicines Commission does a second assessment. It gives its feedback to the Licensing Authority along with its recommendation. Once a drug passes and is given a license, it enters into the U.K.'s list of prescription drugs, which is called the British National Formulary.

There is no official reimbursable drug list in the U.K. Any drug that receives a license to be sold on the market is automatically qualified to receive reimbursement from insurance, except for over-the-counter drugs, prescription drugs that are prescribed by private doctors outside the National Health Service system, and drugs in the two negative lists that are set up in accordance with the General Medical Service Regulations. The two negative lists refer to the 'black list,' for drugs that doctors are not allowed to prescribe, and the 'white list,' for drugs for which only patients with specific indications can be reimbursed.

There are two main ways the U.K. manages and controls the prices of patented drugs. The first is indirect, and seeks to control profits. The second is a kind of non-direct price control that uses the cost-benefit evaluations done by the NICE. A third approach is to use the overall management of spending on drugs as result of the newly added April 2019 cost-budgeting of NICE. Indirect control of prices through controlling profits is done by the Department of Health when it carries out annual profit assessments of the largest pharmaceutical companies. Such assessments look at the relationship between actual profits and a target upper limit of profits. Depending on the results, the Department of Health imposes management requirements, which can involve returning excess profits, or lowering prices. Controls are achieved mainly through the PPRS (prior to 2019) or the VPA (after 2019). Starting in 1993, the PPRS took over responsibility for managing the country's price controls. The scope of its responsibilities covers drugs that go over the NHS 'usage value' by 80%. It signs agreements once every five years, and it controls prices mainly by controlling profits. If drug manufacturers' profits go over the agreed-to amounts, then the excess must be returned to the government. If profits are below the 'excess profits' limit, then companies may raise profits accordingly. (In 2005, the highest profit rate was 140%, the lowest was 40%, and if profits were below 40%, they could be raised to 65%.) This plan has three main objectives. First, it aims to ensure drug quality as well as control prices. Second, it aims to encourage R&D and innovation. Third, it aims to ensure that the market for drugs is competitive. Drug manufacturers enter into agreements voluntarily. Participants must submit their financial reports to the government every year by a specified time. It should be noted that the prices that the PPRS controls are the list price of drugs. Manufacturers may still extend a certain percentage of discount when they sell drugs to wholesalers and pharmacies, that is based on the list price. At this point, they are more concerned about the welfare of patients than they are about the value of drugs. Because of this, on January 1, 2014, the U.K. began experimenting with a shift toward value-based pricing. This was later abandoned due to the way research impinged upon social ethics, but basing pricing on value was a sound concept that was worth exploring.

In contrast to the indirect method of controlling profits, the cost-benefit evaluations that NICE has launched have more direct results. The results of NICE's 'highly specialized technology assessments' are particularly notable. These take into consideration only drugs that are used under extremely rare circumstances (this is discussed in more detail later). Drug manufacturers, in order to guarantee their level of sales, will take into consideration their past levels of cost-effectiveness and will carry out their own price adjustments. They will voluntarily come to fairly reasonable pricing in order to qualify as prescription drugs that NICE recommends. The innovative drugs that NICE recommends come with legal requirements: within three months, they must be implemented by the National Health Service, which means that, within three months, all those patients who need to take new drugs that have been recommended by NICE must be able to have access to the new drugs.

The impact of the new cost-budgeting analysis has not yet been evaluated, but it is expected to have a definite influence on drug prices.

2.3.2 Price-formation for generic drugs

Prior to 2004, the U.K. adopted a Maximum Price Scheme with respect to price controls on generic drugs. The country was moved to adopt this measure in August 2000, given the constant price hikes in 1999, and it stipulated that this measure be protected by law. Given the limitations, drug manufacturers could not exceed certain prices when they sold to pharmacies and doctors. Detailed regulations were now also placed on the price of drug packaging. If the packaging of a given drug was not regulated then the drug used another similar drug on the market as reference. Using that as the basis, the price was figured according to the packaging ratio. Before drug manufacturers released new drugs or their packaging, they had to submit relevant information to the government, which then evaluated and set a maximum price.

The maximum price scheme was able to stabilize prices of generic drugs for a short period, but it was impossible to formulate reasonable prices for new generics. What's more, this scheme severed the connection between tariff prices and market prices. As a result, the scheme was replaced by the New Drug Tariff in 2004. Tariff prices are generally determined by the different concentrations of a drug (quantity of contents), the packaging, and the *ex factory* price (i.e., the average price at which the factory sells the drug after a quantity weighting). Three main types of generic drugs are the focus of tariff pricing. The first type involves generics that are produced by the great majority of drug manufacturers. In this case, the government only takes on a regulatory role while letting market competition lower the price of the drug. If the extent of price change exceeds a certain measurement value during the period of regulatory control, then the manufacturer is required to explain the situation. The second type involves new generic drugs. In this case, the government generally allows the manufacturer to set prices at a certain percentage of the price of the original prescription drug. After the drug has been on the market for a certain period of time, any necessary price adjustments are then required. The third type involves generics that are produced by just a small number of manufacturers. In this case, the government generally allows the enterprise to set a price in its application for the drug, once the maker provides materials that show its profit is reasonable, given a cost analysis (Figure 6.17).

The National Health Service is responsible for setting the reimbursement prices of generic drugs in the U.K., and pharmacies conduct their purchasing based on these prices. Reimbursement prices are related to the type of drugs and, in general, are equal to the average market price of the drug group. When pharmacies purchase generics, the difference between the higher reimbursement price and their purchasing price is their profit. However, by the terms of the profit recovery system

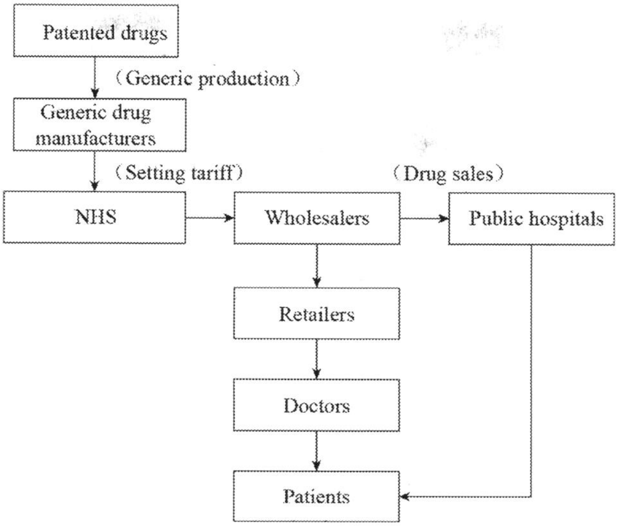

Figure 6.17 Flow Chart of Generic Drugs Circulation in the U.K.

in the U.K., pharmacies must return an average of roughly 9% of their profits to the NHS. If the price at which pharmacies buy in drugs is higher than the reimbursement price, then the pharmacy has to bear the cost of that difference. The General Practitioner system has a function that applies to the prescribing of drugs: if there is a generic for a given drug, the doctor first must automatically indicate the name of the generic when he writes out a prescription. This rule is to remind doctors to give preference to using generics.

2.3.3 The flow of drugs, contracts, and funds

2.3.3.1 METHODS BY WHICH DRUGS ARE DISTRIBUTED

The U.K. currently has two methods of distributing drugs. One is the traditional way and the other is a new way that meets the way times are changing. The traditional way comes in two forms. In the first, the drug manufacturer sells directly to hospitals. In the second, the manufacturer authorizes a wholesaler to sell to agents – the manufacturer can choose a sole agent or a number of agents who then sell on to retail pharmacies or general practitioners before the drug reaches the hands of the patient. The new way comes mainly in three forms. In the first, the drug manufacturer sells directly to community pharmacies. These get prescription information online and provide the drugs to patients based on the prescriptions. In the second, the drugs go directly from the drug manufacturer to the patients. In the third, the patient relies on home-care services to have drugs sent directly from a hospital to the home.

2.3.3.2 SIGNING CONTRACTS FOR DRUGS

First, patented drug companies sign contracts with the National Health Service, and companies join the PPRS on a voluntary basis. The PPRS signs or renews contracts once every five years. Once a company voluntarily joins the plan, it agrees to submit its financial information to the government every year by a prescribed time. After signing a contract, the company must accept the controls that the PPRS exercises over its price list. Right now, this mainly means accepting the pharmaco-economic evaluations of NICE in order to have drugs qualify for reimbursement status. Second, a patent drug company signs sales contracts with either a wholesaler or a retailer, after negotiations. Frequently the company will offer a discount to one or the other parties, based on sales quantity. Meanwhile, generic drug manufacturers must sign new price recovery (or tariff) contracts (with the government). While price-formation is determined by the market, companies must also accept government supervision over changes in their profits. The contracts that generic drug makers sign with wholesalers or retailers can be quite flexible and the profits derived from generics are somewhat less subject to government controls that those of patented drugs.

2.3.3.3 THE FLOW OF FUNDS

Patented drugs: only after patented drugs have been approved by NHS and undergone evaluation (assessment) by NICE are they eligible for reimbursement status. Such reimbursement funds can be received 90 days after receiving reimbursement status. When makers of patented drugs sell to wholesalers or retailers, or in few cases to hospitals and patients, the funds from the transactions go immediately from buyer to seller. At the same time, the wholesaler or retailer may then obtain the reimbursement from the NHS. Generic drugs: only once generic drugs have been sold in competitive markets do they form an initial kind of price. Based on that price, the government either carries out controls or adjustments, and it then dispenses reimbursement funds. Meanwhile, since there is more flexibility in negotiations between the generic drug maker and either wholesalers or retailers as buyers, there is greater room for profit, so the source of funds actually comes more from these buying entities.

2.4 The latest dynamics in price management of drugs in the U.K.

Price management measures are fairly well established in the U.K., and have achieved fairly notable results. In recent years, however, there have been certain developments and innovations. In 2014, the PPRS brought forth the Patient Access Scheme that allows for voluntary participation by drug companies. Participants must submit relevant plans to NHS England and the aim of this is to improve the accessibility (affordability) of high-cost drugs to patients. In January 2019, the VPA was put forward after the expiration of the PPRS. This represents a new form of voluntary plan and it is having a positive effect on controlling drug prices, stimulating drug innovation, and improving drug accessibility.

2.4.1 The 2014 edition of the PPRS and the 2019 VPA

First, two new mechanisms were added to the 2014 version of PPRS as compared to the 2009 version, in order to reflect value more accurately. These were Flexible Pricing and Patient Access Schemes, both of which are still in effect today, with the same substance and values.

On December 30, 2018, the term of the 2014 PPRS expired and the VPA came into effect in January of 2019. This plan's aims are as follows: first, improve the patient's opportunity to get drugs that are the most effective and at the best price; second, enable the NHS to bear the cost of branded drug bills by limiting the increase in sales of branded drugs; third, support innovation in the U.K. and its successful life sciences industry.

The VPA represents a further development of and evolution of the PPRS. In order to accommodate changing circumstances in the U.K., however, it has made corresponding adjustments while still maintaining many of the core aspects and values of the 2014 PPRS. These include Flexible Pricing and particularly Patient Access Schemes – at present, in fact, latter is carried on as set forth in the PPRS (a more detailed description follows). There have been minor adjustments to the Flexible Pricing. As called for in the 2014 PPRS, drug prices could be adjusted after March 1, 2014, but (drug manufacturers) had to notify the Department of Health and Social Security Department 28 days prior to such adjustment and they then had 21 days in which to respond. However, no applications for price adjustments would be allowed within two years of the expiration of this current plan, since that would jeopardize future price neutrality. In contrast, the 2019 VPA says that price increases must be announced eight weeks in advance, and price decreases must be announced 21 days in advance. Meanwhile, plan members must revise the information on their pricing of drugs and equipment within 24 hours of those prices being changed in the NHS price list (through the on-demand portal website).

2.4.2 Patient Access Schemes

Patient Access Schemes are price agreements that are proposed by drug companies, with the aim of enabling sick people to obtain high-cost drugs. These plans incorporate new price agreements, and drug companies participate voluntarily since they enhance the ability of patients to get specific drugs or other technologies.

The Department of Health has authorized NICE to set up a Patient Access Scheme Liaison Unit (PASLU) to cooperate with companies who are considering applying the plan to their drugs, so that this Unit can provide recommendations on the feasibility of company plans. The Unit is a part of the NICE Centre for Health Technology Evaluations. It coordinates the reviews and evaluations of patient access schemes, and submits recommendations to NHS England.

The PASLU evaluates Patient Access Schemes according to the principles set forth in the 2014 PPRS. That is, such plans should have clinical significance, clinical rationality, and appropriateness, and should be able to be monitored. According to the requirements of the 2014 PPRS, a plan may adopt one of two forms, namely complex or simple discount. The procedures for each of these are different and the simple discount plan allows for faster evaluation. A simple Patient Access Scheme can have a fixed price agreement that is set lower than the list price of a given treatment, or it can call for a discount of a certain percent off the list price. Since these plans are simpler than the complex version and also easier for NHS to administer, the PASLU's examination can undertake fairly low-level negotiations on them with the NHS – generally speaking, the PASLU can undertake an examination of this kind within four weeks. In contrast, the complex plans include such things as ceilings on outcomes-based doses, rebates, and upfront free stock. Due to the complexity of these plans, the PASLU's examinations must give them higher priority and negotiations with the NHS are at a higher level. A PASLU expert's group requires at least eight weeks of meetings after the application has been submitted, and the group must also consider whether or not the plan can be implemented in both NHS England and NHS Wales. The PASLU usually submits proposals to the NHS within four weeks of the expert group meeting, so the total review period takes at least 12 weeks. All complex proposals are considered by an independent expert group of the PAS, while simple discount proposals are not normally reviewed by expert groups. Final comments are signed off on by the Director of the NICE Center for Health Technology Evaluations (Complex PAS), or the Director of Technical Evaluations and Highly Specialized Technical Programs (Simple Discount PAS).

2.4.3 The 'highly specialized technology evaluations' of NICE, and its budgeting analysis

2.4.3.1 HIGHLY SPECIALIZED TECHNOLOGY EVALUATIONS

These are recommendations that NICE makes with respect to highly specialized drugs and treatment procedures that are either new to the National Health Service or already being used by the NHS. The subjects of most of these highly specialized technology evaluations are determined by the National Institute for Health Research Innovation Observatory. The goal of this organization is to notify the Departments of Health and Social Security of any key new and emerging medical technologies, and to make these technologies available to NICE within the following timeframes. Newly developed drugs: within 20 months of gaining market approval. New drug components: within 15 months of gaining market approval. The procedures for highly specialized technology evaluations are as follows.

First, according to the interim list of assessment subjects as compiled by DHSC, select interim subjects. Second, have consultants and evaluation experts confirm evaluation subjects. Third, NICE and DHSC cooperate to develop the scope within which the technologies and technology goals with respect to patients and illnesses are defined. Fourth, DHSC submits the HST evaluation subjects to NICE. Fifth, submit evidence: ask the developer of the technology or its funder to submit evidence. NICE also invites all non-developers who are advisers to submit a declaration of potential clinical results and cost-effectiveness of treatment. Sixth, NICE authorizes an independent academic center to do a technical review of the evidence that has been submitted, and it prepares an Evidence Review Group report. Seventh, write the assessment report. This relates to all evidence that will be reviewed by the committee, including any discussion and written statements of personal views by patient experts and clinical experts. Eighth, an independent advisory committee reviews the assessment report and listens to evidence from designated clinical experts, patients, and nursing staff. Discussions are open to the public. Ninth, as necessary, prepare an Evaluation consultation document. In the process of doing this, the evaluation committee presents its initial recommendations. Only when these recommendations are restrictive can the Evaluation consultation document be improved. The restrictive recommendations are more limited than the instructions accompanying the technology. Consultants and commentators will then have four weeks to comment on progress of the Evaluation consultation document. During this process, the document is also available for review on the official website, to facilitate opinions from professionals as well as the public. Tenth, produce a Final Evaluation determination. The evaluation committee takes into consideration opinions expressed on the Evaluation consultation document (if any), and it then makes its own final recommendations on how the technology should be used in the National Health Service (England) system. Consultants may raise appeals against this final proposal. Finally, publish the guidelines. If there are no objections, or if any appeals fail to gain support, then the recommendations are published as NICE guidelines.

2.4.3.2 NEWLY ADDED BUDGETARY ANALYSIS

The National Health Service (England) and NICE conducted a meeting to determine how to achieve certain objectives by using the NICE technology evaluations, the drug evaluations by HST, a number of other health technology evaluations, and, finally, how to handle financial arrangements. The objectives to be achieved were: faster access by patients to new treatment methods that are the most cost-effective; more flexible ways for the National Health Service system to adopt technologies that are cost-effective but have a major impact on budgets; improving the understanding of patients and companies with respect to treatments for rare diseases that are covered in NICE evaluations. After consultation, the Board of Directors confirmed the primary subject that was incorporated in the review and revision of HST methods as approved on July 17, 2019. Within these new methods was one on budget impacts. Specific recommendations were as follows.

First, incorporate a budget impact threshold of 20 million pounds (into decision-making). For technologies that come in below the budget impact threshold (i.e., that have gone through the NICE value evaluation using methods publicly announced by NICE), there is no need to carry out business negotiations. If the threshold is exceeded for any one of the first three years, however, this then triggers business negotiations. If the negotiations are not successful or if they do not completely resolve the budget impact issues, then England NHS will apply to NICE to change its funding requirements in order to be able to incorporate the product into National Health Service plans in stages and thereby control its budget impact.

Second, link together the NICE and NHSE processes of evaluating highly specialized technologies. Introduce the concept of Quality-Adjusted Life Years (QALY) as the standard by which to measure the value of HST plans. Apply the 100,000 pound 'limit' per QALY as a determining factor. Any technology costing lower than the limit would immediately enjoy legal funding mandates. (In the case of no budget impact, these mandates would apply immediately. If the budget impact threshold of 20 million pounds is triggered, then the mandates are gradually used for a period of time.) As for technologies whose calculated costs exceed 100,000 pounds per QALY, there would be an opportunity to consider funding through the relatively more preferential procedures of the Clinical Priorities Advisory Group within the National Health Service (England). This possible consideration takes into account the unique position of a very small number of sick people whose new form of treatment will be extremely expensive.

Third, introduce a new 'high-speed evaluation.' This recommendation recognizes that it should be possible to make a reliable determination about financial value in the early stages of doing an evaluation. This would then allow for a new high-speed evaluation with a shorter process. In addition, if recommendations are positive then the period of extended funding can be shortened to 30 days instead of 90 days. The consultation committee recommended that one of the standards for entering this 'high-speed lane' for approval was 10,000 pounds per every level of QALY. The reason was that, at this stage, they could predict with confidence whether or not a technology would have successful results. The budget impact threshold would still, however, be applicable to products that met the requirements of a fast-track evaluation process.

2.4.3.3 MANAGEMENT OF THE CANCER DRUGS FUND

The U.K. established the Cancer Drugs Fund in 2011 with the aim of providing cancer patients with faster free access to innovative and effective anticancer drugs. When it was first established, all such drugs, without exception, were entered into the list of drugs receiving government funding. Cost-effectiveness was not taken into account, and this situation continued all the way to the end of 2015. Due to the absence of sound scientific selection criteria and clear withdrawal criteria for drugs, however, financial pressures on the CDF were enormous in the years between 2011 and 2016. The unsustainable nature of the project became obvious. The annual budget of the CDF went from 200 million pounds in the 2011–2012 fiscal year to 340 million pounds in the 2015–2016 fiscal year. The actual funding in 2015–2016 came to 466 million pounds, however. That is, spending was in excess of the budget by 126 million pounds (37%). As a result, in October of 2015, the British government began to reform the CDF. It determined that there would no new inclusions of new drugs in the list, starting immediately, and it set up an independent third-party working group to take on the responsibility of doing evaluations. At the end of 2015, the NHS and NICE carried out public consultations with regard to the reform plan of the CDF. On February 26, 2016, the National Health Service gave approval to the reform plan, and on July 29, 2016, the CDF reform was officially implemented.

Once reforms had been implemented, all innovative anticancer drugs had to undergo evaluations by NICE prior to receiving permission to go on the market. The evaluations were based on safety and clinical effectiveness, with the degree of innovation and time sensitivity of a drug being allocated a weighting for purposes of a weighted calculation. Differential weightings were assigned based on the type of drug. In the course of evaluations, policy support might be extended depending on the audience for the drug. Once the drug went through the healthcare technology assessment of NICE, it was subject to three kinds of recommendations. The first recommended it for routine clinical use. The second did not recommend it for routine clinical use. The third recommended that it be used within the Cancer Drugs Fund. If the NICE recommendation did not confirm whether or not the drug conformed to the standards of routine use, then the drug could still be supplied for a short time while ongoing observations and evaluations were taking place. This could go on until there was a clear resolution. Meanwhile, as NICE carried out pharmaco-economic evaluations, it stressed the need to include the participation of multiple parties. All stakeholders were part of the process, including government, companies, the public, patients, and so on – all were invited to be either consultants or commentators, and all participated in decision-making that was transparent and open to the public.

2.5 The centralized procurement situation in the U.K.

The main entities involved in centralized procurement of drugs in the U.K. are public hospitals and community pharmacies.

2.5.1 Public hospitals

The drugs used in public hospitals account for around 20% of the overall drug-cost budget of the National Health Service. The hospitals use different methods of procurement for patented drugs and generic drugs.

First, patented drugs are not only subject to substantial price controls, but their price is essentially fixed and there is only one manufacturer per drug. As a result, patented drugs are not suited to centralized procurement by a bidding process. Generally, they are purchased by the hospital itself. Second, the specific bidding and signing of agreements for generic drugs is carried out by the Commercial Medicines Unit of the Health Department. Selections among companies who are bidding are made by taking into account four considerations, including price, quality, risk of supply disruptions, and the qualifications of the supplier. However, hospitals can decide voluntarily on whether or not to participate, and those that do participate sign their own purchase contracts with suppliers. To take the National Health Service of England as an example: the Department of Health divides the country into six regions, and the hospitals of each region form a procurement team.

The six procurement teams are then again divided into three groups, which generally have a term of two years. Generic drugs take up roughly 60% of the quantity of all drugs that public hospitals use, but just 20% of the funds that hospitals spend on drugs.

2.5.2 Community pharmacies

The drugs that community pharmacies procure (and then are reimbursed for) come to between 70% and 80% of the total NHS budget. Community pharmacies are more flexible than hospitals can be, so their negotiations with wholesalers and drug manufacturers are more flexible and they can obtain higher price discounts. These price discounts are also generally related to the quantity of drugs they buy, so large drugstores can buy in at prices that are below reimbursement prices. The reimbursement amount that they get from the NHS is the list price of the drug less the drug discount.

2.6 Methods of drug price-formation in the U.K.

In the past, the system for determining prices for reimbursement of drugs used in the U.K. attempted to use 'full-price evaluations' as guided by value-based purchasing concepts. Our study group carried out face-to-face discussions with the president of NICE, in order to fully understand the whole story of NICE and value-based purchasing. The system was suggested by the U.K.'s Department of Health in the Social Care Act of 2012 medical reform. After NICE had organized experts to research this subject for a while, it was discovered that this touched upon the bottom line of social ethics and it was inappropriate to continue the research. Research into value-based purchasing therefore stopped some time ago. However, the concepts and terminology of VBP have been retained up to today. The U.K. does not have an independent mechanism for pricing drug reimbursements or for determining prices in general. Once new drugs receive permission to be sold on the market, the drug manufacturer doing the R&D can be reimbursed for the entire amount of the price. The great majority of prescription drug costs can all be reimbursed. Because of this, the conclusions of NICE evaluations and the prices set publicly by the U.K. Medicines and Healthcare Administration are, in reality, an authorization to companies not only to put their drugs on the market but also to access drug reimbursement.

Reimbursement prices for drugs in the U.K. generally go through three necessary procedures. First, there is an examination of the basic issues of safety, quality, and effectiveness, which is completed in the drug warning system. Second, NICE does a VBP-based health technology evaluation (a pharmaco-economic evaluation). Third, an independent scientific committee estimates the cost-effectiveness of the drug using such indicators as quality-adjusted life years (QALYs). Once these three procedures are over, the National Health Service then references the price that the drug manufacturer reports and formulates a final reimbursement price. This price must be lower than the price reported by the manufacturer.

Once NICE carries out an evaluation of value and formulates a price, depending on the results of its discussions with the drug manufacturer, it can come up with five types of recommendations: recommend for reimbursement, reimburse after improvements, restrict use, only use in research, and do not recommend use. The National Health Service then makes its decisions on reimbursement and price based on the recommendations of NICE. Within 90 days of making its decisions public, it pays reimbursement to the drug manufacturer.

After the decision on reimbursement and price is made, and funds are allocated, the drug enters the process of being re-evaluated. In this process, NICE can collect indicators of the real value of observed clinical results. Combining those with non-linear VBP reimbursement, QALY weighting, fund adjustment, and other theories, it does micro-adjustments of the drug price and spending of funds. If any major problems appear at this time, then the reimbursement list is promptly adjusted.

2.7 Drug-pricing mechanisms of the U.K.: a summary

The pricing of drugs is a complex process. In the U.K., once a company making patented drugs has developed a new drug, it can receive a permit issued by LA (the Licensing Authority) only after being allowed to sell on the market by the organizations under the MHRA, CSM, and CPS. When necessary, it also sometimes must go through the MC for re-evaluation. After that, it goes through the pharmaco-economic evaluations of the National Health Service and its evaluating organization NICE, relying on VBP with respect to effectiveness, safety, quality, and so on. Once these processes are completed, a reimbursement price is formed and the drug is qualified to be reimbursed and receive compensation, but it still has to go through subsequent regulatory examination and supervision. Finally, and only then, can it start business relationships with such buyers as wholesalers, retailers, as well as hospitals and patients. The price-formation mechanisms of generics drugs are less complex, in relative terms. Prices are mainly formed through market competition but they are then monitored and regulated by the National Health Service before the drug is allowed to go through subsequent drug distribution.

The price-formation of drugs in the U.K. possesses the following most notable characteristics.

First, the overall orientation is to focus on profit-control mechanisms. From the PPRS to VPA, controls over drug prices in the U.K. are carried out to ensure two main principles, namely to be cost-effective and to keep prices down to the greatest extent. In achieving these principles, the U.K. shows tremendous flexibility.

Second, decisions on market access and price determination for innovative drugs are centered on the patient, using evidence-based decision-making. In the course of determining market access and pricing for innovative drugs in the U.K., NICE's healthcare technology assessments play an indispensable role. All organizations must go through NICE's patient-centered evaluations, whether they are TA, HST, or CDF, and they must be given recommendations on use of the drug. Experience has proven that drugs that have not gone through the evaluation process can very easily lead to waste of financial resources, adding to the burden on public finance.

Third, with regard to healthcare technology assessments and an innovative spirit: the U.K. is relatively experienced in using this methodology, having been through constant explorations and attempts to improve the process. This expresses the country's willingness to try new methods and its innovative spirit in being proactive about new technologies.

Fourth, with regard to open and transparent operations and processes: the U.K. places special emphasis on the openness and transparency of processes, whether they involve the healthcare technology assessments and recommendations of NICE, or the participation of doctors and patients. This spirit of openness is precisely what enables policies to be broadly accepted by the public and what therefore enables smooth implementation.

Fifth, with regard to using guidelines on the clinical use of drugs as a form of end-point management: the U.K. focuses on the 'supply side' in its controls over drugs. By making use of clinical guidelines, it is able to limit behavior on the part of doctors, that is, to control the hand that writes the prescriptions. At the same time, the U.K. welcomes the participation of doctors and the doctors' association in decisions on market access of drugs, which ultimately benefits the degree of enforcement that is needed at the end-point of drug usage.

Sixth, the U.K. is strongly in favor of the participation of patients in decision-making, and takes steps to ensure that such participation actually happens. It has specifically set up a 'citizens' committee' to that end. Having mechanisms that allow for multiple parties to participate in decision-making is beneficial to effective implementation of policies.

Seventh, with regard to making the use of generic drugs the routine and standard option: in the U.K., the quality of generics is able to be guaranteed, which allows for their widespread use. This has even become the standard practice. Within the General Practitioner system, generics are generally prescribed to treat common diseases.

Eighth, the U.K. encourages pharmaceutical innovation. This is particularly obvious in the policy bias when determining prices and considering market access for innovative drugs. The main evidence is allowing innovative drugs to have a higher cost-effectiveness threshold in receiving approvals.

Abbreviations and acronyms

CCG: Clinical Commissioning Group
CPAG: Clinical Priorities Advisory Group
CPD: Continuing professional development
CPS: The Chemistry, Pharmacy, and Standards Sub-committee
CSM: The Committee of Safety of Medicines
DH: Department of Health
DHSC: The Department of Health and Social Care
FED: Final evaluation determination
HST: Highly specialized technology
LA: The Licensing Authority

MC:	The Medicines Commission
MHRA:	Medicines and Healthcare Products Regulatory Agency
NCB:	National Commissioning Board
NHS:	National Health Service
NICE:	The National Institute for Health and Care Excellence
PAS:	Patient Access Scheme
PASLU:	The Patient Access Scheme Liaison Unit
PPA:	The Prescription Pricing Authority
PPRS:	Pharmaceutical Price Regulation Scheme
QALY:	Quality-adjusted life years
QOF:	Quality and Outcomes Framework
RCGP:	Royal College of General Practitioners
VPA:	Voluntary Scheme for Branded Medicines Pricing and Access

3 Case study of Germany

3.1 General introduction to the country

3.1.1 Basic characteristics of the economic structure

Situated in the middle of Europe, Germany covers an area of 357,022 square kilometers and is composed of 16 states, 13,552 towns, and 14,808 districts. It has a population of 80.2 million people and operates as a federation. As the fifth largest economic entity in the world, Germany has high levels of income, high taxes, and high social benefits. In 2018, its GDP was around USD 4.4 trillion, which gave it a GDP per capita of USD 53,089. Healthcare costs constituted 11.5% of GDP – this ranked the country at tenth in the world, lower than the average level of developed countries (Figure 6.18).

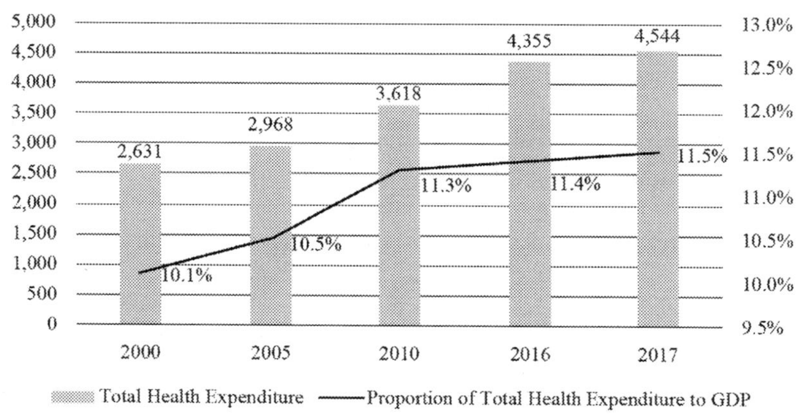

Figure 6.18 Total Healthcare Expenditure in Germany (Million Euro) and Percentage of GDP from 2000 to 2017

Source: German Federal Database

3.1.2 Characteristics of the medical system

Given the plentiful human and material resources of Germany's healthcare and medical system, the citizens of the country have access to excellent care at a relatively low price. In 2018, there were 2.85 doctors per one thousand people, and eight hospital beds per one thousand people. In 2017, the average life expectancy of females was 83.4 years, and of males, 78.8 years, and the infant mortality rate was 3.3%. Levels of health are fairly high.

Outpatient care is mainly provided by individual professionals, including doctors, dentists, psychotherapists, and other such healthcare specialists. Patients generally first see family doctors (Hausarzt), including general practitioners, internists, and pediatricians, and then the family doctor refers them to specialists, such as dermatologists, gynecologists, and so on. Patients may also, however, go directly to specialists without being referred. In addition, outpatient services are offered at clinic alliances and medical health centers (these places generally have two or more doctors). Large alliances of clinics, called 'practice hospitals,' can also provide services that are similar to those of hospitals, such as specialized examinations or outpatient procedures. Hospital-type non-overnight care can also be provided by clinics.

Inpatient care is mainly assumed by hospitals. Germany's large hospitals are subsidized by the government, while other hospitals are run by philanthropies or churches, including those run by the Red Cross or religious groups. Some private hospitals only treat patients who are covered by personal insurance – these are generally small and highly specialized. Hospitalized treatment includes situations that require an overnight stay, but it also includes hospitalized rehabilitation, including physiotherapy, psychiatric treatment, and helping patients learn how to use medical aids and equipment (Table 6.7).

With respect to the market for pharmaceuticals: Germany has a large drug market and a system of clinical trials that is highly efficient and of high quality. Its legal framework and regulations on market entry and reimbursement are quite rigorous. In 2017, the global market for pharmaceuticals came to USD 1.07 trillion. Of this amount, Germany's market totaled USD 43 billion, ranking it fourth in the world and the largest among Europe's markets (Table 6.8; Figures 6.19, 6.20).

Germany's healthcare system is divided into three tiers, federal, state, and autonomous institutions. The federal healthcare departments are responsible for formulating laws and drafting administrative guidelines and policies. Each state is responsible for hospital planning and for investing in and funding hospitals.

Table 6.7 Overview of German Hospitals in 2017

Number of Hospitals	*Number of Ward Beds*	*Number of Health Workers*
1,942	497,182	186,021
Number of ward beds per capita	Number of health workers per capita	
0.006	0.002	

Table 6.8 Size of the Market for Drugs in Certain European Countries, 2016

EU Member Countries	*Business Revenues (Billion)*	
	US Dollar	*Euro*
Germany	$44.20	£ 40.98
France	$33.11	£ 30.69
Italy	$29.03	£ 26.91
The U.K.	$26.41	£ 24.48
Spain	$21.13	£ 19.59

Note: Manufacturers' business revenues refer to drugs' *ex factory* prices

Source: IGES based on BPI e. V. (Federal Association of the Pharmaceutical Industry), Pharmadaten 2017, p. 40

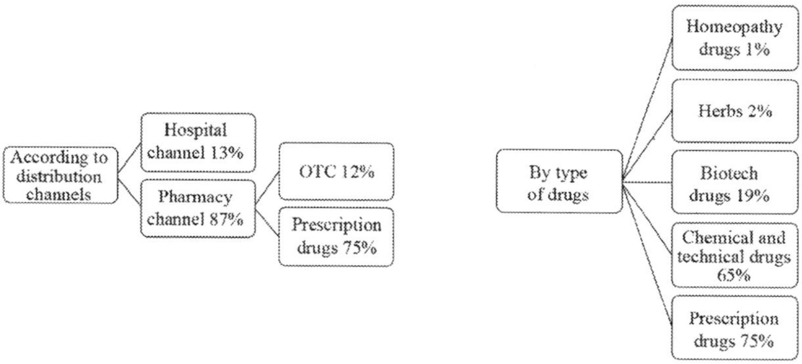

Figure 6.19 Size of the Market for Different Types of Drugs in Germany, 2016 (as Calculated by Profit)

Source: IMS Health Report 2016

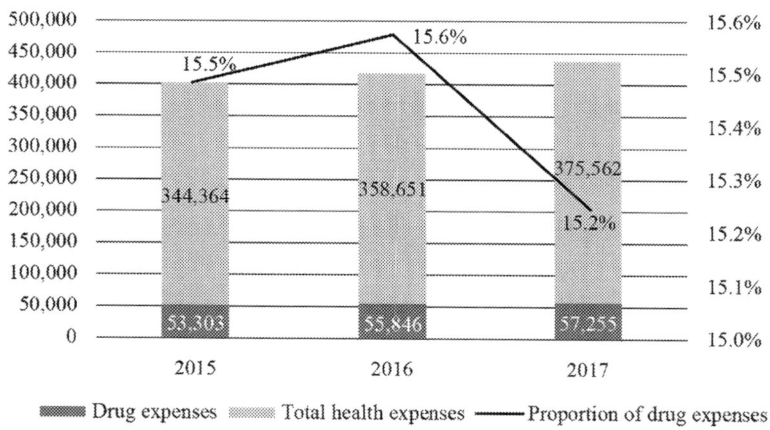

Figure 6.20 Expenditures on Drugs in Germany and their Percentage in Total Healthcare Spending, 2015–2017

Source: German Federal Database

Such autonomous organizations as 'sickness funds' and provider associations are gathered together into a Federal Joint Committee. This committee is responsible for transforming legislative goals into concrete provisions. Regulatory details are determined by the Federal Joint Committee (Gemeinsamer Bundesausschuss, or G-BA). The G-BA is the most important self-governing decision-making body involved in healthcare.

3.1.3 Characteristics of the medical insurance system

Germany established a statutory health insurance system in 1883 (called the GKV, for Gesetzliche Krankenversicherung). It was the first country in the world to set up such a nationwide social insurance system. Together with the alternative private healthcare insurance (Krankenversicherung, or PKV), this social insurance pays for the medical insurance of the country's citizens.

The GKV (social insurance), supported by roughly 100 statutory health insurance funds, provides comprehensive medical insurance services to citizens. GKV covers a package of goods and services that are legally defined at a national level, while the G-BA decides which specific goods and services can be included in the package. The private insurance plan, PKV, also provides a package of services that is similar to the statutory medical insurance, but PKV has more flexibility in expanding or limiting the scope of its safeguards.

All citizens of Germany must purchase health insurance. The GKV is a mandatory insurance plan and under normal circumstances all residents must accept it. Only if certain requirements are met (such as annual income, self-employment, and so on) can a person choose to be covered by PKV. In 2017, 71.2% of German residents were covered by GKV, while 8.8% were recipients of PKV and the national aid insurance (Figure 6.21).

The statutory (social) and private insurance programs, GKV and PKV, must observe different rules and regulations when it comes to financing and payment. The

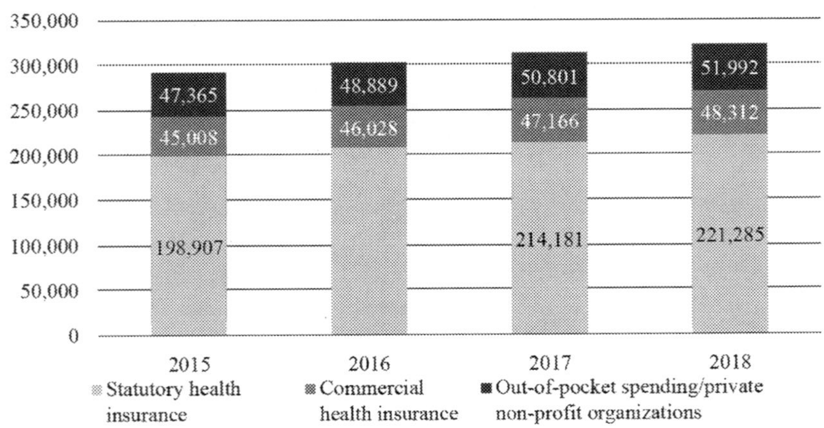

Figure 6.21 Data on Who Pays for Healthcare Costs in Germany, 2015–2018

Source: Federal Statistical Office of Germany

premiums of beneficiaries of GKV are related to wages, so GKV funds are highly cyclical. In 2018, GKV funds realized a surplus of about 2 billion euros, and accumulated financial reserves were in excess of 2.1 billion euros. This was equivalent to over one month's worth of GKV spending, and was more than four times the legally required lower limit of reserves. The medical insurance funds are consolidated or pooled in the country's central fund, and then are re-distributed to various sub-funds according to a risk-balancing plan. The payments made to PKV are determined by the risk preferences of individuals, and the premiums are higher than those of GKV.

3.2 Price-formation mechanisms of drugs

3.2.1 Germany's drug system

3.2.1.1 A REVIEW OF DRUG POLICIES

1998 Germany began using a price-reference system.

2003 The Contribution Safety Act introduced the possibility of having the Federal Health Insurance Fund sign rebate contracts with drug manufacturers for them to obtain rebates.

2004 The GKV and the IQWiG (the Institute for Quality and Efficiency in Healthcare), which is mainly responsible for evaluating any additional benefits of drugs, were established in accordance with the Statutory Health Insurance Modernization Act.

2007 The Medical Insurance Act on Strengthening Competition provided for rules to promote the signing of rebate contracts.

2011 The Pharmaceuticals Market Reorganization Act (Arzneimittel markt Neuordnungsgesetz, or AMNOG) was implemented. This is the key price-regulation mechanism for innovative pharmaceuticals. Its process comprises two phases, starting with health technology assessments by G-BA, and then reimbursement price negotiations between the manufacturer and GKV-SV (Association of Statutory Health Insurance Funds). The Act stipulated that new drugs can still enjoy the right of self-determined pricing in the first year on the market, but a negotiated reimbursement price applies as of the 13th month after the initial product launch of the new pharmaceutical in Germany.

3.2.1.2 CHARACTERISTICS OF GERMANY'S DRUG POLICIES

Germany's social insurance (GKV) uses a negative list in reimbursing for medicines – that is, it lists drugs for which it will not reimburse. Basically all drugs that are allowed on the market can be reimbursed by medical insurance, except for those outside the scope of coverage as defined by regulations (such as over-the-counter drugs), and except for those that have been excluded from coverage after a determination by G-BA.

Germany's drug policies attempt to coordinate two objectives. One is to encourage innovation (prices of drugs are determined by the manufacturer when the drug comes to market), and the other is to ensure that medical funds are being used effectively (drugs are grouped according to equivalent effectiveness, and a maximum reimbursement rate is set for different groups, while generic drugs are procured through a bidding process, and various measures encourage rational prescribing). However, since the end of 2008, medical insurance has been hoping to change its passive function of having to accept the pricing of new drugs that cannot be fit into an equivalent group. Starting in 2007, the Medical Insurance Act on Strengthening Competition asked the Institute for Quality and Efficiency in Healthcare (IQWiG) to carry out cost-benefit assessments. The results then become the basis for determining the reimbursement prices. After many months of work and consultations among experts, the IQWiG issued assessment method, but the AMNOG went into effect in January of 2011 before these methods could be put into practice.

3.2.2 Introduction to entities involved in price-formation of drugs

3.2.2.1 FEDERAL JOINT COMMISSION (G-BA)

The Federal Joint Commission (G-BA) was set up in accordance with the Statutory Health Insurance Modernization Act of 2004. The legal basis of the G-BA is the No. 5 Book of the German Social Code. It is the highest decision-making body in a self-governing system composed of all relevant stakeholders. As a decision-making entity, it participates in pricing new drugs and is responsible for determining the scope of products and services that medical insurance will reimburse. It also formulates regulations for use in actual practice. The most important function of G-BA is to decide on the scope of coverage that insurance will reimburse. It determines specifically which non-prescription drugs may receive reimbursement, and it formulates a list of those innovative drugs for which it is impossible to prove sufficient efficacy. It chooses which products to exclude from the scope of insurance coverage, and it defines a reference-price group. Once a drug is put on the market, drug manufacturers must immediately submit documentation on the value of the drug to G-BA. After this, the G-BA authorizes IQWiG to evaluate any additional benefits of those that are innovative and to organize the grouping of those that are non-innovative.

The G-BA is composed of representatives of the Federal Medical Insurance Fund Association (GKV-Spitzenverband, GKV-SV), the German Hospital Alliance (DKG), the National Association of Statutory Health Insurers (KBV), and the National Association of Statutory Health Insurers (KZBV). The G-BA Plenary Session is a decision-making body that consists of a plenary session chairperson, two plenary session members, two hospital representatives, two doctors' representatives, one dentist representative, and five health insurance fund representatives, all of whom have voting rights. Patient representatives may also participate in G-BA plenary sessions and receive consultation from members. Within G-BA, the drug sub-committee is responsible for drug evaluation. The sub-committee consists of the chairperson, vice-chairperson, three hospital representatives, three doctors' representatives and six representatives of the disease fund. The G-BA Drug Sub-committee is responsible for evaluating the therapeutic benefits of new drugs and asking its working group to prepare an evaluation draft.

3.2.2.2 INSTITUTE FOR QUALITY AND EFFICIENCY IN HEALTHCARE (IQWIG)

The Institute for Quality and Efficiency in Healthcare (Institut für Qualität und Wirtschaftlichkeit im Gesundheitswesen, IQWiG) was established in 2004, and was initially responsible for assessing the clinical effectiveness of drugs. In 2007, its functions were expanded to include cost-effectiveness assessments. The Institute is independent and is authorized by other entities to carry out the actual work of evaluating the quality and efficiency of healthcare services and products. It is the second-most important organization in the process of bringing new drugs to market.

The IQWiG mainly takes on assessments as requested by G-BA, but the Federal Department of Health, patient representatives in G-BA, and the commissioner in charge of patient issues in the federal government can also ask it to conduct assessments. The Institute does not have the authority to formulate regulations or decide on whether or not a given drug can be reimbursed. Instead, as a research organization, it provides the evidence-based results of assessments to decision makers to facilitate their decisions. In the context of the AMNOG process, IQWiG's results are open to external stakeholders and it also takes in external opinions. Doctors, physicians' associations, interest groups, and pharmaceutical manufacturers' academic groups or associations can all submit written responses after IQWiG issues an assessment, and then hold public hearings. Manufacturers can submit other data during this process, and based on this additional information, G-BA can make decisions that are different from the IQWiG assessment.

The IQWiG employs around 140 people, half of whom are experts and scholars. The Institute's governing board is made up of representatives from the Federal Ministry of Health (BMG), health insurance funds, hospitals, physicians, and G-BA.

3.2.2.3 THE FEDERAL MINISTRY OF HEALTH (BMG)

The Federal Ministry of Health (Bundesministerium fur Gesundheit, BMG) is the competent federal authority for all health-related issues in Germany. It drafts bills, decrees administrative regulations on issues in the fields of health, prevention, and long-term care. The Federal Ministry of Health is responsible for supervising a number of government agencies that deal with health systems, including the Federal Joint Committee (G-BA) and the Institute for Quality and Efficiency in Healthcare (IQWiG).

3.2.2.4 THE ARBITRATION COMMISSION

The role of the Arbitration Commission is to serve as arbitrator on prices when no agreement can be reached in price negotiations for new drugs. The commission consists of one impartial chairperson and two impartial members, who serve for a term of four years. In addition, both sides in the dispute must nominate two additional members (the parties include the drug manufacturer and GKV-SV, see next). After the Department of Health solicits the opinions of GKV-SV and people in the industry, it has the authority to fire arbitration personnel if there is good and sufficient reason. Patient organizations are allowed to participate in meetings of arbitration personnel.

3.2.2.5 THE FEDERAL HEALTH INSURANCE FUND ASSOCIATION (GKV-SV)

The Federal Health Insurance Fund Association was established after the medical reform of 2007. It is the federal-level association of all health insurance funds. The GKV-SV is the central lobbying group of GKV (Gesetzliche Krankenversicherung), and it has shaped the basic conditions of medicine and healthcare in Germany.

The CKV-SV (GKV-Spitzenverband) has a short history, but its main function in the process of pricing new drugs is to conclude agreements on reimbursement prices with the relevant manufacturers.

3.2.2.6 THE GERMAN RESEARCH CENTER OF MEDICAL DOCUMENTATION AND INFORMATION (DIMDI)

This Research Center (Deutsches Institution für Medizinische Dokumentation Und Information, DIMDI) is under the jurisdiction of the German Federal Ministry of Health. It provides information via the Internet for all spheres in Germany's healthcare system, and it is responsible for developing and operating Germany's data information system on drugs and Health Technology Assessments (HTA). As authorized by the government, it publicizes the latest information on drug prices, among other data. Making this information public helps guide patients in their choices on what drugs to use and also encourages drug manufacturers to set appropriate sales prices.

3.2.2.7 RESEARCH INSTITUTE ON THE REIMBURSEMENT SYSTEM OF HOSPITALS (INEK)

This Institute (InEK, Institution für das Entgeltsystem IM Krankenhaus), was established in 2001 and is responsible for managing and developing G-DRG. This includes defining G-DRG, processing and updating coding standards, and taking in applications from hospitals for additional reimbursement.

3.2.3 Drug price-formation process

3.2.3.1 PRICE-FORMATION IN THE COURSE OF DRUG ALLOCATION (DISTRIBUTION)

Germany's drug manufacturers initially set their own list prices on drugs. After they do this, retail drugs go through wholesalers and retail pharmacies to reach the hands of patients. The profit markup that retail pharmacies may charge on each kind of drug is fixed.

The profit margin at each link in the retail channel is as follows:

1 Wholesalers' profit margins vary but average 4%.
2 The profit that pharmacists get from each prescription is 8.1 euros, plus 3% of the wholesale price. Profits from non-prescription drugs vary.
3 The federal government charges a 19% value-added tax.

Drugs that go directly into the inpatient departments of hospitals may decide on procurement methods by themselves, but Group Purchasing Organizations also exist and drugs are also procured through them. For details, see Part IV, Group procurement of drugs.

3.2.3.2 PRICE-FORMATION IN THE COURSE OF DRUG PAYMENT

3.2.3.2.1 Outpatient drugs Drug manufacturers may set initial list prices of drugs as they wish in Germany. As for the prices at which drugs are reimbursed, those drugs that are new to the market have prices determined mainly through additional-benefit assessments of the drug, negotiations, and comparison to reference prices. Payment prices for generic drugs are determined directly through reference prices. Statutory health insurance does not reimburse for drugs that are on the G-BA negative drug list.

When a drug enters the market for the first time, drug manufacturers may receive GKV payment according to list prices that they have set themselves. This payment price (reimbursement price) can continue for one year. Around the time a drug is put on the market, its manufacturer must provide documentation on the effectiveness of the drug, and the documentation must have proof of additional therapeutic benefits of any new drug. As for reference prices, these must refer to a drug for which the G-BA has generated prices according to current care standards (Figure 6.22).

Within three months of being on the market, a new drug must have gone through an assessment that compares its therapeutic results to those of a reference drug. The G-BA has the task of issuing evaluations to the IQWiG (the Institute for Quality and Efficiency in Healthcare). The G-BA not only carries out the actual

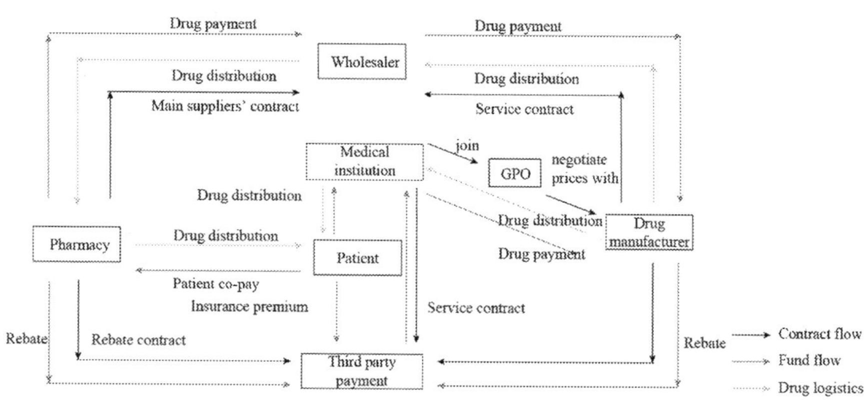

Figure 6.22 Price-Formation Mechanisms for Drug Prices in Germany

assessment but also issues the report. Once reports are published, external stakeholders have the opportunity to present written and oral statements on the results.

Within another three months after the release of the additional-benefits assessment, the G-BA may issue a resolution stating that the additional therapeutic benefits of a given drug are in accord with the treatment needs of a given patient group and the costs of treatment are similar to those of other drugs. This resolution determines the reimbursement price at which the drug will be reimbursed for the first year it is on the market.

Within the next six months, if the drug does indeed show added therapeutic benefits, then the drug manufacturer and GKV-SV will come together again to renegotiate the price of insurance payments. If agreement cannot be reached, then the decision on price goes to arbitration. The price set by arbitrators applies from the 13th month that the drug is on the market.

If, however, the new drug does not exceed the additional therapeutic benefits of the care standard, then G-BA will incorporate the new drug into the existing group of reference prices, and will set the ceiling on reimbursement for the group. If the drug cannot be incorporated into an existing group of reference prices, then there will be a price negotiation that is similar in method to the one for drugs that do have additional benefits, but the goal of the negotiation will be to set a price such that the annual treatment costs of the new drug do not exceed the costs of existing treatment (Figure 6.23).

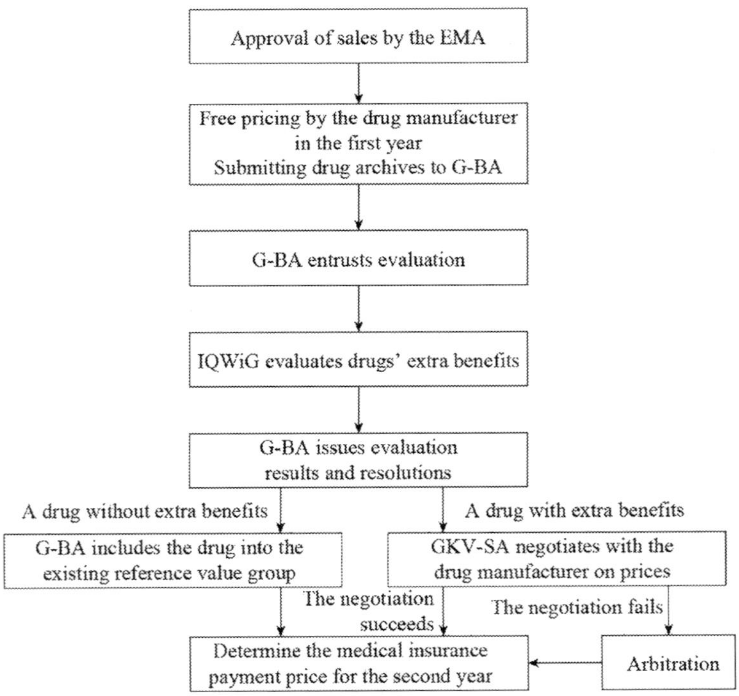

Figure 6.23 'Additional Benefit Evaluation' and the Negotiation Process for New Drugs in Germany

For drugs that do not belong to the reference-price group, the funds of GKV and other medical insurance may require a mandatory rebate from manufacturers. Since 2003, the GKV-SV is allowed to sign rebate contracts with manufacturers that link rebates to sales volume. At present, essentially all generic drugs and some patented drugs have signed rebate contracts, and in the great majority of cases these are exclusive agreements between GKV-SV and the drug manufacturer. In 2011, AMNOG ruled that the statutory mandatory rebate was being raised to 16%.

The term of the rebate contracts is generally between one and two years. Once agreement is reached on a contract, in principle all patients covered by the medical insurance fund may use the drug, but in some cases the fund designates use within a certain geographic area to a particular manufacturer. A medical fund may ensure sales quantity of a given rebate drug by taking one of the following measures:

The 2007 Statutory Health Insurance Strengthening-Competition Act requires that pharmacists give preference to dispensing the rebate drug, in the event there is such a drug. Once a pharmacist receives a doctor's prescription, he or she is obliged to fulfill the prescription with the rebate drug if there is one and if it has the same active ingredients, even if the doctor has not prescribed the rebate drug.

With respect to doctors' prescriptions: doctors have prescribing authority and are not required to choose the rebate drug. The doctors' prescribing system may inform the doctor of information on rebate drugs, however, and since every doctor in Germany has an upper budgetary limit on prescriptions, doctors are motivated to prescribe rebate drugs.

In addition, the Statutory Medical Insurance Strengthening-Competition Act allows GKV funds to sign incentive contracts with doctors, pharmacists, or pharmacies, so they will prescribe more drugs with rebates.

Patients may no longer need to pay out-of-pocket (self-pay) amounts for rebate drugs.

Generally speaking, patients must pay between 5 and 10 euros of self-pay per prescription. Drugs whose prices are 30% or more lower than reference prices, however, can be exempted from this requirement. If a drug is within a reference-price group, then the maximum reimbursement price of the group must be taken into consideration – the patient must pay the difference between the market price and the maximum reimbursement amount.

The following example (Figure 6.24) of a particular drug describes the allocation of benefits to the various entities involved in distributing and paying for the drug. The hypothetical list price of the drug is 50 euros.

3.2.3.2.2 Inpatient drugs GKV funds reimburse for the entire amount of inpatient costs of a sick person, rather than reimbursing by care items. Reimbursement is made according to a system of costs associated with specific illnesses – payment is therefore made by referring to 'Germany's Diagnosis Related Groups,' or G-DRG). Germany defines roughly 1,300 different diagnosis related groups. All costs associated with inpatient treatment of a given group, including drugs, use a unified rate that is based on the cost of the group. Every

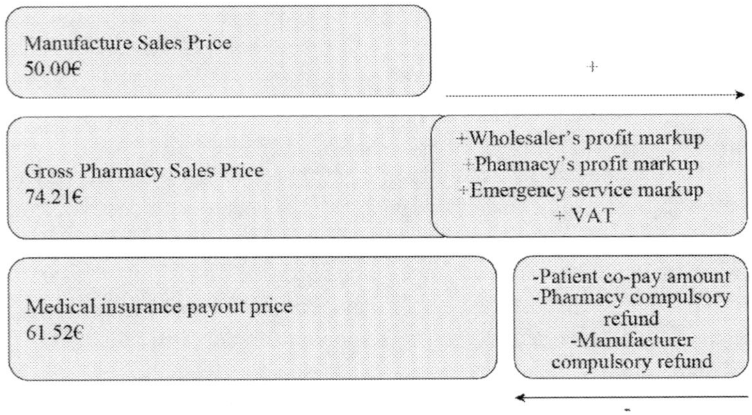

Figure 6.24 Composition of Prescription Drug Prices in Germany

Source: IGES based on ABDA (Federal Union of German Associations of Pharmacists), Zahlen, Daten, Fakten 2016, p. 26

year, InEK revises the contents of the DRG system. The payment amounts are based on actual statistics collected continuously from hundreds of German clinics. There is a time gap between obtaining the new DRG codes and use of the DRG, so InEK's updates are based on empirical data from the previous several years.

With respect to high-priced drugs used in hospital treatments that the DRG is unable to reimburse for at the present time, there are two alternative ways to subsidize these.

First, obtain additional fees or payments (Zusatzentgelt). In 2018, a total of 205 such additional payments were approved. Applications to receive these come from hospitals and the medical association. Under appropriate circumstances, InEK may also take the initiative in setting up additional fees. In most cases, the amounts of payments are based on a confirmation of the empirical costs that hospitals incur.

Launch a request for funding of 'New Methods for Treatment and Screening (NUB),' which target new technologies or procedures. Hospitals may issue one electronic request per year to InEK to inquire whether or not negotiations have been opened for temporary extra-budgetary assistance (NUB payments) for the hospital. If the answer is positive, then the hospital may enter into negotiations with the local health insurance payer. Each hospital must apply on its own, and the extra-budgetary funds are only for hospitals whose negotiations have been successful.

InEK carries out regulatory supervision over NUB applications that have been successful. It incorporates the corresponding new technologies or procedural methods into the Diagnosis Related Group system of standards in the future. These procedures are widely used. However, if the technologies or methods are already included in existing DRG standards or are not considered innovative, then the NUB procedures will not be successful. It is worth noting that InEK has no decision-making authority over the financial amount of extra-budgetary funds. That figure is the result of direct negotiations between the hospital and GKV.

3.2.4 Micro-methods of pricing drugs

3.2.4.1 ADDITIONAL THERAPEUTIC BENEFITS ASSESSMENTS

3.2.4.1.1 Scope of assessments Article 35a of the No. 5 Book of the German Social Code (FünftesSozialgesetzbuch-SGB V) stipulates that additional therapeutic benefits of drugs must be evaluated under the following circumstances:

A drug has adopted new active ingredients or a new combination of existing active ingredients;

A drug that is currently on the market is targeting new applications, or the therapeutic goal of such new applications aims at a different patient group than the drug's existing applications, or a new application can be attributed to different therapeutic realms (such as prevention, treatment, or diagnosis);

The G-BA or drug manufacturers request a new evaluation for a drug. This may be done by both sides due to new scientific discoveries, requiring a new evaluation, but the G-BA is not obliged to accept the request for a redone evaluation. G-BA may also request that (the manufacturer) submit the existing drug's documentation;

A drug for which G-BA has already issued a temporary determination has a new combination of active ingredients.

If the annual GKV spending on a given drug is not expected to exceed 1 million euros, then the drug's manufacturer may request that it be exempt from an assessment.

3.2.4.1.2 Contents of additional therapeutic assessments Investigating the addition benefits of a new drug is done in order to improve a patient's health condition, reduce the duration of a disease, increase life expectancy, reduce negative side effects, and improve quality of life. The G-BA requires that evidence be produced that is as detailed and valid as possible. Its bias is in favor of direct comparisons, but when necessary, it allows for flexibility (for example, when a company is unable to obtain evidence based on randomized controlled trials).

To prove their 'additional benefits,' new drugs with new active ingredients and additional benefits in terms of their pharmacology or their therapeutics, must be compared to the comprehensive materials on drugs in a reference-price group. Other drugs with new active ingredients must be compared to drugs that are 'an appropriate comparison' as legally defined, in order to evaluate the additional benefit for each kind of 'appropriate indication' (or symptom). The documentation must include an estimate of the likelihood of improved benefits.

The results of additional therapeutic benefits assessments must be measured according a six-point scale.

Major additional benefits. In treating patients, the new drug shows tremendous and ongoing improvement over an 'appropriate comparison' drug, for example, it restores health to a sick person, or extends lifespan, or relieves severe symptoms for a long period of time, or it is able to avoid a wide range of negative side effects.

Considerable additional benefits. The new drug shows 'a fairly large improvement' over an 'appropriate comparison' drug, with particular regard to relieving serious symptoms, extending life, providing observable relief to the patient, and ability to avoid serious or other side effects.

Relatively minor additional benefits. The new drug has not been able to show significantly moderate or mild improvement over the appropriate comparison drug, particularly with regard to relieving severe symptoms, or avoiding side effects.

Additional benefits are hard to quantify. Due to the limitations of current scientific data, the drug's additional benefits are impossible to quantify.

The drug has not proven it has any additional benefits.

The benefits are fewer than those of the appropriate comparison drug.

Since orphan drugs can be put on the market without any similar drugs being available, the additional benefits of such orphan drugs are tacitly accepted. However, the manufacturer must demonstrate additional therapeutic benefits. G-BA will not do a comprehensive evaluation of orphan drugs unless its expected sales volume exceeds 50 million euros.

3.2.4.1.3 Determination of evaluation Within three months of the release of the evaluation report, G-BA will formulate a binding determination on the benefits evaluation, which it puts on the Internet for open viewing by the public. This then forms the basis for price negotiations, since it presents the drug's quality, efficiency, and reference-price group for distribution (for drugs that do not have additional therapeutic benefits). This determination includes the following information:

The therapeutic results of the new drug;

Its additional benefits as compared to an appropriate comparison;

The number of patients that can be treated by the drug, and the definition of the patient group;

Special requirements for ensuring accurate use;

Cost of treatment as compared to an appropriate comparison drug.

3.2.4.2 NEGOTIATIONS ON THE PAYMENT PRICE (REIMBURSEMENT PRICE)

If the new drug has some specific additional therapeutic benefits, then GKV-SV must negotiate with the manufacturer regarding the reimbursement price at which insurance reimburses for the drug. The basis for this negotiation is the additional benefits evaluation of G-BA and the prices of similar drugs. In addition, the annual cost of treatment of similar drugs is taken into account, as well as the payment price that other countries in Europe or other regions pay, as reported by the drug manufacturer.

An appendix that lists reference prices of other countries or regions is attached to the agreement signed between GKV-SV and the pharmaceutical industry. Countries that are included in the list must have satisfied three standards: each country must be a member country of the European Economic Area (EEA), all of the countries on the list must reach at least 80% of the population of the EEA (excluding Germany), and they must have a level of development that is equivalent to that of Germany. Drug manufacturers must provide overseas *ex factory* prices. If a company cannot provide the actual payment price in a given country or region, then all parties together must estimate the actual price. The drug manufacturer must also provide information on the expected sales quantity.

This list is reviewed annually by the negotiators and may be modified as necessary. In 2012, it included 15 countries of the European Union: the U.K., France, the Netherlands, Italy, Austria, Belgium, Sweden, Greece, Czech Republic, Denmark, Portugal, Sweden, Spain, and Slovak Republic. Although Greece was listed as a reference country in the renewal of the framework agreement between GKV-SV and the pharmaceutical industry in 2016, it has temporarily been excluded from this list.

No relevant information about the price negotiations is open to the public. Negotiations must be concluded within six months of the release of the G-BA determination, during which time four meetings must be held in principle. Representatives of private insurance companies may attend these meetings. The results should be summarized in written form, and should be shared among all parties. The GKV-SV must advise the parent company of the private health insurance company of the final reimbursement price. Unless otherwise stated, the agreement has no term limit. The price as determined by the negotiation starts being effective in the second year that the drug is put on the market (that is, the 13th month); during the first year, the drug manufacturer may itself determine a price. One year after the agreement takes effect, either side may choose to withdraw from it, but must give notice of this action three months in advance.

With regard to drugs that have no additional therapeutic benefits and cannot be grouped according to any existing reference-price group: price negotiations should also be conducted, but the annual total reimbursement spending for such drugs should not be higher than the annual spending for an appropriate comparison drug.

If parties do not reach an agreement within six months of the release of the G-BA determination, then arbitration proceedings begin. Decisions are made by a simple majority vote, and no waiver is allowed. If there is no majority, then the vote of decisive significance is the one that the chairperson of the board believes will pass. According to article 130, item b, paragraph 4, of the 5th Social Security Act (SGB V), the arbitration board must make a decision within three months. After arbitration, any party within G-BA may request a cost-benefit evaluation by IQWiG. This evaluation does not have the effect of suspending action, but it means that price can be renegotiated after the evaluation.

One year later, any part to the arbitration may raise doubts about the agreement or the arbitration decision. However, already existing drug prices remain valid until a new agreement is reached. If a new evaluation shows additional therapeutic benefits or if the composition of the reference price cluster leads to price changes, then renegotiation shall be carried out within one year.

3.2.4.3 METHODS OF DETERMINING REBATES

Drug rebates are generally determined through one of two different methods. One is to have manufacturers bid for each active ingredient separately. The second is to have a combination contract: drugs are put into groups, and an assessment is made of the rebate levels that companies can provide for each group.

Bidding within the Europe is published on three websites, those of the European Union, the industry association, and the GKV-SV. The granting of contracts is determined not only by the lowest price of special drugs, but also by the quantity of drug types that the winning bidder (will take) as based on measurements (that is, the degree to which the winning bidder consolidates drug groups). Given that not all companies are able to assemble a fairly complete combination of drugs, at times they may join together to compete as an alliance. Relatively speaking, the standards of assessments are not transparent but they generally include prices and the completeness of a product grouping. They may also take into account whether or not the bidder has established relationships with doctors, whether or not they notify pharmacies and provide training to relevant parties.

3.2.4.4 REFERENCE PRICES

The main idea behind reference prices is to divide drugs into a number of groupings according to specific criteria, and set a maximum reimbursement price for each group (that is, the 'reference price'), then to place drugs that have not yet been classified into existing drug groups and apply the same maximum reimbursement price to them. Drug manufacturers may still set prices freely, but if their prices are higher than the reference prices then the patient is responsible for covering the difference. Patients are inclined to choose drugs for which their self-pay amount is minimized. This reference price mechanism thereby forces drug manufacturers to lower their list prices.

The main criterion by which drugs are grouped defines comparability in terms of pharmacology and therapeutic value. Groupings depend on the degree to which drugs conform to this criterion, which is defined more specifically at three levels. The first level is that drugs in the same group have the same active ingredients; the second is that drugs in the same group have similar active ingredients and the same or similar pharmacological effects; the third is that drugs in the same group have different active ingredients but their therapeutic results are comparable. The most common way of grouping is classification by the first level.

In principle, reference prices may not be higher than the actual price of the top one-third of drugs with the highest prices in a given group. In addition, at least 20% of drug prices should be lower than the reference price.

3.3 The current situation with regard to the management of drug prices in Germany

The German government passed the Pharmaceuticals Market Reorganization Act in 2011 (known by the acronym AMNOG, for Arzneimittelmarkt Neuordnungsgesetz). This was done in response to the urgent need to resolve financial deficits, and was aimed at reducing the government's spending on drugs. In order to generate results that would have a real impact, the government put a price freeze on drugs already being sold in the market and it raised the mandatory rebate on CKV drugs (those covered by statutory health insurance) from 6% of list price to 16%. At the same time, the law called for innovative drugs to undergo 'additional therapeutic benefits assessments' as a way to seek long-term price reductions. For manufacturers, the reforms meant an increase in competition, and it meant that they could not longer freely determine prices. Instead, they had to find a balance through direct negotiations on reimbursement prices with GKV-SV (Association of Statutory Health Insurance Funds). At the same time, the Pharmaceuticals Market Reorganization Act relaxed certain regulatory policies. The heart of this was the abolishing of incentives and punishments system, and the requirement to have a medical practitioner ask another medical practitioner for his or her advice prior to prescribing a high-priced drug. Efficiency audits were simplified. Regulatory supervision of the exclusion of certain treatments and prescriptions is more clear-cut. Moreover, the Act did away with a large amount of unnecessary paperwork on the part of insurers and medical services providers.

In April 2015, in an 'additional pharmaceutical benefits assessment,' the G-BA for the first time awarded (a drug with) the highest level of classification. (G-BA = Federal Joint Committee.)

In July 2017, the G-BA strengthened its cooperation with the European Medicines Agency (EMA, an agency of the European Union).

3.4 Centralized procurement of drugs in Germany

The primary retail channels for drugs in Germany are social (private, or community) pharmacies and pharmacies within hospitals. Social pharmacies get their products mainly through wholesalers – the largest five wholesalers in Germany hold around 85% of the market. It has not yet been determined whether there should be Group Purchasing Organizations as intermediaries between these retailers and wholesalers. Chains of hospitals generally carry out direct procurement, while independent hospitals go through Group Purchasing Organizations. Over 80% of hospitals choose to go through GPOs in making purchases, and GPOs may sign contracts on discounts with a number of individual drug manufacturers or they may sign a rebate contract with just one manufacturer. In order to increase quantity and thereby get a higher discount, a GPO may well choose to sign an exclusive rebate contract. Starting in 2017, the negotiated price for drugs has become the ceiling price or upper limit at which hospitals buy drugs.

3.5 The situation with regard to price-formation of the reimbursement price for drugs

Germany administers reimbursement prices for drugs according to a system of drug categories. Reimbursement prices for innovative drugs are generally determined by the additional benefits assessments, then negotiations and reference prices. Reimbursement prices for generic drugs are determined directly by reference prices. For specifics on price-formation methods, see parts 'Price-formation mechanisms of drugs,' 'Drug price-formation process,' and 'Micro-methods of pricing drugs' earlier.

3.6 Lessons China can learn from Germany's price-formation mechanisms

1 Focus on pharmaceutical benefits in the pricing of drugs, and seek a balance between drug benefits and (China's requirements with respect to) economic reporting

Germany has professional research organizations carry out its 'additional pharmaceutical benefits assessments.' It also has flexible mechanisms that allow for consultation. Decisions and assessments are kept separate, in order to safeguard the objectivity and fairness of the results of evaluating clinical benefits.

2 Manage drug prices by classifying drugs into categories, and differentiate between innovative drugs and generic drugs in administering price controls

Like other industries, the pharmaceutical industry suffers from the problem of strangling initiative if controls are too stringent, but allowing prices to soar if controls are too loose. To a degree, managing drugs according to different categories can resolve this contradiction. Implementing a reference-price system can effectively control the prices of generic drugs while also increasing the rate at which they are used, which raises the efficiency with which insurance funds are used. Meanwhile, Germany's systems of additional pharmaceutical benefits assessments, and its negotiated reimbursement prices, can also, to a degree, improve a willingness to innovate (among pharmaceutical companies).

Abbreviations and acronyms

BMG: Bundesministerium fur Gesundheit
CKV-SV: GKV-Spitzenverband
DIMDI: Deutsches Institut für Medizinische Dokumentation und Information
DKG: Deutsche Keramische Gesellschaft
G-DRG: Germany Diagnosis Related Groups
GKV: Gesetzliche Krankenversicherung
GPO: Group Purchasing Management
InEK: Institut für das Entgeltsystem im Krankenhaus
KBV: Kassenärztliche Bundesvereinigung
KZBV: Kassenzahnärztliche Bundesvereinigung
NUB: New Methods for Treatment and Screening
PKV: Private Krankenversicherung

4 Case study of Japan

4.1 Japan's medical and healthcare system

In 2018, Japan achieved a GDP of roughly USD 4.97 trillion, which ranked it third in the world, and its per capita GDP was USD 48,919.60. In the World Health Reports that the WHO has issued over the years, Japan has consistently ranked first in terms of 'high-quality medical services,' 'low levels of medical burden on its people,' and 'high average life expectancy.' All hospitals in Japan are not-for-profit, and indeed Japan prohibits the operation of for-profit hospitals. Japan took steps to lighten the burden of medical costs on its people back in the 1950s, when it began the establishment of a universal health insurance system. It was through this system that the country realized the highest level of average life expectancy in the world, as well as the highest level of medical insurance. By the 1980s, average life expectancy was first in the world, and by 2018, the overall life expectancy of Japanese people had reached 86.6. Within this, the figure for men was 81.7, and that for women 87.26. On average, lives were roughly five years longer than they had been 30 years earlier. Meanwhile, the infant mortality rate was 1.7%, lowest of any OECD country. There were 2.4 doctors for every one thousand people, and 11.3 nurses for every one thousand people. There were 13.1 hospital beds per one thousand people. People's ability to access medical services is quite high. In 2018, overall spending on healthcare in Japan was 10.9% of GDP. Spending on drugs was roughly 21% of healthcare spending.

Medical insurance in Japan is centrally administered by the Medical Insurance Administration, which is under the jurisdiction of the Ministry of Health, Labor, and Welfare. Nevertheless, specific types of insurance and classified according to the type of employment of the insured person: 1) employees of ordinary companies generally are covered by 'Health Insurance'; 2) people who operate private businesses, freelance workers, and retired corporate employees are covered by the

'National Health Insurance; 3) civil servants in either the national or regional parts of the government and teachers in private schools, among others, are covered by 'Mutual aid associations'; 4) medical insurance that covers people who are age 75 and above (senior citizens are generally covered by national the municipal, village, and town national insurance); and 5) maritime insurance, which covers a small number of people. The two main forms of insurance are the Health Insurance and the National Health Insurance, which together cover 90% of the Japanese population.

There are two main sources of funding for Japan's medical insurance, namely insurance premiums and public-finance subsidies from the central and local governments. In consideration of the issue of fairness when it comes to payments, the reimbursement percentage of medical insurance in Japan is determined only by differences in annual income. (Since income is correlated with age), the following four main levels of reimbursement are the result: medical expenses of children under the age of 6, when compulsory education begins, are reimbursed at 80% of costs; children age 6 and people up to the age of 69 are reimbursed at 70% of costs; people age 70–74 are reimbursed at 80% (or at 70% if taxable income is over 1.45 million yen); people over the age of 75 are reimbursed at 90% (or 70% if taxable income is over 1.45 million yen). Japan follows the practice of seeing the doctor first, and then paying the bill. See Figure 6.25 for a description of the health insurance reimbursement system.

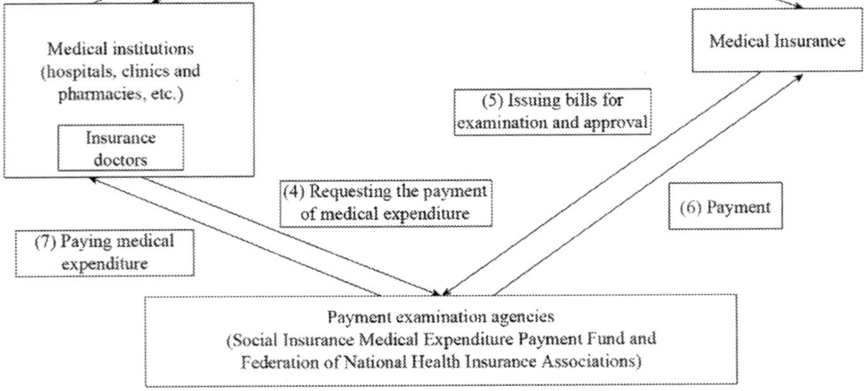

Figure 6.25 Japan's Medical Insurance Payment System

4.2 Drug price-formation mechanisms in Japan

In recent years, the problems of an aging population and a population that bears fewer children are intensifying, which means that the problem of ferocious increases in medical costs is also intensifying. In 1998, Japan's healthcare spending was 6.6% of GDP, whereas it was 10.9% in 2018. Spending by health insurance rose swiftly as well. In 2018, spending on medical safeguards was roughly 42.6 trillion yen, or 8.3% of GDP, while ten years earlier it had been 6.4% of GDP. The two main factors leading to an increase in medical costs have been the aging of the population and the development of medical technology, such as advanced medical equipment and innovative drugs. Since 1958, when Japan set up a pricing system for drugs and medical services under its universal medical insurance, the task of drug pricing has been the responsibility of the Ministry of Health, Labor, and Welfare. The government sets prices on all drugs that are included in the medical insurance list. As noted earlier, drugs were already approaching 40% of medical spending in the 1970s. In the 1980s, however, the Ministry of Health, Labor, and Welfare began conducting price surveys and adjusting prices once every two years. The new pricing system focused on reducing the margins when medical institutions bought drugs.

Meanwhile, in 1974 the country began to separate out the business of drugs from the business of medicine. Through mandatory implementation of this policy, the interest relationships among hospitals, doctors, and drugs were severed. While prices of medical services kept going up, drug rebates as a percentage of the income of doctors and hospitals went down. As a percentage of medical spending, spending on drugs went from 38.2% in 1980 to 20.2% in 2000. Once at that level, spending on drugs remained at roughly 21% to 22% on average (in 2018, the OECD average was 17%). The main subject of this study is, therefore, to determine how Japan achieved price control over drugs, and how it has maintained a fairly low level of drug spending as a percentage of total spending on medical costs.

4.2.1 Main entities and processes involved in price-formation of drugs in Japan

Japan classifies drugs into two categories, medical drugs, most of which are prescription drugs, and over-the-counter drugs, drugs that can be purchased by patients as they wish, in pharmacies. Like most countries in the world, the Japanese government only intervenes in the pricing of prescription drugs. It regulates their prices and includes almost all of them in the reimbursable drug list of medical insurance. The prices at which drugs are put on the market, as determined by government, are the prices at which medical insurance reimburses for drugs. The process by which drugs are priced is therefore also the process by which drugs are entered into the reimbursable drug list. However, at the same time, Japan's drug-pricing system has unique features that combine market pricing with government pricing. That is, the price at which drugs can be put on the market, as determined by the government, and the price at which insurance reimburses for drugs, is not in fact the actual market price. The actual market price is formed in combination with market adjustments, as described next.

Before being priced and allowed into health insurance, innovative drugs as well as generic drugs must go through a review and approval process to be put on the market. Those that pass this process, that is, those that can be put on the market as well as automatically enter health insurance (reimbursement), express the synchronized nature of market and health insurance.

Putting innovative (new) drugs through a secondary course of reviews helps fill in the gap between (inadequate) information on the effectiveness of a drug prior to its appearance on the market and the complexities of clinical usage after it has been on the market. For generic drugs, Japan applies a double set of safeguards to ensure quality – that is, it requires a second evaluation process that evaluates both effectiveness and quality. Three such re-evaluations have been carried out since 1971 in three overlapping time periods. These were the first re-evaluation (1971–1995), the second re-evaluation (1985–1996), and the new re-evaluation (1900–the present). Re-evaluation of quality also means assessments for consistency. This is mainly done through in vitro dissolution tests to test the internal quality of drugs. The assessment process is thorough, meticulous, and rigorous.

The entities involved in administering innovative drug prices in Japan include the MHLW; entities authorized to represent manufacturers and the market; experts from the fields of medicine, pharmacology, and pharmaco-economics; and the medical committee of the Central Social Insurance (Chuikyo). The Chuikyo committee itself is composed of a diverse group of people who include eight representatives of insurers, representing health insurance companies and pharmaceutical companies; eight people who represent doctors, dentists, and pharmacists; four people who represent public interests; and a number of other people who are specialists in various fields. The entities that administer generic drug pricing are similar to those involved in innovative drug administration, but the specific methods of determining prices are different (see later for details).

After going through the review and approval process for being put on the market, authorized representatives of manufacturers or the market submit an application for including the drug in the reimbursement drug list. As the main administrative department handling healthcare, the MHLW determines the reimbursement price of drugs and medical equipment, which applies nationwide on a uniform basis. The Economics Section of the Health Policy Bureau under MHLW is the main authority governing drug prices, and is responsible for such matters as drug price surveys and surveys of certain medical materials that are reimbursed by insurance. It also convenes the initial meeting on drug pricing. At this meeting, the economics department of the medical bureau first presents its draft proposal on pricing as determined by its own research. Parties authorized by the manufacturer or market then may express their opinions directly (as needed), and experts from the fields of medicine, pharmacology, and pharmaco-economics express their opinions as well and also look into several aspects: are there similar drugs on the market, is there a need to apply for insurance premiums, what is the estimate of cost-pricing, and so on. The Economics Section of the Health Policy Bureau then revises the pricing of the draft proposal, depending on the majority opinion of members. It formulates a list price and submits this to Chuikyo and it also informs the authorized representatives of manufacturers and market. If the manufacturer does not accept this price, it can submit a request for re-evaluation to Chuikyo, who then organizes a second meeting. The organization under Chuikyo that calculates drug pricing then compares the price that is in the draft proposal with the principles on pricing as set by the Economics Section of the Health Policy Bureau, and takes into consideration the majority opinion of representative members, and it then holds a second discussion and reappraisal of the drug price. After informing the authorized representatives of the manufacturer or market, it resubmits this to Chuikyo. Chuikyo then proceeds to grant approval to the price proposal. Generally there is no need to undertake any revisions. The specifics of this process are described in Figure 6.26.

Innovative drugs have the opportunity to be entered into the drug pricing list four times a year, in February, May, August, and November. These times correspond to the approval schedule as determined by the Drug Administration Law. In principle, once a drug is entered into the schedule, it should be approved within 60 days or at the latest within 90 days. As for generic drugs, the frequency of approvals for the NHI drug pricing list was once every two years prior to 1994, but this was changed to once a year in 1994, and since 2008 it has been twice a year, in June and December.

4.2.2 Methods of price-formation

4.2.2.1 METHODS OF PRICE-FORMATION FOR NEW DRUGS

Unlike in other countries, the Pharmaceutical Affairs Law, promulgated in 1961, determined that the government sets prices of prescription drugs in Japan, and the Law set forth detailed rules on how to calculate official prices. The pricing of the official price of innovative drugs is done through two main methods, namely 'comparison with similar drugs,' and 'cost-accounting.' In addition, referencing international prices is important but is not considered a separate pricing method. Japan has developed a pricing system that is a combination of a markup on a benchmark price, cost pricing, and comparison with international prices. (See Figure 6.27.)

When pricing a new drug, the methodology of 'comparison to similar drugs' is used if similar drugs are already in the list. If such things as drug efficacy, pharmacological characteristics, composition and chemical structure, usage method, preparation type, dosage form, and mode of administering the drug are all the same, then pricing the new drug at the same price as the existing drug will ensure fairness in market competition. If a new drug is rated as an 'innovative drug,' then the Ministry of Health, Labor, and Welfare will add a premium to the price which can range from 5% to 120% of the price of the similar drug. The degree to which a drug is regarded as innovative depends on the four following determinations: 1) new active mechanism, 2) higher therapeutic results or safety, 3) improved treatment of target disease, and 4) favorable pharmaceutical formulation. The

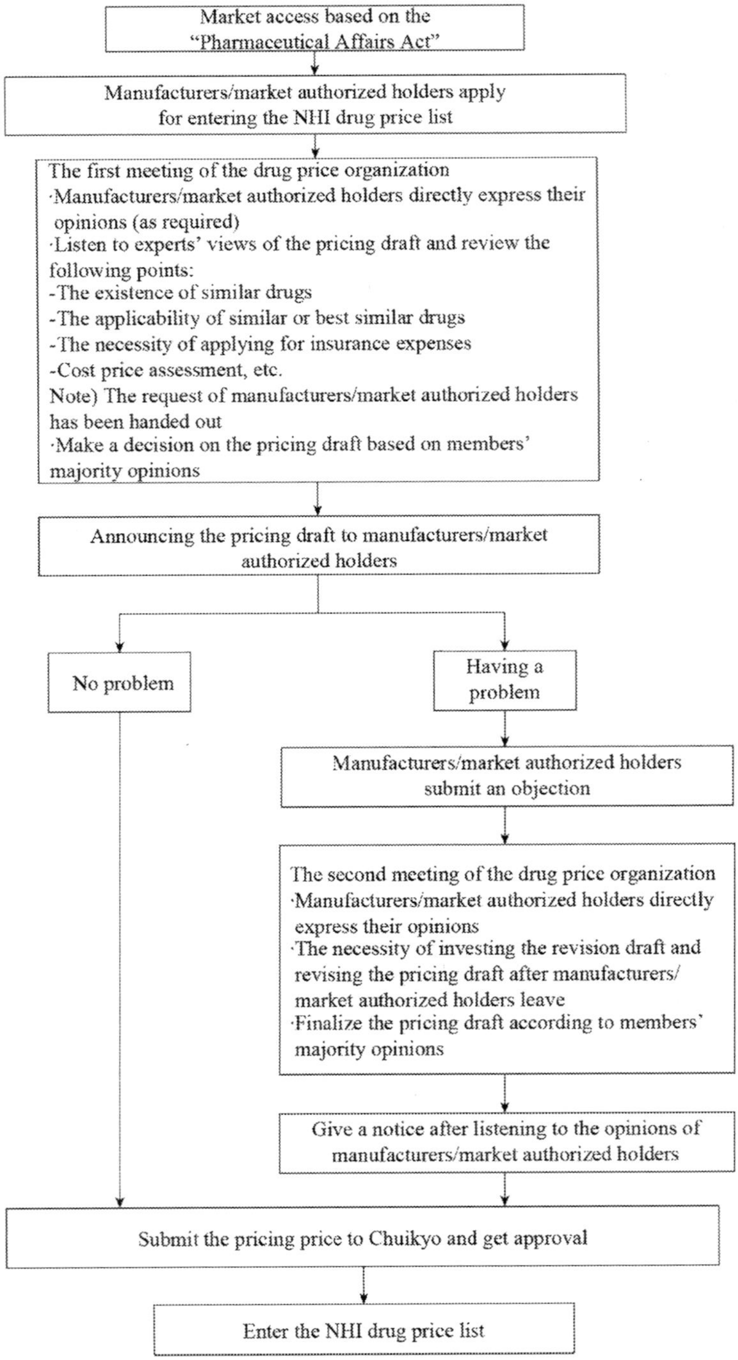

Figure 6.26 Drug Pricing Process in Japan

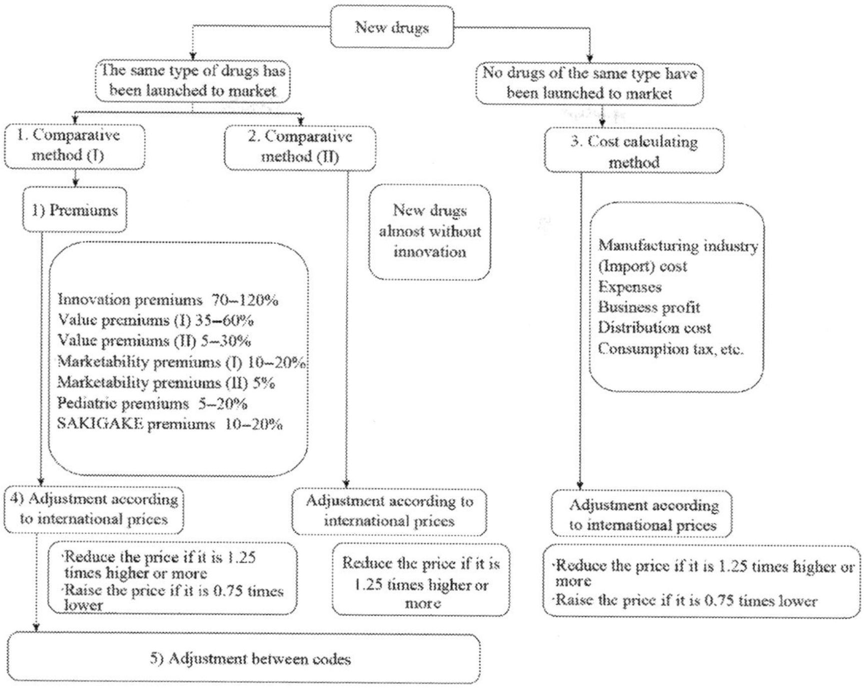

Figure 6.27 Pricing Methods of New Drugs in Japan

percentage of the premium depends on the degree of innovation, which is what can give the manufacturer an extra 5% to 120% in price. If a certain new drug is regarded as an 'orphan drug,' according to the definition of PAL, or if it has a very small market, or if it potentially can be used on children (including infants, infants during lactation period, newborns, and low birth-weight infants), and is also defined as an 'innovative targeted drug,' this status can also gain the manufacturer a premium of a certain percentage.

If no similar drug can be used for comparative purposes, then pricing is done by a cost-accounting method. Cost is figured by adding up the various sums of production, management, marketing, profit, and value-added tax, which incorporates costs of raw materials, labor, selling costs, research and development, operating profit and tax. As of fiscal year 2016, Japan's operating profit margin for pharmaceuticals was set at 14.6%, which refers to the average profit margin for the entire industry. Depending on the degree of innovation in a drug, however, as well as its effectiveness and safety, this margin may be adjusted relative to the standard profit margin by as much as 50% less to 100% more.

In addition, after determining price through these methods, it is also necessary to compare prices of the same class of drugs in other countries. Japan's system for comparing international reference prices is quite complex. It includes many different aspects, including the varieties of international reference pricing, determinations by reference countries, obtaining reference prices, methods of calculating prices, and methods of adjusting prices. 1) Japan has explicit rules on the principles behind selecting international reference drugs: the referenced drug must have the same ingredients and dosage form as the new drug being priced in Japan, or the specifications and scope of application must be similar to the new drug and must be in the relevant drug price list of the reference countries. 2) Japan has selected four countries to serve as reference countries, given such factors as level of economic development, exchange rate fluctuations, and market size. Those four are the United States, the U.K., Germany, and France. 3) The reference prices that Japan uses are mainly the retail prices openly published in price lists in the reference countries. 4) Japan mainly uses an arithmetic average of the retail prices of the four reference countries in determining average price levels of international drugs. 5) After arriving at the average prices of the international reference drugs, Japan must use this to adjust drug prices within the country. If the calculated price of the new drug in Japan is more than 1.5 times the international reference price, then a price-lowering adjustment is made. One thing worth noting is that Japan began pricing new drugs based on health technology assessments in April 2019. Key points regarding this are described later.

4.2.2.2 METHODS OF PRICE-FORMATION FOR GENERIC DRUGS

Japan mostly sets prices of generic drugs according to a certain percentage of the price of the original drug. In the 2016 price reform, the country decided that from 2021 onward generic drug prices that had been 60% of the original drug price would now be 50% of the original. (For certain oral preparations that included more than ten varieties, the figures went from an initial 50% to 40% of the original.) Bio-similar generic drugs maintained the percentage of 70% of the original-drug price. (For oral preparations that included more than ten varieties, the figure went to 60%.) If the same type of generic drug was already in the reimbursable drug list, the newly added generic drug price was set at the same level as the lowest-priced alternative. In 2005, generic drugs constituted 32.5% of the pharmaceutical market in the country. By 2017, this had gone up to 65.1%, and in 2020, the goal is to make it reach 80%. Prior to this, in order to encourage their use, Japan promoted generics by regulating product quality and providing insurance reimbursement. In 2002, the country began to pay an additional bonus for generics delivered by pharmacies. It also changed the way in which prescriptions were fulfilled, such that patients and pharmacies now had the authority to choose generics for a given prescription. In 2007, Japan included the effort to 'promote the use of generic drugs' as part of national policy in the reform program.

4.2.2.3 *Adjustment of prices and reformulating prices*

Japan began to implement a 'drug price benchmark' in 1950, by which is meant the reimbursable drug list system. This list shares two functions, in that it is both a list of products and a list of prices. Only once the government determines the retail price of a drug for insurance purposes can medical insurance reimburse for the costs of that drug. Administering the reimbursable drug list includes incorporating drugs into the list, setting their prices, adjusting their prices, and reformulating prices. After MHLW has confirmed prices for new drugs, that is, has entered the new drug into the reimbursable drug list, the procurers of drugs and dealers in drugs are allowed to carry on secondary negotiations that allow for buying drugs at a unit price that is lower than the medical insurance settlement price. Any surplus may be retained. In specified intervals of time (originally this was once every two years, but in 2021 it started being once every year) the government carries out price adjustments that are based on the difference between these two prices. Price adjustments use market price information as evidence, derived from drug price surveys. Chuikyo conducts these surveys, which cover all items in the national reimbursable drug list (currently about 16,000 items). They go to a certain percentage of all drug distributors that supply medical institutions directly, in order to obtain valid price information.

Price adjustments that are made on the basis of information from surveys mainly rely on specific formulas. These formulas include the '90% Bulk-line method' in 1953, the '81% Bulk-line method in 1982,' and the 'reasonable-zone method' since 1992. The latter means that the new reimbursement price is equal to the calculated weighted-average market price plus a certain percentage of the current reimbursement price. (The percentage has been 2% since 2000.) This method more correctly reflects market prices and corrects unnatural price fluctuations.

In addition to adjustments based on the reasonable-zone method, in 1994 the Japanese government determined that price renewals could be made on drugs that meet the following four conditions (with the possibility of an increase in price). These four are an expansion of market sales, changes in drug efficacy, changes in drug usage and dosage, and drugs that are now defined as showing a loss. In 2010, in order to encourage research and development in pharmaceuticals and also avoid excessive usage of drugs, the government ruled that new drugs that had been on the market less than 15 years could raise prices in the course of price adjustment, provided the difference between the actual price and reimbursement price was not greater than the average market price. In 2014, during the adjustment of drug prices, a proposal was made to adjust prices of original drugs based on the rate at which generics were being substituted for them – the aim of this was to go a step further in reducing the price gap between generic drugs and their originals.

4.2.2.4 *New directions in price reform of medical insurance (reimbursable) drug prices*

In order to deal with the constant increase in exorbitant medical-technology costs, and their impact on public finance, in addition to regular price surveys and adjustments, in 2012 the MHLW started considering adopting a new system for evaluating the cost-effectiveness of innovative drugs, medical equipment, and intervention procedures. That is, it considered using the results of Cost-Effectiveness Assessments (CEA) in carrying out adjustments of drug prices in the reimbursable drug list.

Japan's explorations into using health technology assessments (HTA) began in 2012 when the cost-effectiveness special committee was set up. Only in April of 2016 did these get started on a trial basis, however. In April 2018, the MHLW carried out some adjustments based on the results of seven pilot projects dealing with seven kinds of drugs. In April 2019, Japan began to formal implementation of Cost-Effectiveness Assessments. Companies that already have drugs in the list must submit economic data. Companies whose drugs are newly entering the list must similarly submit data for future discussions.

The Cost-Effectiveness Assessment process in Japan is mainly divided into four parts: selection of the targets for assessment, analytical procedures, comprehensive assessment, and price adjustment.

1 Selection of targets for assessment. The main objectives of a Cost-Effectiveness Assessment include evaluating the impact of a drug on the medical insurance funds, so targets are those drugs and equipment that are both highly innovative and have a strong impact on the funds. The Chuikyo makes specific selections of items to assess.
2 Analytical procedures. The entire analytical process is divided into two stages, analysis of the company and official analysis. Based on the framework of parameters in the Cost-Effectiveness Assessment model, as determined by Japan's National Institute of Public Health, the analysis of the company takes around nine months, while the official analysis takes around three months (if a second analysis is carried out, then around six months).
3 Comprehensive assessment. The comprehensive assessment mainly does a scientific analysis of the incremental cost-effectiveness ratio (ICER) of a drug. For example, when there is a tremendous amount of data that is suitable for analysis, and using ICER is difficult, a broader assessment is allowed. After the comprehensive assessment, the main results of the analytical framework and ICER are reported and made public.
4 Price adjustment. When a specific adjustment is made depending on the CEA results, and when ICER exceeds the benchmark value, an impartial experts organization discusses and decides which level of price adjustment rate should be adopted. Depending on the current level of reimbursement and the results of past payment intentions, on the per capita GDP and each country's benchmark value, during the trial period three separate values are used: 5 million yen/QALY, 7.5 million yen/QALY, and 10 million yen/QALY. The benchmark values for drugs for difficult and severe diseases, hemophilia and HIV infection, rare diseases and pediatric diseases, cancer and other drugs are set at 7.5 million yen/QALY, 11.25 million yen/QALY, and 15 million yen/QALY.

4.3 Summary of Japan's experience in administering health insurance-reimbursed drugs

Japan has had considerable success in maintaining its percentage of drugs to total healthcare costs at a stable 21%–22% over time. This has been achieved through building the systems described earlier and institutionalizing the whole process from having drugs go to market, managing them by category, determining prices, determining access to the reimbursement list, to ongoing price adjustments.

1 Drugs are launched on the market while simultaneous procedures go forward to enter the drug in the reimbursable drug list. The importance of access to this list is emphasized.

The moment a new drug is authorized to be sold on the market, it may apply for admission to the reimbursable drug list. This allows for the simultaneity of the two processes and also strengthens the importance of gaining access to health insurance. Pricing of the drug is being realized by the process of allowing entry into the reimbursable drug list. Such entry into reimbursable status, in addition to having a drug on the market, is of enormous importance to the accessibility of drugs to the country's citizens. It improves the quality of life of patients. As for those who are authorized to represent the drug manufacturer or the market, the simultaneity of the two processes of listing on the market and access to insurance reimbursement signifies that the marketing of the drug must be based on the value of the drug itself. There is more emphasis on whether or not the drug has innovative mechanisms, obvious therapeutic results, and can be used safely. A drug company will start considering whether or not insurance will cover the drug at the stage of research and development, not after the drug has already launched on the market. Japan includes all prescription drugs in its reimbursable drug list. On the one hand, new drugs thereby gain the possibility of a larger market share, but on the other they face competitive pressures from similar drugs. Natural price reductions can be realized under market competition.

2 Drug innovation is encouraged by managing drug pricing by categories.

The method by which Japan prices new drugs gives full expression to the degree of innovation in the drug. It thereby improves willingness to develop new drugs. Depending on whether or not there is already a drug of the same category, Japan first divides drugs into two classes and then determines pricing by either a 'comparative method for similar drugs' or a 'cost-accounting' method. In the comparative method, drugs are again divided into various categories by using assessment criteria to evaluate the degree of innovation and effectiveness, and the premium rate is determined by these criteria. As innovation increases, the premium rate goes up. The cost-accounting method is adopted for new drugs that have no comparable on the market. Once the price of a drug has been determined by using one or the other of these methods, adjustments to price still need to be made by referencing international prices. Japan attempts to be in alignment with international levels as much as possible, and this in fact is a way to use international price comparisons as a way to express the degree of innovation in a new drug. Whether the comparative method or the cost-accounting method is used together with comparative international prices, all go through a scientific accounting process to determine final price. Price determination and adjustments are done by explicit formulas and ratios. This method of pricing by category not only incorporates the extent of innovation in the price of a drug, but it allows Japan to form a set of price-control methods that aligns the country's domestic realities with the international track of drug prices.

3 Even as the government controls prices, it also focuses on allowing the market to play its role.

With respect to price controls on drugs, although Japan implements price controls on essentially all prescription drugs, it does not regulate prices at the distribution stage. Instead, it leaves it to the entities that carry out market transactions to negotiate for and determine distribution margins. When medical institutions carry out procurement of drugs, they often use group procurement through hospital alliances as a means of getting better discounts. Negotiations with distributors result in procurement at wholesale prices, and the margin between the procurement price and the price at which insurance reimburses for drugs become a legal profit that the hospital is allowed to retain. Medical institutions therefore have an incentive when they negotiate with manufacturers and distributors since the larger the margin they can negotiate, the greater their profits. By releasing controls over the price of market transactions, the government can constantly keep drug prices down, squeeze out the excess water in prices as it were, thereby taking full advantage of the role of market mechanisms.

4 Japan carries out regular adjustments to prices and allows for dynamic readjustment of reimbursement prices.

Japan conducts market surveys every two years in order to carry out adjustments of drug prices. Doing this gives it a thorough understanding of the actual market-price situation and allows it to grasp the dynamics of market prices. Such grasp of actual market prices is useful to the government when it implements macro-controls and makes proper use of 'the unseen hand of the market.' When doing specific price adjustments, Japan puts in place scientifically sound price-adjustment formulas in order to ensure the stability of drug supply. In addition, regular surveys of the market price of drugs serve as a form of monitoring and regulatory supervision, to ensure that the market is developing in a sound way.

5 Japan actively explores new methods by which to adjust drug prices and is constantly updating its systems design.

Japan began to experiment with health technology assessments in 2012 and by now the country has achieved a measure of success in applying Cost-Effectiveness Assessments to some of its pricing adjustments for drugs on the reimbursement list.

It will be strengthening the institutional basis for such assessments in the future by improving the training of human resources, who are the main consideration. More specifically, in order to cultivate personnel who can carry out assessments, Japan will be launching a new human resources educational program. At the same time, Japan is undertaking a complete upgrading of the institutions within MHLW and NIPH. Although the industry holds different views on Japan's current proposal to adopt health technology assessments in a comprehensive way, since they feel that these work against innovation and limit the ability of patients to access innovative drugs, exploring such assessments should be affirmed in order to maintain long-term stability of Japan's health insurance funds.

Abbreviations and acronyms

CEA: Cost-Effectiveness Assessment
Chuikyo: Central Social Medical Insurance Council
EFPIA: European Federation of Pharmaceutical Industries and Associations
FNHIA: Federation of National Health Insurance Associations
HTA: health technology assessment
ICH: International Conference on Harmonization
IFPMA: International Federation of Pharmaceutical Manufacturers & Associations
JMA: Japan Medical Association
JPMA: Japan Pharmaceutical Manufacturers Association
MDC: Medical Devices Center
MHLW: Ministry of Health, Labor, and Welfare
NHI: National Health Insurance
NIPH: National Institute of Public Health of Japan
OPSR: Organization for Pharmaceutical Safety and Research
PAFSC: Pharmaceutical Affairs and Food Sanitation Council
PAL: Pharmaceutical Affairs Law
Paying Fund: Social Insurance Medical Fee Payment Fund
PHRMA: Pharmaceutical Research and Manufacturers of America
PMDA: Pharmaceuticals and Medical Devices Agency
PMDEC: Pharmaceuticals and Medical Devices Evaluation Center
PMDL: Pharmaceutical and Medical Device Act/Law
SCCEA: Special Committee on Cost-Effectiveness Assessment

5 Case study of the Republic of Korea

5.1 Summary of relevant circumstances

5.1.1 Economic structures

The full name of the country is the Republic of Korea (Daehan Minguk) (shortened to the ROK). It is a republic, located on the southern part of the Korean peninsula in East Asia. It has a total land mass of 100,210 square kilometers and in 2018 it had a total population of 51,635,256 people. With a fairly advanced economy, the ROK ranks in the forefront of levels of development in Asia. In 2017, its GDP was USD 1.73 trillion, and its per capita GDP was USD 27,090. The country's health services system operates efficiently. In 2018, medical and healthcare costs were roughly 8.1% of GDP, or average healthcare spending per person of USD 734.9. The cost burden on the population is relatively light. Healthcare resources are allocated reasonably within the country – in 2017, there were 2.34 doctors per one thousand people and 12.27 hospital beds per one thousand people. In 2017, the average life expectancy of women was 85.7 years, and 79.7 years for men; the infant mortality rate was 2.8%. The level of people's health in the country is quite high.

5.1.2 The medical services system and provision of healthcare resources

5.1.2.1 SPECIAL FEATURES OF THE ROK'S MEDICAL SERVICES SYSTEM

The country's medical services system is divided into a number of tiers. The total number of medical institutions in all tiers comes to around 62,000, which can be divided into categories depending on size and function. These include Level Three hospitals (the top level), comprehensive hospitals, small-scale hospitals, long-term care institutions, and clinics. Among these, private medical institutions account for 95%, while public medical institutions account for just 5%. Healthcare institutions in the country are responsible for disseminating knowledge and education on health, for family planning, for prevention of chronic diseases, and so on, and for providing a small number of routine clinic services. Such institutions are composed of a three-tiered network that includes healthcare centers, quasi-healthcare centers, and primary healthcare stations. In addition, the ROK has a combined total of around 21,000 community pharmacies and hospital pharmacies.

5.1.2.2 CHARACTERISTICS OF THE PROVISION OF HEALTHCARE RESOURCES IN THE ROK

The provision of healthcare resources in the ROK is directly related to the evolution of the country's healthcare policies, which include roughly the following three stages. The first was when Korea was a colony of Japan and that government guided healthcare policies (1910–1945). During this period, under colonial influence, western medicine was dominant in the overall pattern while Korean medicine served as a supplement. Resources were mainly provided by the state, which was a primary feature of colonization. The second stage was a period of laissez-faire after New China was established (1945–1977), during which time there was essentially no intervention in the sphere of medicine and healthcare. Korean medicine developed to the point that the pattern allowed both Korean and western medicine to advance, while the provision of healthcare was clearly market-driven. The third stage came after the implementation of Korean medical health insurance policies. This 'managed-style' stage (1977 to the present) involves stronger government intervention in the field of medicine and healthcare. While based on market-driven liberalism, the government is increasing administrative controls and the pattern is more of a tripod that combines western medicine, pharmacology, and Korean medicine. Healthcare resources are provided by the cooperative efforts of both government and the market.

5.1.2.3 DRUG SUPPLY IN THE ROC

As one form of healthcare resources, drugs and the provision of drugs went through a difficult reform in the ROC, namely the transition from a system in which drugs and medicine were combined as a business to a system that separates out the business of drugs from the business of medicine. Prior to this separation, given the over-development of a market-driven system, all levels of medical institutions carried out disorderly and even vicious competition. Although the country had established a referral system, this operated more in name than in reality since each tier of medical institution had not defined its own position and was not handling just its own functions. The manufacturing of and provision of drugs had no rules to guide them in this chaotic market. First, this meant that quality could not be guaranteed. The Korean government's attitude toward quality control was extremely relaxed. Drug companies were asked to discipline themselves, so they typically paid fees to medical institutions and then sold the institutions substandard drugs. The overall quality of drugs circulating in the Korean market was poor. Second, this meant that drugs were prescribed unreasonably. Prior to the separation of drugs and medicine, Korea's pharmacists and doctors formed two opposing interest groups that competed with each other for large prescriptions, given the seduction of huge profits to be made from the drug industry. As this situation intensified, the Korean government formulated a law in December 1953, called the Pharmacists Act, which began to embody the idea of separating out medicine from drugs. Given the massive obstructive power of stakeholders, however, this policy was not truly put into effect until July 2000.

5.1.3 The medical safeguards system

5.1.3.1 FORMATION OF THE SYSTEM

The ROK passed the Medical Insurance Act in December 1963, marking the establishment of a medical safeguards system in the country. In 1977, large companies with over 500 employees formally set up medical insurance systems and then expanded the scope of their coverage in 1979. Insurance for rural residents of Korea was set up in 1988, and medical insurance for residents of cities and towns was set up in 1989; in 1989, the country basically achieved universal health insurance coverage. In 2000, the more than 300 insurance companies that had operated independently were merged into one entity under the jurisdiction of the Ministry of Health and Welfare. The name of this entity, the National Health Insurance Corporation, was later changed to the National Health

Insurance System, which then marked the establishment of a unified nationwide system of health insurance.

5.1.3.2 RESPONSIBLE ORGANIZATIONS

The first responsible organization is the National Ministry of Health and Welfare. The National Ministry of Health and Welfare is the competent authority governing the medical safeguards system. It is responsible for the management and regulatory supervision of the operations of medical insurance. Its functions include formulating medical insurance policies and guiding principles, which include policies that cover food hygiene, healthcare, medical insurance and pensions, and maternal and child welfare.

The second responsible organization is the National Health Insurance Corporation (System) (NHIS). NHIS is the only insurance company in the ROK that is responsible for providing all national medical insurance and for operating the insurance system. Non-profit in nature, NHIS is specifically responsible for collecting premiums, negotiating fee contracts, paying medical insurance allowances, and so on.

The third responsible organization is the Health Insurance Review and Assessment organization (HIRA). Also under the Ministry of Health and Welfare, HIRA is mainly responsible for reviewing medical expenses, controlling medical quality, evaluating the rationality of medical services, and carrying out pharmaco-economic assessments. HIRA has set up a national medical insurance payment database in the ROK, which contains all medical and drug payment records covering almost the entire Korean population. In other words, HIRA can use a value-based medical insurance system to generate synergy through rule-making, infrastructure management, monitoring and feedback procedures to finally realize medical insurance control.[7] Additionally, HIRA's Drug Welfare Evaluation Committee is responsible for evaluating the efficacy and cost-effectiveness of drugs, so as to make decisions on whether or not to include them in the national drug reimbursement list. HIRA also manages the standardized coding of drugs.

5.1.3.3 FUNDING OF THE SYSTEM, AND MEDICAL TREATMENT

First, with respect to the funding of the ROK's medical insurance: the NHIS is responsible for collecting the premiums on this insurance. Of these premiums, government subsidies cover 14.7%, while individuals and employers pay 85.3%. People with a fixed place of employment must pay 5.8% of their monthly income to medical insurance, with the employer and the employer each responsible for one half. People without a fixed place of employment, such as those who operate small businesses, pay at a level that is commensurate with indicators of their financial

7 Feng Chang, Ji Meiyan, Lu Yun, Cui Penglei, and Zhu Xiaorui. Research on the ROK Medical Security System and Its Operation Mode [J]. *China Health Policy Research*, 2015, 8 (12): 41–46.

situation, such as age, income, household assets, and so on. Adjustments are made annually in line with levels of economic development and per capita income. Second, with respect to the process of receiving medical care for those who are covered by insurance: After a patient who is covered by insurance receives medical care, the patient needs to pay only the self-pay part of the bill, as prescribed by insurance policies. The remaining part will be covered initially by the medical institution. After HIRA receives an application from the medical institution, HIRA reviews the costs and actions of the institution and gives feedback within two weeks of getting the results of the review. Depending on the results of the feedback, and whether or not the actions of the medical institution are in line with regulations, NHIS then decides whether or not to pay the medical costs to the medical institution. If actions are deemed unreasonable, then NHIS may lodge a complaint as per relevant rules and regulations. At this point, the HIRA organizes experts to undertake a second review.

5.2 Drug price-formation mechanisms in the ROK

In 2017, the volume of drug sales in the ROK came to USD 32.619 billion, or a per capita figure of USD 634. The industry is market-driven, as shown by the 54% of retail spending that was due to government procurement, lower than the 58% average of OECD countries. The self-pay (out-of-pocket) portion of residents was 45%, higher than the OECD average of 39%. The number of licensed pharmacists in the country is gradually increasing and went from around 60 per 100,000 people in 2000 (close to the OECD average) to 72 per 100,000 people in 2017 (less than the OECD average of 83).

5.2.1 Overview of the drug market in the ROK

The speed at which the drug market in the ROK has grown is quite remarkable, as well as the way the market is being consolidated. In 2015, the market ranked 14th in the world in size and held a 1.5% share of the global market. Seoul ranked first in the world in terms of clinical-trial cities, and was tenth in terms of new drugs approved by the FDA. The ROK has roughly 894 pharmaceutical factories that produce close to 27,000 different kinds of pharmaceuticals, valued at close to USD 16 billion. In the pharmaceuticals sector there are also 393 manufacturers who are making 7,200 different kinds of pharmaceuticals for overseas companies, valued at USD 1.24 billion. The country has 1,895 manufacturers of cosmetics, producing close to 9,000 different products that are valued at USD 6.38 billion, and it has 2,607 manufacturers of medical equipment, producing more than 10,000 different products that are valued at USD 3.4 billion.

The pharmaceutical industry is highly regionalized – the manufacturing of and also trade in drugs is concentrated in the Gyeonggi region of the ROK. In 2015, 288 drug manufacturing factories were concentrated in this area, plus 38 makers of plant extracts for drugs, 209 makers of quasi-drugs, 1,081 makers of medical devices, and 572 manufacturers of cosmetics. From a municipal perspective, Seoul is still central when it comes to the drug manufacturing industry. In 2015, the city had 29 drug manufacturing factories, 75 makers of plant extracts for drugs, 26 makers of quasi-drugs, 601 manufacturers of medical equipment, and 346 manufacturers of cosmetics.

The most important drug manufacturers in the ROK are Dong-A Pharmaceutical Co., Ltd.; Hanmi Pharmaceutical Co., Ltd.; Yuhan Co., Ltd.; and Daewoong Co., Ltd. Among these four, Dong-A Pharmaceuticals is currently the largest. It produces prescription drugs, non-prescription drugs, and health supplements, as well as biological products and medical equipment. It is primarily aimed at the domestic market and has only in the past few years begun to explore overseas markets with a limited number of drugs for export. In contrast, Hanmi Pharmaceuticals ('Korea-America') has gone international faster than any other Korean company. In 2015, this company ranked second in the pharmaceutical industry in the ROK.

5.2.2 The drug system in the ROK

'Drugs' covers a broad range of subjects, including production and distribution, price formulation and price controls, wholesale and retail, and so on. The main legal and policy aspects relating to drugs in the ROK include the following.

1 Regulations relating to pharmacies

The ROK law governing the establishment of pharmacies is called the 'Pharmaceutical Affairs Law,' which stipulates that only licensed pharmacists can open a pharmacy and each legally licensed pharmacist may only be allowed one license for an independent storefront. Under this regulation, pharmacists are not allowed to open chains of pharmacies. Pharmacies that are set up in supermarkets or chain stores are generally operating under special permits. These are required to pay rent to the store, but the amount of deposit they put up generally bears no relationship to the sales volume of the franchise.

2 Systemic regulations regarding the separation of the business of drugs from the practice of medicine

First, the initial idea for realizing a separation of 'drugs' from 'medicine' came in the Pharmacists Act of December 1953. This stated that 'non-pharmacists are not allowed to fulfill (concoct) drugs, and pharmacists must only fulfill drugs in a pharmacy.' This regulation went on to say that 'pharmacists may not change or revise prescriptions without the approval of a doctor, dentist, Korean-medicine practitioner, or veterinarian.' However, it was very hard to satisfy this requirement due to conditions at the time, such as the low levels of both quantity and quality of doctors and pharmacists, inadequate medical infrastructure and so on, which meant that the regulations had no effect whatsoever in reaching the desired outcome. Both doctors and pharmacists in fact fulfilled prescriptions directly. Second, the ROK revised the Pharmacists Act in December 1963. This explicitly separated out the roles that doctors and pharmacists were to play and stated that 'pharmacists must "concoct drugs" (fulfill prescriptions) (only) according to the prescriptions of doctors, dentists, and veterinarians.' The policy guidance about separating drugs and medicine was more explicit. Nevertheless, the results of this were also not apparent, given that the government had not done sufficient preparation in explaining detailed and specific procedures on how to achieve the separation. Next, in 1994 the ROK passed the 'Amendment to the Pharmacists Law,' which declared that reforms to separate out medicine from drugs would be instituted over the next three to five years. This Act was triggered by a sudden conflict between the two large interest groups, Korean-medicine doctors and pharmacists, over the right to concoct medicines. The Act explicitly ruled that the Korean-medicine pharmacists system would be re-established, but it also said that within three years drugs and medicine would be separated out as two different businesses. After this, Kim Dae-jung came to power in 1998 and the reform separating out medicine from drugs began to be implemented in earnest. Although the reform process encountered opposition and obstruction from all interest groups, including vicious strikes that extended the process for a full year, in the end a separation of drugs and medicine was truly realized in July 2000. The ROK thereby achieved a pattern that separated the business of drugs from the business of medicine.

5.2.3 Regulations regarding the price-formulation system

First, with regard to regulations on pricing innovative drugs: the ROK has transitioned from pricing through reference to external prices to pricing through negotiations. The external pricing method relies on international drug prices as the criteria and disregards the cost and quality of drugs, as well as any unique qualities determined by a country's specific conditions. Its defects gradually become obvious. The ROC therefore later focused its reforms on a negotiated method of pricing, and also supplemented that with quantity-based adjustments. Cost-effectiveness became the main criterion for pricing, which was more scientific relative to pricing according to reference prices.

Second, with reference to price controls over generic drugs: prior to April 2012, the ROK used a linked-price system for both generic drugs and original-research drugs. After April 2012, the country adjusted its pricing method for generic drugs and began to use a single-price system. These two methods apply different rules regarding the generic's percentage of price, depending on (the generic's market-entry status and quantity). This is to accommodate the way the drug market is developing (details are given later).

5.2.4 Regulations on the drug reimbursement system

Prior to 2007, the ROK employed a negative list in managing its drug reimbursements. That is, it would only reimburse for drugs that were not on the medical insurance list. This system, however, was regarded as the cause of overly high drug spending and the main reason for an enormous burden on public finance. Given this insupportable burden, in May of 2006, the country issued a *Plan to rationalize spending on drug costs*, and in November of the same year, it passed and began to implement the *Health insurance reform act*. One of the provisions of this Act determined that a positive list of reimbursable drugs would be implemented from 2007. This meant that drug manufacturers now had to submit pharmaco-economic reports on their drugs, and only after the drugs passed an evaluation could they be entered into the reimbursement list. Meanwhile, negotiations were among the follow-on procedures in order to determine the prices at which medical insurance would reimburse for drugs.

5.3 Entities involved in the price-formation of drugs in the ROK

The pricing of drugs is highly complex and of necessity involves multiple parties. In overall terms, these include government, drug manufacturers, wholesalers, retailers, doctors, and patients (Figure 6.28).

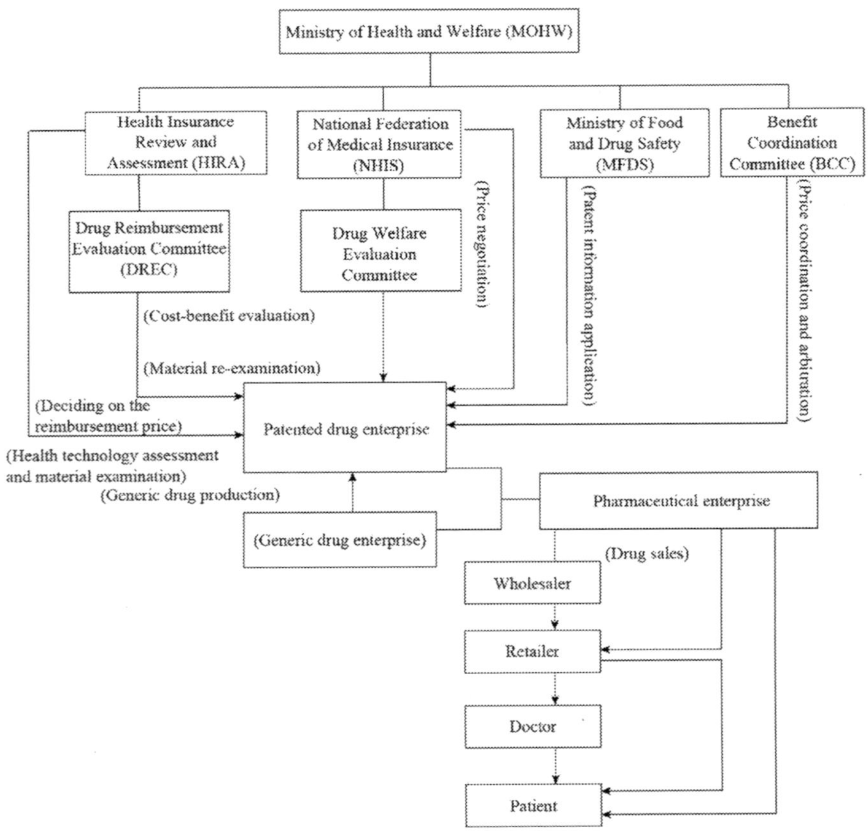

Figure 6.28 Inter-relationships of Entities Involved in the Pricing of Drugs in the ROK

First, with respect to government bodies. The main government institutions that play a role in the process of drug price-formation in the ROK are the following: the Ministry of Health and Welfare (MOHW), the National Health Insurance System (NHIS), the Health Insurance Review and Assessment organization (HIRA), and the Drug Welfare Assessment Committee. The ROK's Ministry of Health and Welfare (MOHW), as the competent authority of the national medical security system, plays a role in the process of drug pricing mainly by formulating macro policies and principles. It thereby carries out overall management and supervision. The former National Federation of Medical Insurance (NFMI) was later split into two main bodies, the National Health Insurance Corporation (NHIS) and Health Insurance Review and Assessment organization (HIRA). These two now assume the two roles that were once held by the NFMI, namely providing statutory medical insurance, and serving as an independent third party that provides health technology assessments and project research support for the government. They also now assume the two functions of the previous body, namely medical insurance decision selection and funds operation, and medical insurance selection index standard formulation and review. By dividing up the original entity, the medical technology assessments and the decision-making on health insurance selection were separated from the operations of health insurance funds, thus ensuring the independence and scientific nature of the technology assessments.

The Drug Welfare Evaluation Committee is specifically responsible for evaluating the efficacy of drugs and their cost-effectiveness. It is under the jurisdiction of the HIRA, and it decides whether or not a drug should be entered into the reimbursement list. At the same time it is responsible for establishing a national standard coding system and managing the information-technology aspects of the ROK's drugs.

Second, with respect to drug manufacturers, wholesalers, and retailers. The ROK divides drug manufacturers into those that make innovative drugs and those that make generics. Once an innovative drug manufacturer has developed a drug, this is put on the market after a review and approval process and it is granted a certain period of patent protection. Generic drug manufacturers reproduce the ingredients in innovative drugs to develop generics, also known as commonly used drugs or over-the-counter drugs. These are put on the market once the patent of a new drug expires. The therapeutic results of new drugs and generics differ very little.

Third, with respect to doctors and patients. Doctors make decisions on behalf of patients on what kinds of drugs to use and in what quantity, while patients are the ultimate consumers of drugs. The drug-prescribing behavior of doctors and the drug needs of patients have a key influence on drug pricing.

5.4 The process and methods by which drug prices are formed in the ROK

Prices for innovative drugs and those for generics are formed via different methods.

5.4.1 Price-formation of innovative drugs and patented drugs

Before 2007, the ROK used external reference prices to determine the pricing of innovative drugs within the country. It referenced the average drug prices of seven specific countries in formulating the domestic price, that is, in forming the initial price of the innovative drug within the ROK. Only once the new drug of an innovative drug company had gone through the review and approval process could it be put on the market as a patented drug, but the price-formation of patented drugs prior to 2007 relied on the negative-list system, that is, drugs on the list within the country were not reimbursed, while drugs not on the list would all be reimbursed. At the time, there were actually very few drugs on the negative list. This form of reimbursement system led to soaring levels of government spending on drugs, far beyond the carrying capacities of public finance. As a result, the ROK reformed the system in 2007. First, the pricing of innovative drugs now relied mostly on price negotiations as informed by pharmaco-economic assessments. Second, the patented drug-pricing system was changed to a positive-list system, that is, only drugs included in the list would be reimbursed and all drugs not on the list would not be reimbursed (Figure 6.29).

Meanwhile, the prices at which innovative drugs will be reimbursed are decided by negotiations between the NHIS and the drug manufacturer. The five main aspects taken into consideration during these negotiations are as follows. 1) Pharmaco-economic evaluations that the drug manufacturer submits to NHIS; 2) consideration of the impact that admitting this type of drug to the list will have on health insurance funds; 3) the international price of this type of drug; 4) the patent situation for this type of drug; and 5) the domestic outlay that went into researching and developing this kind of drug. In addition, the NHIS might also undertake negotiations on the drug's expected quantity of usage. This figure can be adjusted as appropriate later, once actual usage figures are known. If the drug's sales are more than 30% over what was originally expected, then the reimbursement price is lowered by a certain percentage, but the degree of adjustment can be no more than 10%. The specific formula for such adjustments is:

$$\text{Price after adjustment} = 0.9 \times P_0 + 0.1\times [P_0 \times (V_e/V_a)]$$

In this formula, PO is the price of the drug as determined by negotiations; Ve is the expected volume of sales; Va is the actual volume of sales (usage).

5.4.2 Price-formation of original-research drugs and generic drugs

Before April 2012, the ROK used the 'linked-price system' (LPS) to set prices on original-research drugs and generic drugs. (Note: original-research drugs are known as Reference Listed Drugs in the U.S.) By LPS rules, if the patent protection on an innovative drug has expired, and generics are already on the market, then the 'innovative drug' becomes an 'original-research' drug and its price will automatically fall to 80% of the innovative drug's price. The first five generic drugs to be put on the market will be priced at 68% of the original price, while the 6th generic,

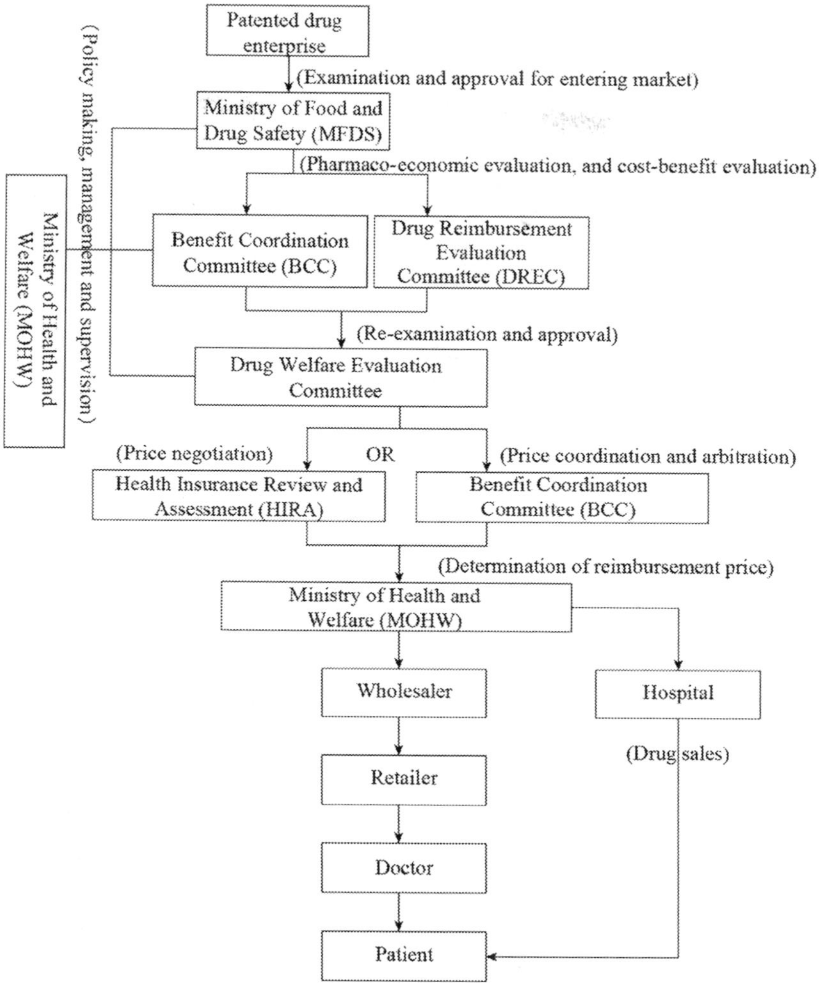

Figure 6.29 Price-Formation of the Prices of Patented Drugs in the ROK

or any generics after this, will be priced at 90% of the lowest price on the market. After April 2012, the method of setting pricing on generics was changed to become a 'single-price system' (SPS). Under SPS rules, once the first generic drug that reproduces an original-research drug is entered into the reimbursable drug list, its price automatically falls to 70% of the original-research drug. Within one year after this, all prices of generics must, by regulations, be priced at 59.5% (of the price of the innovative drug), that is, at 85% of the original-research drug after its price has been reduced. Pricing is not subject to the number of generic drugs on the market. After one year goes by, the prices of all original-research drugs as well as generics must be reduced to 53.55% of the original (innovative drug) price (Figure 6.30).

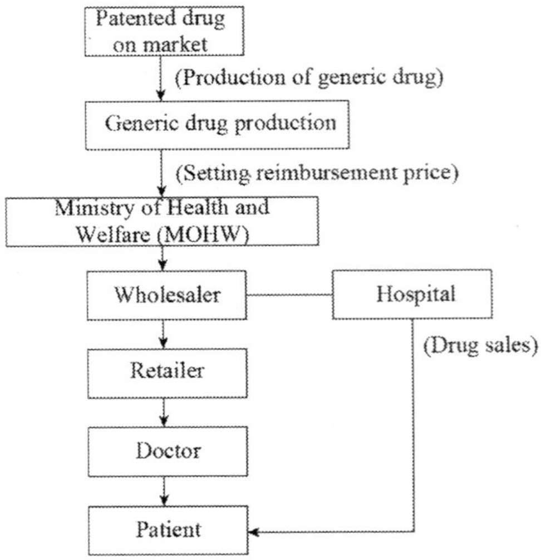

Figure 6.30 Price-Formation of the Prices of Generic Drugs in the ROK

5.4.3 Latest dynamics of managing drug prices in the ROK

Starting on March 15, 2015, the ROK began implementing a comprehensive 'patent-linking system' in the country. Specifically, this included public announcements on patent information, patent declarations, suspension periods, and the exclusive-period system for the first generic on the market, as described next.

5.4.3.1 PUBLIC ANNOUNCEMENTS ON PATENT INFORMATION

A public announcement of a patent symbolizes to the pharmaceutical industry that a given drug enjoys patent protection, and this is the foundation of the patent-linking system. First a drug company applies (for such an announcement) to the Ministry of Food and Drug Safety. If this application passes, then the drug's patent information is posted on a public list, which in the ROK is known as the 'Green List.' The ability of a drug to be put on the Green List is not only directly related to its active ingredients, called-for indications, methods of usage, and so on, but is directly related to such quality indicators as safety and efficacy. The ROK has specifically set up a system for the review of applications to the Green List. That is, once the MFDS receives a patent-listing application from an original-research drug manufacturer, it carries out a review and determines whether or not the drug meets requirements for listing and whether or not it has sufficient comparability, and only when the information on the drug meets requirements will the patent be included in the Green List. This is to prevent the manufacturer of the original-research drug from illegally putting patents that are not directly comparable into the Green List, which leads to unnecessary delays in the ability of generics to come to market. Finally, the original-research drug manufacturer may revise the application or have it deleted from the list, even after the patent information has been included in the Green List.

5.4.3.2 PATENT DECLARATION

A patent declaration is submitted by the manufacturer of a generic drug when it applies for an 'abbreviated' new drug to be put on the market. Once an original drug is put on the Green List, its maker needs to make one of the following declarations in applying for the 'abbreviated' form of the drug to be put on the market. One, the patent protection of the patent listed in the Green List has expired. Two, the generic drug will be sold only after the patent protection period has expired. Three, both the patent holder of the original patent and the research company making the original drug agree that the applicant for the non-patented drug does not have to submit a patent declaration. Four, the scope of patent protection that is on the Green List does not include preventing the non-patented drug from being put on the market. Five, the patent listed on the Green List is no longer effective, or the list of non-patented drugs does not infringe upon the patent. If the drug falls under this fifth provision, then the applicant seeking to put the generic drug on the market needs to issue a 'patent challenge notification' to the holder of the patent and the original-research drug manufacturer within twenty days of submitting its application.

5.4.3.3 SUSPENSION PERIOD

After a patent holder receives a patent challenge notification from the person or entity applying for a generic drug, the patent holder may present a request for a limited period of suspended activity to the Ministry of Food and Drug Safety. This is called the suspension period. The patent holder needs to submit this request within 45 days, and the suspension period can only prevent the generic drug from being sold on the market for this period – it has no impact on the ability of the generic drug maker to receive ultimate approval to go on the market. The patent holder must declare certain things in its request for a suspension period. First, the request must be based on holding a patent that is already listed on the Green List and that is legally valid and reasonable. Second, the request must be in line with the principles of honesty and trustworthiness, it must have at least the prospect of being successful, and it must guarantee that the patent holder will not draw out proceedings unreasonably. After the Ministry of Food and Drug Safety reviews the request and confirms that it is in accord with legal requirements, the patent holder is granted a nine-month suspension period.

5.4.3.4 EXCLUSIVE PERIOD GRANTED TO THE FIRST GENERIC DRUG TO GO ON THE MARKET

To stimulate competition in the drug market and encourage generic drug companies to put forward patent challenges, the ROK has stipulated that generic drug companies that are the first to apply for a generic drug market and whose patent challenges are successful can obtain a 'First Exclusivity period' which lasts for nine months. Obtaining this exclusivity period signifies that the generic drug manufacturer has the right to prevent other generic makers from selling drugs on the market that have active ingredients that are the same as those of the original drug, as well as the same content, dosage form, and efficacy. Only the generic-drug applicant who is first to submit patent challenges and applications is eligible for the First-generic market exclusivity period. If another generic drug applicant also makes a request within 14 days of the First application, or obtains the earliest decision that declares a patent invalid or no longer within the scope of patent protection, this applicant may also be regarded as the 'earliest applicant.'

5.4.4 Price-formation methods of reimbursement prices for drugs in the ROK

In 2006, reimbursement payments for drug costs in the ROK came to 26% of all spending on drugs in the country. This ranked the ROK fourth among OECD countries. Moreover, the speed at which this spending was going up was twice the average of OECD countries. Not only was this putting enormous pressure on public finance, but it posed a grave threat to the sustainability of the country's insurance funds. It was in this context that the ROK formally proposed implementing a positive list in the management of its reimbursable drugs, in 2007.

Under a 'positive-list' system, the price-formation of drugs that are admitted into the reimbursement drug list works as follows. First, a company submits an application to HIRA, requesting permission to put a patented drug that is allowed to sell on the market into the medical insurance list. At a minimum, the information that the drug company must provide when it submits the application will include a pharmaco-economic assessment and an evaluation of the impact on the budget. The application materials must conform to the guidelines that HIRA promulgated in 2006, called Guidelines to Pharmaco-economic Assessments. They must provide a comprehensive evaluation of the impact on spending once the drug has been entered into the medical reimbursement list, which mainly will depend on epidemiology statistics, drug clinical results, and data on cost-effectiveness. The report results are best presented in the form of cost-effectiveness analysis (CEA) or cost-utility analysis (CUA), and an incremental cost-effectiveness ratio must be submitted. In addition, the process of collecting report materials needs to be reflected, and the relevant cost-effectiveness indicators need to be indicated. Second, the HIRA conducts a preliminary examination of the application materials it receives. This is carried out by the organization's internal personnel and takes about 150 days. After the examination, the application is further reviewed by the Drug Reimbursement Evaluation Committee (DREC) under HIRA, which makes a concluding recommendation after the review. It may 'actively recommend,' 'recommend with reservations,' or make 'no recommendation.' The NHIS then holds price negotiations with companies that have been actively recommended, a process which takes around 60 days. If negotiations reach an agreement, the ROK

Ministry of Health and Social Welfare (MOHW) makes the ultimate decision on price within 30 days.

If the negotiation fails to reach an agreement, the company may apply to the Benefit Coordination Committee (BCC) for price coordination and arbitration of this drug. Additionally, BCC has the authority to directly include clinically necessary drugs into the national drug reimbursement list to effectively protect the medical and health needs of patients. For example, BCC once directly included two anticancer drugs, imatinib and dasatinib, and an anti-AIDS drug, enfuvirtide, into the medical insurance reimbursement list when the price negotiations were inconsistent. Meanwhile, drugs must go through a reassessment process, using pharmaco-economics, after they enter the medical insurance reimbursement list. This reassessment follows the same standards as before. If the drug is judged not to have economic advantages after reassessment, it will be removed from the health insurance list unless it voluntarily reduces its price.

5.5 Drug-formation mechanisms in the ROK: a summary

The price-formation of drugs is a complex process. In the ROK, after a maker of patented drugs develops a new drug, this drug must undergo review and approval by HIRA and the results of that process determine three kinds of results with respect to whether or not the drug will be recommended. Once this takes place, the NHIS holds price negotiations with the drug company that are based on pharmaco-economic assessments in order to formulate the reimbursement price. Follow-on procedures may include further price adjustments depending on such information as sales volume. Only after these procedures have been followed may the drug manufacturer initiate business relationships with such buyers as wholesalers, retailers, hospitals, and patients. Price-formation of generic drugs is relatively simple. Prices are formed and adjusted according to the Single-Price System before subsequent drug distribution.

Price-formation of drugs in the ROK possesses the following features.

First, the country has progressed from a simple and extensive mode of pricing and reimbursement to a mode that makes use of assessments. The process has required constant experimentation and learning from mistakes. The determination of innovative drug prices in the ROK has transitioned from being based on reference to external prices to being based on price negotiations. Pricing of generics has transitioned from a Linked-Price System (LPS) to a single-price system (SPS). The formation of reimbursement prices has transitioned from reliance on a negative list to reliance on a positive list as the criteria for admission. The ROK's price-formation of drugs has therefore become ever more scientific in the course of reforms and trial-and-error experimentation.

Second, although the processes of price-formation of drugs are now fairly clear on paper, in actual practice, processes are fairly chaotic. That is, the evidence that two government organizations, the HIRA and NECA, provide on drug prices is not consistent. The division of functions between these two is unclear when it comes to supplying pricing evidence on the supply side. This leads to unclear processes, since mechanisms are not completely established. In addition, the CEA and BIA provide evidence that plays only a minor role in price negotiations, according to information derived from face-to-face discussions with ROK experts.

Third, changes under the ROK's market-oriented policies continue to be turbulent. Between 1945 and 1977, the ROK went through a laissez-faire period after liberation from colonialism. During that period, inadequate supervision of the medical and healthcare sphere led to the country's pronounced market orientation. Later, although the government strengthened interventions, coordination between the roles of market and government was inadequate. Mechanisms that harmonize the two are not yet completely established, which means that the potential for triggering chaos is concealed within the system.

Fourth, as two large stakeholders, doctors and patients do not participate adequately in decisions on drug pricing. Since their opinions are not adequately expressed, policies that result are not supported by the public and implementation encounters problems.

Abbreviations and acronyms

BCC: Benefit Coordination Committee
DREC: Drug Reimbursement Evaluation Committee
HIRA: Health Insurance Review and Assessment
LPS: Linked Price System
MOHW: Ministry of Health and Welfare
NFMI: National Federation of Medical Insurance
NHIS: National Health Insurance System
SPS: Single price system

6 Case study of Taiwan, China

6.1 General introduction to Taiwan's medical system

Taiwan is situated on the continental shelf along the southeast coast of the Chinese mainland. It is made up of two large island groups, the largest island in China, Taiwan Island, together with its surrounding islands, and the Penghu archipelago with more than 80 islands and islets. The total area of Taiwan is 36,192.8155 square kilometers, and in 2018 it had a population of 23.58 million people. Since the 1960s, Taiwan has promoted an export-oriented industrial strategy which has led to soaring economic development and rapid social advances. In the 1970s and 1980s, Taiwan was ranked as one of the Four Little Dragons of Asia, along with Hong Kong, Singapore, and the ROK. In 2018, Taiwan's annual GDP grew by more than 2.6% in real terms over the previous year. The total GDP came to NT$ 17.77 trillion (about RMB 3.9 trillion), which put Taiwan eighth among China's provinces in GDP. Although this is considerably different from Guangdong province, which by comparison has the highest economic volume of any province in China, when it comes to GDP per capita, Taiwan is still the bellwether among

China's provinces. A comprehensive medical services system and a sound system of medical safeguards have created quite high health standards among Taiwan's residents. In 2016, the average life expectancy in Taiwan had already reached 80 years, up from 77.9 years in 2006. Male life expectancy in 2016 was 76.8, while that of females was 83.4.

6.1.1 Introduction to the medical services system

In 1986, the Ministry of Health in Taiwan proposed a plan to build a 'medical network' in Taiwan that would provide all people with access to sound medical services by improving the balanced distribution of medical resources. By the time this plan was completed, in 2000, Taiwan basically had a complete and relatively reasonable medical and healthcare services system that was composed of medical centers, regional hospitals, local hospitals, and grassroots healthcare units. In terms of size and services, medical centers are roughly equivalent to third-tier hospitals on the Mainland (the top level), while regional hospitals are equivalent to second-tier and first-tier hospitals. By the end of 2018, Taiwan had a total of 473 hospitals, of which 80 were public hospitals and 393 were private (non-public), or 83% private. It had 400 public clinics and 20,419 private clinics, or 98% private. The Taiwan region's medical and healthcare system is therefore predominantly run by the private sector. With regard to the level of medical care, the documentary *New Horizons in Asia: Taiwan's Medical Miracle* by the National Geographic Channel of the U.S. noted that Taiwan's medical technology was renowned worldwide, and this was already back in 2012. Taiwan ranks first in Asia and third in the world in a listing of the world's top 200 hospitals, which includes 14 of its hospitals. Its levels of medical care are known as 'Asia's miracle.'

6.1.2 Introduction to the medical insurance system

Since Taiwan began instituting a system of universal health insurance coverage in 1995 (called 'universal coverage' later), its well-designed system has been able to provide health insurance that has both low premiums and high quality. However, this is now facing extremely large challenges given the aging of the population, advances in medical technology, the reduced pace of economic growth, and the expectations of the public for quality medical care.

6.1.2.1 THE HISTORY OF DEVELOPING UNIVERSAL COVERAGE

Taiwan's medical insurance has gone through three stages: the old form of health insurance starting in the 1950s; 'first-generation' insurance, starting in 1995; and 'second-generation' insurance, starting in 2013. The old form of insurance included four main categories with 11 types of insurance. The four main categories were workers' insurance, implemented in the 1950s; civil servants' insurance, implemented in 1958; farmers' health insurance, implemented in 1985; and low-income household insurance, implemented in 1990. The 'universal coverage' plan began in 1995. This consolidated the previous insurance, combining four categories into one, and it set premium rates at 4.25%. The first-generation insurance not only resolved the problem of health insurance for the entire body of people in the Taiwan region but it became a social policy that enjoyed the public's highest degree of satisfaction. However, universal coverage began to experience a severe crisis with the expansion in coverage, advances of modern technology, and aging of the population, all of which led to an increase in medical costs. In order to resolve this financial crisis, Taiwan's second-generation insurance was launched in 2013. The differences between first- and second-generation insurance mainly related to such things as people returning to Taiwan for medical care, care quality, the calculations on premiums, linking income and expenditures, disclosure of financial information, and so on. According to the 'Introduction to universal health insurance coverage 2016–2017,' by the end of June 2016, a total of some 23.72 million people were participants in 'second-generation' coverage, which meant that the coverage rate was 99.6%.

6.1.2.2 ADMINISTERING HEALTH INSURANCE IN TAIWAN

Looking at the administration of health insurance from top to bottom, Taiwan adopts a single-party publicly operated system with the Central Health Insurance Department carrying out funding under unified (centralized) planning that also covers medical administration and pricing of drugs. The actual provision of medical services is carried out by medical institutions. Looked at in horizontal terms, the Healthcare and Benefits Department is the governing authority handling universal coverage. As per the principle of setting up a balance of power, the Healthcare and Benefits Department has set up the Universal Health Insurance Association, the Universal Health Insurance Committee on Dispute Resolution, and the Health Insurance Department. The first of these assists in the planning process on policies, and it oversees the implementation of those policies. The second is responsible for handling disputes relating to health insurance. The third, as 'insurer,' is actually the core entity in the whole operation. This entity, the Health Insurance Department, employs 3,400 people in six regional bureaus. It is responsible for taking in premiums, for managing medicine, and for administering medical insurance reimbursements. Its administrative expenses are a line item in the central government's budget.

6.1.2.3 THE TARGETS OF HEALTHCARE SAFEGUARDS

According to the provisions of Articles 8, 9, and 10 of the *Taiwan Universal Health Insurance Law*, persons who have been missing for six months or who have no household registration, have lived in Taiwan for less than six months, and do not have a specified employer, cannot participate in the universal health insurance program. All other persons (including foreigners who have lived in Taiwan for more than six months) who meet the conditions for the establishment of household registration must participate in the universal health insurance program, which at the present time covers 99.6% of Taiwan's residents. Compulsory participation in medical insurance can effectively prevent adverse selection and ensure the fairness of access to medical insurance for all residents. Participants in the universal health insurance program are called 'insured persons,' who are divided into insured persons and their dependents. As shown in Table 6.9, insured persons are further divided into six categories or 'types.'

6.1.2.4 HEALTH INSURANCE SAFEGUARDS

Universal health insurance provides specifically defined services via contracts that are signed between medical institutions and Taiwan's Health Insurance Department. The rate at which hospitals sign up for these contracts is 100%, whereas for clinics it is 92%, giving an average sign-up rate of 96%. Specific terms of the contracts are negotiated between the Health Insurance Department and four public associations, while at the same time negotiations are carried out among stakeholders and various experts and scholars on the medical services that are to be reimbursed. Taiwan reimburses for a wealth of covered items that include hospitalization under western medicine practices, clinic services for western medicine, imaging and examinations, laboratory tests, prescription drugs and some non-prescription drugs, dental care (straightening, false teeth, and implantations must be self-paid), preventive health measures, and so on.

6.1.2.5 FUNDING AND REIMBURSEMENT

The funding of Taiwan's medical insurance comes mainly from monthly premiums that are based on regular wages and from subsidized premiums. Monthly premiums based on regular wages are set at 4.67% of wages (prior to 2003, this was 4.25%; in 2013 it was raised to 4.55%; then to 5.17% in 2010; in 2012, it was adjusted back to 4.91%; and in 2016 it was again adjusted down to 4.67%). Of this 4.67%, the company bears the cost of 60%, the individual 30%, and the government 10%. Subsidies include funds derived from the value-added tax on tobacco, allocations of earnings from financial instruments, and taxes levied on stock dividends, interest, rent, bonuses, income from part-time jobs, and so on. In 2018, the government and individuals paid for 36% of the funding of Taiwan's health insurance, while companies paid for another 28%. All those who are insured receive the same benefits from medical insurance. The 'basic' cost burden of outpatient (clinic) services depends on the level of medical institutions, and is NT$ 420 for medical centers, NT$ 240 for regional hospitals, NT$ 80 for regional clinics and NT$ 50 for primary clinics. These figures are reduced to NT$ 170, NT$ 100, and NT$ 50 respectively upon referral. The self-pay portion of a patient's hospitalization costs depends on the number of days – it is 10% of costs for stays that are within 30 days, 20% for stays between 31 days and 60 days, and 30% for stays over 61 days. There is no deductible for hospitalization expenses, but there is a ceiling on the self-pay of patients. The self-pay for each hospitalization for the same disease cannot exceed NT$ 39,000, while the cumulative total of self-pay

Table 6.9 Classification of Insured Persons and Insured Units under Taiwan's Universal Health Insurance

Type	*Insured Persons*		*Insured Units*
	Themselves	*Their Family Dependents*	
Type I	Public officials, volunteer servicepeople, civil servants, teaching staff in private schools, employees of public and private enterprises, and institutions with certain employers, employers, self-employed owners, specialized professionals, and technicians who work on their own	Non-professional spouse of the insured Non-professional lineal relatives of the insured The lineal relatives of the insured within the second degree of kinship, who are under 20 years old and have no occupation, or who are over 20 years old and have no ability to earn a living or are still studying and have no occupation.	The organ, school, company, organization, or individual of the insured person
Type II	Professional trade union members, external crew members	The same as the first type of family dependents	The trade union of the insured person
Type III	Farmers, fishermen, members of water conservancy association	The same as the first type of family dependents	Farmers' Association, Fishery Association, and Water Conservancy Association
Type IV	Compulsory servicepeople, military cadets, dependents in pension, substitute servicepeople, and inmates of correctional institutions	None	Designated units of the 'Ministry of Defense,' the 'Ministry of Interior,' and the 'Ministry of Legal Affairs'
Type V	Members of low-income households that meet the social assistance law	None	户籍地的乡（镇、市、去）公所 Offices of townships (towns, city, and district)
Type VI	Representatives of the families of the veterans and their families left behind by the veterans	Non-professional spouse of a veteran Non-professional lineal relatives of a veteran The lineal descendants of the second degree of kinship of a veteran, who are under 20 years old and have no occupation, or over 20 years old and have no ability to earn a living or are still studying and have no occupation.	Offices of townships (towns, city, and district)
	General household head or household representative	The same as Type I	

for hospital costs may not exceed NT$ 65,000 per year. Some portion of costs for both clinics and hospital stays may be exempted for major injuries and illnesses, low-income households, retired military personnel, and children under 3 years old.

Taiwan's system for reimbursing medical costs has gradually transitioned from the previous way of paying after the fact according to volume to the current way of paying mainly in advance by total volume in addition to other reimbursement methods. Payments of medical costs mainly use a budgeting system of total-amount payment, but a portion of inpatient diagnosis and treatment costs are according to type of illness. Under the pre-payment system, settlement is made by converting points to amounts. This has had good results in terms of checking the rise in medical costs. In September of every year, the Health Insurance Department negotiates annual total-amount costs that will be covered by insurance with premium payers such as companies, as well as experts, scholars, and stakeholders. An increase in rates of 6% to 9% over the previous year's actual expenditures has been the general rule, but this percentage may drop to 3% to 5% given negotiations and disputes between the public association and hospitals. In 2018, Taiwan's spending on medical insurance came to 3.5% of GDP. Of this amount, spending through hospitals was 68.8% (inpatient costs came to 30.2% of this and outpatient costs came to 38.6%). Spending through clinics came to 20.3%, dentists 6.4%, Chinese medicine 3.7%, and home-care and other came to 0.8%. Taiwan implements a system of controls over the items covered by insurance and the reimbursement prices. Negotiations between the Health Insurance Department and representatives from all stakeholders have resulted in the *Medical-cost items to be covered by insurance and payment standards*, and *Drug-cost items to be covered by insurance and payment standards*. These have set prices on 4,200 items described as medical services, 9,000 items described as special materials, 1,600 items described as drugs, and 401 items described as types of illness. Between 1999 and 2018, the drug costs that are covered by health insurance in Taiwan have maintained a stable percentage of around 25% of total health insurance costs. In 2018, medical costs were 6.3% of GDP, and per capita healthcare spending was NT$ 10,419. Within total medical costs, drug costs accounted for 26.5%.

Taiwan's health insurance has achieved a nearly 100% rate of coverage, and close to 80% of the population is satisfied with the results. In comparison to OECD countries, Taiwan's universal healthcare coverage has made four great achievements: high medical accessibility, low medical expenses, high medical quality, and a high degree of medical satisfaction. Nevertheless, even as it achieves these things, Taiwan's health insurance is facing the challenges of a shortage of funds brought on by the constant rise in medical costs. These can be attributed to the aging population and high-tech medical technologies. The aging population is contributing 0.5% to 0.6% to the rise in medical costs, while new technologies are contributing 40%. The main driving force behind rising medical costs is therefore high-tech medical technologies.

6.2 Drug price-formation mechanisms in Taiwan

Taiwan's drug-pricing mechanisms have a pronounced Japanese flavor to them. This is because Taiwan took Japan's price-determination mechanisms into account when it started to set up its own policies. In the actual process of price-formation, however, Taiwan does not use Japan's levels of innovative drugs when it does its own classification, and Taiwan has its own independent ways of adjusting reimbursement prices. In overall terms, Taiwan has taken lessons from Japan in its pricing, but it has independently come up with its own system of mechanisms.

6.2.1 Introduction to the entities involved in drug price-formation

6.2.1.1 MINISTRY OF HEALTH AND WELFARE

In July 2013, Taiwan undertook an institutional reorganization that combined a number of previous administrative units into a new ministry called the Ministry of Health and Welfare. The entities that were combined included 21 units and task forces and five agencies previously under the jurisdiction of the Department of Health. These included the Social Affairs Department, the Children's Bureau, the Domestic Violence and Sexual Abuse Prevention Committee, and Residents Pension Supervision Committee of the Ministry of Internal Affairs, and the Institute of Traditional Chinese Medicine under the Ministry of Education. The Ministry of Health and Welfare is a new agency with unified powers including eight departments and six offices. It is responsible for administrative affairs as they relate to health and social welfare in Taiwan. Its subordinate agencies include the Disease Control Department, the Food and Drug Administration, the Central Health Insurance Department, the National Health Department, the Social and Family Department, and the Institute of Chinese Medicine. The Ministry of Health and Welfare directly manages 26 hospitals that are affiliated with the Ministry.

6.2.1.2 THE HEALTH INSURANCE DEPARTMENT

The Health Insurance Department is the primary body governing issues to do with medical insurance and drugs. Under it, the Medical Examination and Medicinal Materials Group is responsible for the registering of drugs, for formulating their reimbursement prices, and for adjusting those prices. Its regulations, contained in the 'Drug Reimbursement Items and Payment Standards' (simplified to 'Standards' later) divide drugs that are registered under health insurance into two categories, new drugs, and new items. Different regulations are applied to pricing each category.

6.2.1.3 ASSOCIATIONS AND SOCIETIES

These include the Taiwan Hospital Association, the Republic of China Public Hospital Association, the Republic of China Medical Consulting Association, the Taiwan Private Medical Institutions Association, the Taiwan Medical Management Association, and the Taiwan Medical Records Information Management Association.

6.2.2 Price-formation process

6.2.2.1 REVIEW AND APPROVAL OF NEW DRUGS

All drugs sold in Taiwan must be reviewed and are then managed by the Food and Drug Administration for their safety, effectiveness, and quality. Risk management is used to ensure sound, whole-life-cycle, management of drugs. Prior to being put on the market, every drug is subjected to technical reviews, on-the-spot examinations and product inspections. On-the-spot and product inspections must conform to the precepts of *Good Laboratory (non-clinical) Practices of Drugs*, *Good Clinical Practices of Drugs*, and *Good Manufacturing Practices*. After going on the market, drugs continue to be monitored for safety and quality. Safety considerations mainly include applying the reporting system on adverse reactions, regular reporting on the safety of new drugs during the monitoring period, advisory monitoring of the safety of foreign and domestic drugs, and other proactive monitoring mechanisms relating to drug safety. Quality considerations mainly include notification of defective drugs, advisory monitoring of domestic and foreign drug quality, plans for inspection and testing of drugs on the market, and inspection of manufacturing operations. Safety and quality is ensured by dynamic monitoring both before and after drugs go on the market.

6.2.2.2 PROCESS OF PRICING NEW DRUGS

In the Taiwan region, both wholesale and procurement prices are mainly formed through market forces. The government applies controls only to the reimbursement prices for drugs covered by medical insurance. The drug manufacturer submits an application to the Health Insurance Department, and the National Institute of Health Technology Assessment (NIHTA) then carries out an assessment of the drug. This institute is an impartial third-party health technology assessment organization that is independent from government. In order to ensure that medical payments are being used rationally and medical services are of sufficient quality, this body mainly assesses the cost-effectiveness, financial impacts, and ethical, legal, and social impacts of the drug. The assessment report does a comparison of the drug and reference drugs, based on clinical trials and a systematic literature review. Before the 'second generation' of health insurance in Taiwan, this work was carried out by the Division of Health Technology Assessments within the Center for Drug Evaluation. After the second generation insurance began, the NIHTA replaced the original body and became the decision maker with regard to coverage and prices under the new health insurance. It provides professional advice to the joint drafting committee on whether or not innovative drugs should be included in the reimbursable drug list and how they should be priced. The joint drafting committee then discusses the recommendations and makes the final decision. The members of the joint drafting committee are elected by stakeholders. Drug companies, doctors, pharmacists, medical insurance, patients and their representative organizations can submit proposals and present relevant opinions at the meeting.

Members of the joint drafting committee vote to decide on the prices of new drugs and the pricing program. Administrative departments send people to participate in and supervise the meeting, but have no authority to vote. If the committee fails to reach a consensus on the prices and pricing program, it is submitted to the Ministry of Health and Welfare for approval. If that body does not reach agreement, then the case is closed or returned for further discussion. If the committee reaches a consensus of 'disagreement,' then the case is closed. If the committee reaches a consensus to agree, the pricing program is temporarily included into the reimbursement list. It is formally made public only after the Ministry of Health and Welfare approves it.

6.2.2.3 PRICING METHODS FOR NEW DRUGS

Taiwan classifies drugs into different categories in order to price them. The categories mainly depend on the degree of innovation in the drug, their clinical effectiveness, and their quality. Using these standards, drugs are put into three categories. The first consists of 'breakthrough drugs' that show significant improvement in clinical effectiveness over the best existing commonly used drugs. The second consists of new drugs of a 'runner-up' or second-best nature. These include 2A category new drugs ('Me-better'), and 2B category new drugs ('Me-too'). 2A new drugs refer to those that show a moderate improvement in clinical effectiveness over the best existing commonly used drugs. 2B new drugs refer to those that are similar to existing reference drugs. The third category consists of extended new drugs, that is, drugs with the same varieties and dosage forms, but different specifications as those already in the reimbursable drug list (Figure 6.31).

Breakthrough new drugs adopt a pricing method that uses international reference prices. Specifically, the reimbursable price in Taiwan is based on the median price of the drug in ten countries, the U.S., Japan, the U.K., Canada, Germany, France, Belgium, Switzerland, and Australia.

Runner-up new drugs are priced with reference to similar drugs. Depending on the improvement in the actual clinical value of the drug, one of the following five methods is chosen. 1) The lowest price of the drug in ten countries; 2) the price of the drug in the country of origin; 3) a method that looks at the dosage percentage in the course of treatment; 4) a method that uses a percentage of international prices; 5) a method that prices at 70% of the reimbursement price of single-party health insurance for when the drug is used in compounds, or that prices as a single principal ingredient. Extended drugs are priced according to dosage percentages and international price percentages.

6.2.2.4 PRICING OF GENERIC DRUGS

In Taiwan, the differential in pricing between a generic drug and the original-research drug (RLD) once a patent has expired is between 10% and 20%. The price of the First generic is 80% to 90% of the price of the original-research drug, and generics that come on the market after that are priced at the lowest price for drugs with the same ingredients.

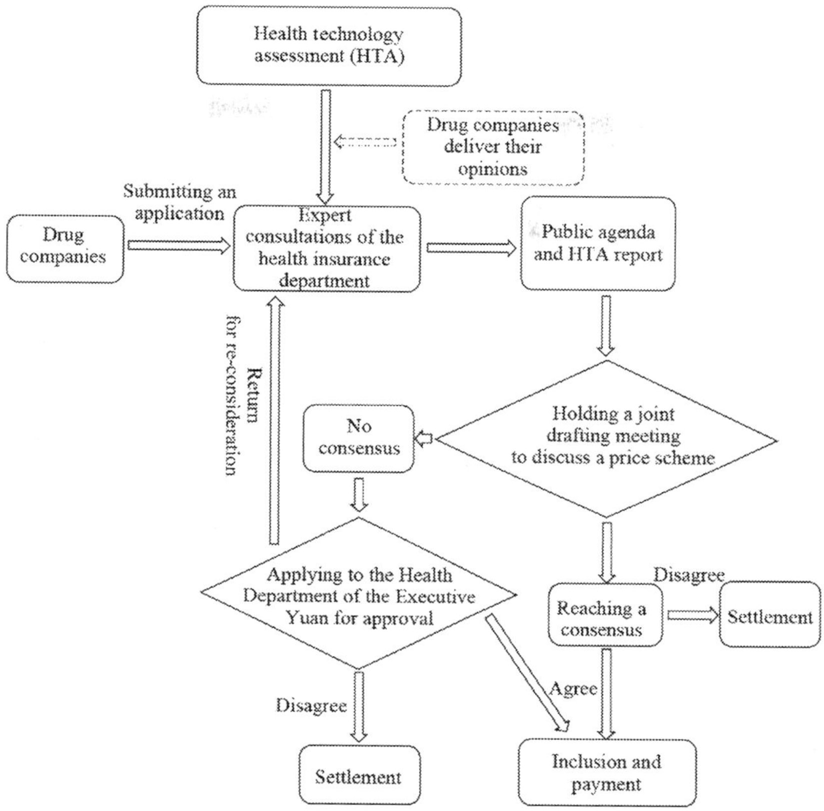

Figure 6.31 Flow Chart Showing Inclusion and Pricing of Drugs Covered by Health Insurance in Taiwan

6.2.3 Health technology assessments in Taiwan

Due to the appearance of an increasing number of new medical technologies, in order to avoid wasting financial resources but still provide new services and technologies, Taiwan's universal health insurance has been conducting health technology assessments since 2007. These are aimed at items that will be reimbursed by insurance and are intended to help with policy-oriented decisions and payment practices with regard to new drugs, special materials, and innovative medical services.

Taiwan's progress in this area can be divided into three stages. The first was from the start of health insurance in 1995 to 2007. During this period, all payment prices were reviewed and decided upon by a committee composed of experts and scholars. The second stage was from 2007 to 2012, when the introduction of health technology assessments began to help guide decision-making with respect to insurance payments. Pharmacists applied to the then Health Insurance Bureau for admission to medical insurance. The Health Insurance Bureau sent the materials of the pharmacists to the health technology assessment group under the jurisdiction of the Center for Drug Evaluation (as legal-person representative of the financial group) for evaluation and for submitting a report on the results. This report was then forwarded to the then Drug Benefit Committee (DBC) for decision-making at a joint drafting meeting. Generally speaking, the review process took about 90 days. The third stage began after Taiwan started implementing its second-generation health insurance in 2013. At that time, the Ministry of Health and Welfare established an independent health technology assessment institution, namely the NIHTA, as an impartial third-party professional agency that is independent of both the government and the public. Once the NIHTA was set up in compliance with the Second Generation Health Insurance Law, it became the decision maker on inclusion and payment decisions for Taiwan's health insurance. The NIHTA replaced the original health insurance drug panel and is composed of 29 people from Taiwan's medical and healthcare systems, including representatives from drug makers, officialdom, and consumers. These determine payment items covered by universal health insurance and payment standards.

Under Taiwan's universal coverage system, the NIHTA, as an impartial third-party organization, assists the Health Insurance Department and other organizations in assessing new drugs, and its results are highly valued as a reference in making decisions. The health technology reports have also become key reference documentation at the joint drafting meeting of the Drug Benefit Committee and the Pharmaceutical Benefit and Reimbursement Scheme.

6.2.4 Drug procurement in the Taiwan region

6.2.4.1 DISTRIBUTION AND PROCUREMENT OF DRUGS

Taiwan follows a policy of having medical institutions do their own procuring of drugs. They do not have to participate in centralized procurement through bidding that is organized by the government. Each institution determines its own procedures and methods of procurement, based on its own drug requirements, but the general practice is to use joint bidding. For small entities such as community pharmacies, decisions on drug purchases are made by the owner of the pharmacy. These have a greater degree of freedom. Large-scale medical institutions, in contrast, have a pharmaceutical affairs management committee and their drug procurement must be carried out in accordance with rules prescribed by the institution. Although Taiwan began to implement a policy of separating out (the business of) medicine from (the business of) drugs in 1997, this was only realized with respect to the division of labor between doctors and pharmacists. Hospitals still have their own pharmacies, and the profits from drugs are still the primary source of income to hospitals. The price difference between the procurement price of drugs and the reimbursement price does not belong to the individual doctor.

Instead, it is 'owned' by the medical institution and then paid out to doctors in the form of salaries. Hospitals therefore have plenty of incentive to negotiate on price with manufacturers when they are procuring drugs. In most situations, the procurement price of drugs will be far below the price at which medical insurance reimburses. The Health Insurance Department allows this kind of price differential for two or three years, but after that it begins to adjust the reimbursement price, in order to reduce the gap. This adjustment of the reimbursement price is based on surveys of the market price of drugs (which are conducted once every two years). Hospitals and drug manufacturers are obliged to submit accurate data on their drug transactions. If they do not use accurate data in the reports they submit, or if there is any fraudulent behavior, the Health Insurance Department may use its authority to cancel the reimbursement status of the institution, or it may lower its reimbursement prices as a punishment.

6.2.4.2 THE SEPARATION OF THE BUSINESS OF DRUGS FROM THE BUSINESS OF MEDICINE IN TAIWAN

Universal health insurance started to be implemented in 1995, and the provisions of Article 2 of Taiwan's Pharmaceutical Affairs Law then went into force which started that drugs and medicine would be separated out as two different lines of business within two years. In 1997, the Taiwan region therefore began pushing forward this policy. At the beginning, it was applied mainly to western-medicine clinics and the pharmacists in ear-nose-and-mouth clinics. The aim was to standardize the behavior of pharmacists in fulfilling prescriptions, and to increase the transparency and safety of prescriptions. For a long time, however, drugs and medicine had not been separate businesses. Given the impact of this historical aspect, but also the interference of various stakeholders, the policy of separating drugs from medicine was implemented in stages. It adopted a 'two-track' method of implementation. What this meant was that hospitals and clinics were allowed to set up pharmacies and hire pharmacists to fulfill prescriptions. At the same time, pharmacy-based pharmacists were allowed to carry on a business of dispensing drugs. Although there was no violent opposition to the policy of separating drugs from medicine, doctors did not completely follow the policy requirements in their actual handling of the matter. Instead, they found legal loopholes. They continued to monopolize their dispensing authority by employing pharmacists in their own clinics or by opening a new pharmacy next to their clinic. As a result, 'front door pharmacies' run by hospitals and clinics were ubiquitous at that time. Through surveys, Tzeng-Ji Chen et al. (2006) discovered that between 1997 and 2004, after Taiwan had started the separation of drugs and medicine policy, many pharmacies were still maintaining very close business relations with this or that clinic. This was directly counter to the idea of developing a fair and competitive drug market. In 2008, some scholars pointed out that 93% of the prescriptions in Taiwan's hospitals were dispensed through 'front door pharmacies.' Only 7% of the total volume of prescriptions flowed through the community health insurance pharmacies.

6.2.5 Drug reimbursement prices and adjustments in the Taiwan region

Taiwan's health insurance reimburses for prescription drugs as well as some 'instructed' drugs (drugs that doctors or pharmacists indicate should be used). It does not reimburse for non-prescription drugs, vaccines, non-medical necessities, and drugs that lack any economic benefits. In addition, manufacturers or medical institutions are not allowed to apply for reimbursement for drugs that do not conform to the good manufacturing practices of the International Drug Inspection Treaty Organization. The reform of Taiwan's reimbursement system for drugs can be divided into roughly three stages. The first stage, before universal health insurance was implemented, paid reimbursement according to the procurement price plus a fee. The second stage began in the early period of universal health insurance, and the reimbursement price was determined through internal examination and approval. The third stage, which came after payment standards began to be implemented, reimbursed according to payment standards and then also adjusted reimbursement at regular intervals. This last stage could also be divided into three periods. The first is the early days of the establishment of the drug price. The second is the period when the benchmark price was revised. The third is the second-generation health insurance period. Those are described as follows.

In the early days of the establishment of the drug price, the Principles of Drug Price Verification for Universal Health Insurance and the Key Points of Drug Payment Price Adjustment for Universal Health Insurance were formulated. The overall framework for managing drug pricing and payment was basically formed. During the period when the benchmark price was revised, the administrative measures for drug payment standards were improved to enhance the transparency of reimbursement pricing and price adjusting, as well as the accessibility of new drugs for patients. During the second-generation health insurance period, the Universal Health Insurance Drug Payment Items and Payment Standards and the Universal Health Insurance Drug Payment Price Adjustment Procedures were revised. As a result of these three periods, Taiwan's drug reimbursement system achieved a step-by-step improvement from the markup on prices as drugs entered hospitals, to pricing by classification of benchmark prices, and adjustment by dividing drugs into groups and classifications.

On October 2, 2013, Taiwan formulated and implemented the *Measures for adjusting prices on drugs under universal health insurance*, as according to Taiwan's *Universal health insurance law*. The main objectives of this were as follows. First, it was done to gradually adjust reimbursement prices so that procurement could be closer to actual market transaction prices. Second, by means of grouping and classification, it was done to gradually reduce differences in price with the reimbursement prices for drugs whose patents had expired and which had been on the market for a long time (generic drugs). Grouping and classification was also done to take into consideration the differences in quality among drugs. Third, it was done to monitor changes in transaction prices for patented drugs or drugs that do not have adequate competition, and to take timely intervention measures in case of major changes.

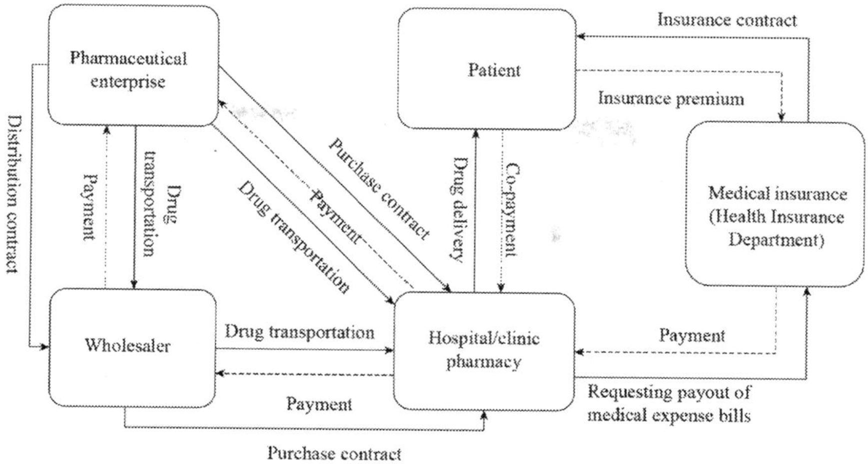

Figure 6.32 Distribution of Drugs in Taiwan, Along with the Flow of Capital and the Flow of Contracts

6.2.5.1 BASIS FOR PRICE ADJUSTMENT

The actual price at which drugs are exchanged on the market is the basis for adjusting reimbursement prices in Taiwan. That is, the basis is the buying and selling price between drug suppliers and medical institutions. The method of obtaining this price is through routine and also special surveys that the Health Insurance Department carries out on a regular basis of products with abnormal prices or quantities. The routine surveys are again divided into three categories, A, B, and C. The targets of A-category surveys are pharmacies and looks at the drug categories included in the reimbursement payment standards. The targets of B-category surveys are medical institutions. Categories of drugs with payment standards are surveyed, and special drugs as publicly announced by the Health Insurance Department. C-category surveys relate to abnormalities in existing declaration materials which are being investigated. The Health Insurance Department cooperates in this process by doing on-site inspections. Special surveys are ad hoc and generally occur when someone makes an incident report about an actual circumstance. Moreover, they occur with respect to items when

> the selling price of a pharmacy or a drug maker is more than 50% lower than the reimbursement price of insurance, there are more than three items with the same ingredient groups, and medical institutions declared [requested reimbursement of] more than NT$ 100 million in the past year.

As the basis for adjusting reimbursement prices, price information must be authentic and objective. Hospitals and drug manufacturers must report truthfully, including basic information on drugs and drug factories, quantity of drug sales, financial volume of sales, and other related information.

6.2.5.2 CLASSIFICATION OF PRICE ADJUSTMENTS

Adjustment of reimbursement standards in Taiwan is mainly based on the degree of innovation in a drug, and Taiwan has set up multiple methods to ascertain this. Drugs are first divided into three categories, depending on whether or not the patent period has expired, how long the drug has been out of patent protection, and how many years (hospitals) have been collecting reimbursement payments on it. The first category includes drugs that are still within the patent period, that is, those whose single or compound preparations contain active ingredients that are still within the patent period. The second category includes drugs that have gone beyond the patent protection period by five years, that is, those whose single or compound preparations contain active ingredients that exceed the patent protection period by five years. The third category includes 3A (the end of the first drug term in the payment standard has not exceeded 15 years) and 3B (the end of the first drug term in the payment standard has exceeded 15 years). The schedule for adjusting prices for each major category of drugs is different. The first and third categories are adjusted once every two years or once every year under the influence of DET (Drug Expenditure Target, see later). The second category is adjusted once a year.

6.2.5.3 PRICE ADJUSTMENT METHODS

Taiwan adjusts reimbursement standards by combining two objectives, namely overall control of costs and adjustment of individual prices. The overall consideration is holding down total insurance costs but various factors also influence the adjustment of drug categories. The first and third categories of drugs started experimenting with a 'Drug Expenditure Target' in 2013. The amount spent on drug costs in a given year is checked to see whether or not spending has been affected by budgeted target set the previous year. If the amount does not exceed the target value, this means that spending on that drug was not affected by the DET. If it does exceed the target value, then spending was affected by the target value. Specific methods of adjusting prices of the three categories of drugs vary. Moreover, lower adjustment limits are set for various drugs to ensure that low-priced drugs maintain a certain market. Drug prices that have not passed PIC/S GMP may not be higher than those of a drug that passes PIC/S GMP, so as to protect high-quality drugs. (See list of acronyms.)

1 Adjustment methods of the first category of drugs

For drugs whose prices are not affected by the DET system, a Weighted Average Price (WAP) is calculated based on data collected from a survey of actual transaction prices in the drug market. If the Weighted Average Price is greater than or equal to 0.85 times the original medical insurance reimbursement price, no adjustment is made. Otherwise, the reimbursement price is adjusted to 0.15 times the 'original medical insurance reimbursement price,' plus the drug's Weighted Average Price.

For drugs that are affected by the DET system, if spending on a given drug exceeds the preset target value of the previous year, the reimbursement price of that drug in the following year is adjusted to the extent that spending exceeded the target value. (The method of verification looks at the previous three quarters of spending, while the fourth quarter is a calculated figure that is based on the first three quarters.) Based on the results of adjusting prices that are not affected by the DET system (called provisional prices), the overall price adjustment for each item in the first and third categories of drugs is calculated as follows: take the difference between the payment price before adjustment and the provisional price and multiply it by the sum of the medical expenses declared in the previous year. The amount exceeding the target value is allocated according to the percentage of the overall amount of adjustment.

2 Adjustment methods for the second category of drugs

In the second category of drugs, the post-adjustment reimbursement price must not be higher than the pre-adjustment reimbursement price. Generic prices must not be higher than prices of original-research drugs (prices of RLDs). If, however, drugs have standard packaging and are in compliance with PIC/SGMP, and if their reimbursement price is the basic price, there is no such restriction. Second-category drugs are adjusted depending on how long their patent-protection status has expired. For those whose patents expired within one year, and for drugs with the same class of ingredients, if the price of the class exceeds the reimbursement price of drugs still under patent, then the new reimbursement price is the lower of either the lowest of prices among ten countries or the group weighted average price times 1.15. The percentage of adjustment that applies to expired-patent drugs is then applied to drugs in the same ingredient class. If there are no such drugs whose patent has expired, then the reimbursement price is adjusted according to the group weighted average price of the same group, multiplied by 1.5.

Regarding drugs whose patents have expired for more than one year but less than five years and their same-ingredient class of drugs, the following holds: if the price of such drugs is more than the price of similar drugs that are still under patent protection, then the price is adjusted to be the group weighted average price of the grouped products, multiplied by 1.5. The percentage of adjustment is then applied to drugs in the same class whose patents have expired. If there are no such drugs, then drugs in the same-ingredient class are adjusted to the group weighted-average price times 1.15.

3 Adjustment methods for the third category of drugs

Adjustment of reimbursement prices of the third category of drugs is divided into three main steps: choosing a target value, calculating a provisional price, and calculating the extent of adjustment. For Type 3A drugs, whose patents have not been expired for 15 years, the target value that is not affected by DET system is usually selected with GWAP of the same group of classified items as the target value of the temporary adjustment price of the item. The temporary adjustment price is 105% of WAP and the target value, and 90% of the target value is the lower limit of the temporary adjustment price. The temporary adjustment price shall not be higher than the payment price before adjustment. The percentage of the difference between the temporary adjustment price and the pre-adjustment payment price is calculated. If the extent of adjustment is less than 15%, the drug payment price will not be adjusted. If the extent of adjustment is greater than 15%, the 'extent of adjustment minus 15%' will be compared with the set 'maximum extent of reduction' and the original payment price will be adjusted if the lower is selected. If the DET system needs to be adjusted, the target value, and temporary adjustment price, etc. shall be calculated according to the 'price adjustment not affected by the DET system,' but not affected by the mentioned maximum reduction range: if the drug is a new drug as mentioned in the drug payment standard, and the time interval between the receipt and collection of drug dealer sales data is within four years, the adjustment shall be made, if the extent of adjustment is less than 5%; if the extent of adjustment is greater than 5%, the payment price shall be adjusted based on the value with the extent of adjustment minus 5%, and the payment price before adjustment shall be the upper limit. Other drugs will not be adjusted if the extent of adjustment is less than 3%. If the extent of adjustment is greater than 3%, the payment price shall be adjusted based on the value with the extent of adjustment minus 3%, and the payment price before adjustment shall be the upper limit.

For drugs over 15 years (Type 3B), the target value of payment price adjustment of the drugs in this type is GWAP of the same type of items in the same group. The temporary adjustment price is 1.15 times the target value of the grouping classification of individual items, and is not higher than the highest payment price before the same grouping adjustment. If DET system adjustment is not required, the last temporary adjustment price is the final adjustment price. If the DET system adjustment is needed, the DET system adjustment will be carried out on the basis of the previous temporary price adjustment. The specific adjustment method of the DET system is the same as that of the first category of drugs.

It can be seen from the previously mentioned that Taiwan adopts different measures for adjusting the reimbursement prices of generic drugs and patented drugs. Stricter price controls are applied to generic drugs. New drugs may be allowed a certain markup if they satisfy specified conditions.

6.2.6 A summary of drug price-formation mechanisms in Taiwan

Taiwan has been remarkably successful in maintaining the percentage that drugs occupy in healthcare spending at a stable 25% over a long period of time. This has been due to the management systems described earlier, and to institution building. Looking back over the series of reforms that Taiwan has undertaken with respect to drug pricing and health insurance management, we have discovered considerable similarities to the way Japan has handled such things as reimbursement pricing, medical insurance access, and the pricing adjustment system. At the same time, however, Taiwan has come up with a number of innovations, as described next.

6.2.6.1 A SYSTEM OF DRUG REIMBURSEMENT SAFEGUARDS THAT PROVIDES FULL COVERAGE

Judging by the policy objective of 'focusing on people as the essential aspect,' Taiwan has already reached quite high levels of coverage in its medical insurance system. Not only does it provide coverage to nearly 100% of residents, but at the same time it gives full consideration to the needs and interests of patients. Essentially all prescription drugs are included within the scope of reimbursement, which broadens the benefits of new drugs and improves their accessibility, while giving people a sense of being able to receive medical care.

6.2.6.2 PRICE-FORMATION MECHANISMS THAT ARRIVE AT ACTUAL MARKET-DERIVED PRICES

Taiwan's medical insurance is a social medical insurance system, but the provision of healthcare services takes full advantage of the vitality of market mechanisms. The main providers are social (i.e., private, as opposed to government). The pricing of drugs places a similar focus on the role of the market. By having hospitals and pharmacies negotiate with drug companies, prices are constantly forced down while at the same time it is possible to get reliable statistics. The margin between the price at which medical institutions procure drugs and the price at which they are reimbursed by medical insurance is retained by the medical institution. It is then released on to doctors in the form of salaries. The systems design that allows for retaining such surpluses gives medical institutions plenty of incentive during their procurement negotiations with drug manufacturers.

6.2.6.3 A PRICING SYSTEM FOR DRUGS COVERED BY INSURANCE THAT ALLOWS FOR DYNAMIC ADJUSTMENTS

Like Japan, Taiwan conducts regular surveys of actual prices in the drug market and then conducts regular adjustments. Taiwan's price surveys and adjustments are more refined than those of Japan, however. Japan carries out surveys of all items that have drug pricing standards and the target of surveys are all retailers plus a certain percentage of medical institutions. Taiwan does regular price surveys of category A, B, and C drugs, but in addition to surveying retailers and medical institutions, the Health Insurance Department also does on-site inspections for abnormal situations. This includes making ad hoc investigations of drugs on which complaint reports have been filed. In terms of price adjustment methods, Taiwan's methodology is quite refined. Japan generally uses a 'reasonable-range' method, whereas Taiwan mainly looks at the extent of innovation and then constructs a multi-method system of reimbursement price adjustment. It formulates three main categories, depending on whether or not the patent period has expired, for how long, and how many years health insurance has included the drug in its reimbursement. Based on that determination, Taiwan then distinguishes whether or not pricing has been influenced by DET and different adjustment cycles and methods are then adopted. This dynamic method of adjusting insurance reimbursement prices is used as a kind of market-based supervision, to ensure the healthy development of the drug market.

6.2.6.4 INNOVATIVE PRICING METHODS FOR DRUGS INCLUDED IN MEDICAL INSURANCE REIMBURSEMENT

Health technology assessments and pharmaco-economic evaluations are already used in many developed countries and some developing countries to determine access to insurance reimbursement and the pricing of reimbursement. Taiwan began experimenting with health technology assessments in 2007 as a way to assist in policy decisions about payment for new drugs, special materials, and innovative therapeutic services. While Japan is only using the results of health technology assessments as the basis for adjusting insurance reimbursement prices, Taiwan has already set up the NIHTA, an impartial third-party professional organization that includes government and public participation. It uses the assessment reports and results as key reference documentation for decision-making by the 'health insurance and pharmaceutical affairs team' and the 'joint drafting meeting PBRS.'

Abbreviations and acronyms

CDE: Center of Drug Evaluation
DBC: Drug Benefit Committee
DET: Drug Expenditure Target
DHTA: Division of Health Technology Assessment
GCP: Good Clinical Practice
GLP: Good laboratory practice of drug
GMP: Good Manufacture Practice
GWAP: group weighted average price
HTA: Health Technology Assessment
NIHTA: National Institute of Health Technology Assessment
PBRS: Pharmaceutical Benefit and Reimbursement Scheme joint committee
WAP: Weighted Average Price

Bibliography

[1] World Bank Database. https://data.worldbank.org.cn/
[2] AMA Database. www.aha.org/data-insights/health-care-big-picture
[3] CDC Database. www.cdc.gov/DataStatistics/
[4] Patricia Van Arnum. Biopharmaceutical Innovation: Which Countries Rank the Best? [EB/OL]. 2016-4-13/2019-12-3

[5] https://dcatvci.org/250-biopharmaceutical-innovation-which-countries-rank-the-best

[6] APEC Database. https://data.oecd.org

[7] Adam J. Fein. The 2019 Economic Report on U.S. Pharmacies and Pharmacy Benefit Managers[R]. Philadelphia: Drug Channels, 2019.

[8] U.S. Census Bureau. 2016 Annual Retail Trade Report[R] U.S. Census Bureau, 2019.

[9] Alex Azar. How Team Trump Is Bringing Drug Prices Down[EB/OL]. 2019-2-7/ 2019-12-3

[10] www.hhs.gov/about/leadership/secretary/op-eds/how-team-trump-is-bringing-drug-prices-down.html

[11] Healthcare Supply Chain Association. *A Primer on Group Purchasing Organizations Questions and Answers.* [R] Washington: Healthcare Supply Chain Association, 2019.

[12] Overview of the UK. Embassy of the People's Republic of China in the United Kingdom of Great The UK and Northern Ireland, 2019. www.fmprc.gov.cn/ce/ceuk/chn/zl/t687647.htm.

[13] OECD.stat. https://stats; Stat. https://stats.oecd.org/Index.aspx#

[14] Shen Shili and Yu Xiaosong. Basic Medical and Health System and Its Improvement on the Development of Chinese General Practitioners [J]. *Chinese General Practitioners*, 2019, 22 (19).

[15] Liu Yongjun, Liu Na, Zhang Qi, Wang Chao, Gu Yingli, and Li Ziyang. Salary Incentive Policy for General Practitioners in the UK and Its Reference Significance [J]. *Chinese General Practitioners*, 2018, 21 (25).

[16] How Are General Practitioners Are Motivated in the UK? [EB/OL]. (2017-09-04) [2018-01-05]. www.sohu.com/a/169348804_454478

[17] Mike H. *General Practice and the NHS: Past, Present and Future [R].* Shenyang: Fifth China General Practice Conference, 2018.

[18] Xie Chunyan, He Jiangjiang, and Hu Shanlian. The Health Service Payment System in the UK: Experiences and Implications [J]. *Chinese Health Economics*, 2015, 34(1).

[19] *Exploring the Early Workings of Emerging Clinical Commission Groups: Final Report.* 2012(12).

[20] Li Tao, Xiufeng Wang, and Zhao Kun. Enlightenment of the UK Health System on China's Medical Reform [J]. *Chinese General Practice*, 2015,18 (34).

[21] Wang Yun. Current Situation, Experience and Implications of Drug Production and Circulation System in UK [J]. *Economic Research Reference*, 2014 (32).

[22] Gao Lianke and Yang Shuqin. Changes in the British Medical Security System and Its Implications [J]. *The Northern Forum*, 2005 (04).

[23] Department of Institutional Reform. Briefing by the Leading Group of the State Council on Deepening the Reform of the Medical and Health System (No. 51) *Summary of Research on Universal Health Coverage*. www.nhc.gov.cn/tigs/ygjb/201904/625c83f073a0412dadf4d5af2a3d6810.shtml

[24] OECD. *Health at a Glance 2019 OECD INDICATORS*, 2019, PDF.

[25] NICE. *Patient Access Schemes Liaison Unit*. www.nice.org.uk/about/what-we-do/patient-access-schemes-liaison-unit

[26] Li Ying. Study on Drug Economic Evaluation Model of Drug List Selection: Based on Comparison of Australia, the UK, Germany and France [J]. *Journal of CPC Central Committee Party School*, 2009,13 (05).

[27] Dong Xinyue, Zhang Lingli, and Shao Rong. The Connection between the Value Pricing Concept and Drug Compensation System in the UK and Its Implications [J]. *Health Economics Research*, 2018 (10).

[28] Ye Lu and Hu Shanlian. Drug Price and Management Policy in the UK: Experiences and Implications [J]. *Chinese Pharmacy*, 2005 (09).

[29] Department of Health and Social Care. *The 2019 Voluntary Scheme for Branded Medicines Pricing and Access – Annexes*, 2018 (12).

[30] NICE. *Patient access schemes (PASs) [EB/OL].* www.nice.org.uk/The_pharmaceutical_price_regulation_scheme_2014

[31] NICE. *Voluntary Scheme for Branded Medicines Pricing and Access (2019)[EB/OL].* www.nice.org.uk/voluntary-scheme-for-branded-medicines-pricing-and-access-chapters-and-glossary.PDF.

[32] Patient Access Scheme Liaison Unit at NICE. *Procedure for the Review of Patient Access Scheme proposals*, 2018 (1).

[33] NICE. *NICE Highly Specialised Technologies Guidance [EB/OL].* www.nice.org.uk/About/What-we-do/Our-Programmes/NICE-guidance/NICE-highly-specialised-technologies-guidance

[34] NICE. *Changes We're Making to Health Technology Evaluation[EB/OL].* www.nice.org.uk/board-paper-TA-HST-consultation-mar-17-HST-only.PDF

[35] Lu Lanting and Yu Liujie. A Comparative Study on Anti-cancer Drug Policies between China and the UK [J]. *China Health Policy Research*, 2019, 12 (02): 15–21

[36] IGES. *Reimbursement of Pharmaceuticals in Germany 2018[R].*IGES, 2018.

[37] OECD. *The European Observatory on Health Systems and Policies, European Commission. European Commission. State of Health in the EU Germany Country Health Profile 2019[R].* OECD, 2019.

[38] Lu Lanting, and Fu Ronghua. Analysis on the Transformation Path and Method of Health Technology Assessment Decisions in Germany [J]. *China Health Policy Research*, 2017 (4).

[39] Su Hong. Analysis on Drug Price Control Systems in the UK, Germany and Switzerland [J]. *Pharmaceutical and Clinical Research*, 2016, 24 (5): 353–356.

[40] CBI. *CBI Market Survey: The Pharmaceutical Products Market in Germany[R].* CBI, 2010.

[41] Hogan Lovells. *EU Pricing & Reimbursement – Pricing & Reimbursement Schemes in Major European Countries*[R]. Hogan Lovells, 2014.

[42] Chen Jing, Zhao Xizi, and Zhao Liang. Experience and Implications of Drug Price Regulation in Germany, Japan and Taiwan [J]. *Chinese Pharmacy*, 2017, 28 (25): 3464–3467. doi:10.6039/j.issn.1001-0408.2017.25.03

[43] Sebastian Sieler, *Thomas Rudolph, Carola Brinkmann-Sass, and Richard Sear. AMNOG Revisited [EB/OL].* 2015-5/2019-12-4. www.mckinsey.com/industries/pharmaceuticals-and-medical-products/our-insights/amnog-revisited

[44] Hinrichs S, Jahagirdar D, Miani C, et al. *Learning for the NHS on Procurement and Supply Chain Management: A Rapid Evidence Assessment[J].* www.ncbi.nlm.nih.gov/books/NBK269149/doi: 10.3310/hsdr02550

[45] Julia Graf. The Effects of Rebate Contracts on the Health Care System[J], 2012. *The European Journal of Health Economics*, 2014 (5): 477–487.

[46] IMF: World Economic Outlook Databases, Oct., 2019.

[47] Fullman N, Yearwood J, Abay SM, et al. Measuring Performance on the Healthcare Access and Quality Index for 195countries and Territories and Selected Subnational Locations: A Systematic Analysis from the Global Burden of Disease Study 2016[J]. *Lancet*, 2018, 391 (10136): 2236–2271.

[48] Ministry of Health. *Labour and Welfare [EB/OL].* www.mhlw.go.jp/policy/health-medical/health-insurance/index.html,2019-10-21

[49] Organisation for Economic Co-operation and Development [EB/OL]. www.oecd.org/. www.oecd.org/health/health-at-a-glance-19991312.htm,2019-11-01

[50] Chen Jinkui. *Implications of Japan's Medical Insurance System to China [D].* Northeast University of Finance and Economics, 2018.

[51] Feng Zeyun, Wang Haiyin, Chen Duo, Yan Yang, Fang Liang, and Jin Chunlin. Japanese Medical Insurance Payment Policy and Its Implications: A Case Study of Laboratory Projects [J]. *China Health Quality Management*, 2018, 25 (01): 104–106.

[52] Qian Yongfeng. Enlightenment of Japan's Medical Security Model on Improving China's Medical Security System [J]. *Modern Hospital Management*, 2012, 10 (02): 24–26.

[53] Qian Yongfeng. Implications of Japan's Medical Security Model on Improving China's Medical Security System [J]. *Modern Hospital Management*, 2012,10 (02): 24–26.

[54] Liu Lu, Yan Jianzhou, and Shao Rong. Research on Japanese Innovative Drug Policy Environment-Empirical Analysis Based on Thrombomodulin α [J]. *Chinese Journal of New Drugs and Clinical Medicine*, 2017, 36 (12): 717–722.

[55] Chen Cheng. Study on Japanese Drug Pricing Method [A]. Pharmaceutical Affairs Management Committee of Chinese Pharmaceutical Association. *Proceedings of the 2013 Annual Meeting of Pharmaceutical Affairs Management Committee of Chinese Pharmaceutical Association and Academic Forum on "Pharmaceutical Safety and Scientific Development" (Volume II)* [C]. Pharmaceutical Affairs Management Committee of Chinese Pharmaceutical Association: Chinese Pharmaceutical Association, 2013: 5.

[56] Li Lei. Japan's Innovative Drug Price Management and Its Implications to China [J]. *China New Drugs*, 2013, 22 (05): 502–504.

[57] Feng Chang, and Li Sihan. Implications of the International Reference Pricing System for Drugs to China-Taking Canada, Netherlands and Japan as Examples [J]. *Price Theory and Practice*, 2013 (07): 62–63.

[58] Zhang Xing, Tatsuo Oyama. Measuring the Impact of Japanese Local Public Hospital Reform on National Medical Expenditure via Panel Data Regression [J]. *Technological Forecasting & Social Change*, 2016, 113.

[59] Japan's Central Social Security Medical Committee Discusses NHI Drug Price Reform and Market Expansion [J]. *Chinese Pharmacoeconomics*, 2009 (06): 96.

[60] Gao Yan. Japan's Drug Price Management System and Its Implications [J]. *Macroeconomic Management*, 2015 (10): 84–85+92.

[61] Guo Ying, Zhang Huiling, Chen Jing, and Yuan Hongmei. Research on Japanese Drug Price Policy and Its Implications for China [J]. *Chinese Pharmacoeconomics*, 2010 (04): 63–67.

[62] Feng Chang, and Sun Jie. Implications of the International Reference Pricing Method in China for New Drugs to China [J]. *China New Drugs*, 2014, 23 (05): 510–512+522.

[63] Chen Jing, Zhao Xizi, Zhao Liang, and Shi Luwen. Experience and Implications of Drug Price Regulations in Germany, Japan and Taiwan [J]. *China Drug Store*, 2017, 28 (25): 3464–3467.

[64] Wang Liang, Li Aihua, Yue Xiaomeng, and Wu Jiuhong. Research on Japanese Drug Price System and Implications for Drug Price Management in China [J]. *Chinese Health Economics*, 2017, 36 (10): 87–91.

[65] Guo Liyan. Japan's Medical Insurance System and Drug Price Management System and Its Implications for China [J]. *Chinese Prices*, 2013 (07): 60–62.

[66] Shen Jing. *Study on Drug Pricing Mechanism and Medical Insurance Payment Standard* [D]. Capital University of Economics and Business, 2017.

[67] OECD.stat. https://stats.oecd.org/Index.aspx#.

[68] Tan Jingchen, Zhu Kongdong, and Niu Yan. Understanding of the ROK's Health Care System and Using it as a Reference [J]. *Chinese Health Economics*, 2008 (07): 79–80.

[69] Feng Chang, Ji Meiyan, Lu Yun, Cui Penglei, and Zhu Xiaorui. Research on the ROK Medical Security System and Its Operation Mode [J]. *China Health Policy Research*, 2015, 8 (12): 41–46.

[70] Bulletin of the Leading Group of the State Council on Deepening the Reform of the Medical and Health System (No. 11): Overview of the ROK's National Medical Insurance System. www.nhc.gov.cn/tigs/ygjb/201310/740634c646414614b6e567b22d6fb83e.shtml

[71] OECD. *Health at a Glance 2019 OECD INDICATORS*, 2019, PDF.

[72] Guo Xiaodan. Pharmaceutical Market in the ROK: an Overview [J]. *Import and Export Manager*, 2017 (01): 41–43.

[73] Pharmaceutical Retail Reform in the ROK: a Prospect [J]. *China Drug Store*, 2009 (06): 46–47.

[74] Li Songhua. The Reform on the Separation of Medical Treatment and Drugs in the ROK and Its Implications to China [J]. *Chinese Health Economics*, 2009, 28 (08): 75–78.

[75] Feng Chang, Liu Hongqiang, and Xi Yue. The Reform of the Positive Drug List and Price Negotiation System in the ROK: Experience and Implications [J]. *Price Theory and Practice*, 2015 (05): 97–99.

[76] Qiu Fu'en. Introduction of the Drug Patent Linking System in the ROK and Its Implications to China's System [J]. *Electronic Intellectual Property*, 2019 (03): 22–28.

[77] Taiwan Statistical Bureau. *Taiwan Statistical Yearbooks 2008–2019*, 2019.

[78] Fu Chen, and Zhang Gang. Enlightenment and Reference from Taiwan's Medical and Health Management System [J]. *China Health Resources*, 2007 (01): 24–26.

[79] Huang Guowu and Wang Mengting. Study on the Development and Changes of Health Care Drug Reimbursement List in Taiwan [J]. *China Social Security*, 2018 (05): 76–79.

[80] Li Yincai. Equity and Evaluation of the Universal Health Insurance System in Taiwan [J]. *Medicine and Philosophy*, 2019,40 (16): 55–58.

[81] Yang Wan. *Taiwan's Universal Health Insurance Financial Research* [D]. Wuhan University, 2017.

[82] Taiwan's "Ministry of Health and Welfare, Central Health Insurance Department". Introduction to "2016–2017" Universal Health" Insurance (EB/OL). [2019-011-08]. www.nhi.gov.tw/nhi_e-librarypubweb/custompage/p_detail.aspx?CP_ID =129

[83] Liao Xiaoyan. *Taiwan's Universal Health Insurance on the Improvement of China's Basic Medical Insurance System* [D]. Southwest University of Political Science and Law, 2015.

[84] Taiwan's "Ministry of Health and Welfare, Central Health Insurance Department" [EB/OL]. [2019-11-09. www.nhi.gov.tw/nhi_e-librarypubweb/custompage/p_detail.aspx?CP_ID=129

[85] Hou Yan, Dai Tao, Zheng Ying, Zhuang Ning. Experience and Enlightenment from the Medical Service System management in Taiwan [J]. *China Health Policy Research*, 2015, 8 (05): 13–18.

[86] National Health Administration, Ministry of Health and Welfare, Executive Yuan. www.hpa.gov.tw/BHPNet/Web/Index/Index.aspx

[87] Taiwan's "Central Health Insurance Department of the Ministry of Health and Welfare" [EB/ol]. [2019-11-11 [EB/OL].[2019-11-11]. www.nhi.gov.tw/Nhi_E-LibraryPubWeb/CustomPage/P_Detail.aspx?CP_ID=129

[88] www.hatw.org.tw/

[89] You Shuhua, Chen Yanyu, and Jiang Dongying. Taiwan's Drug Supervision and Administration System: An Exploration [J]. *Lishizhen Med Mater Med Res*, 2013, 24 (08): 2008–2009.

[90] Ren Lei, Jiang Rong, Yuan Han Shipi, and Shao Rong. A Study on the Management System of Innovative Drug Payment Standards in Taiwan: An Empirical Analysis Based on Apixaban Tablets [J]. *China Medical Insurance*, 2018 (06): 63–67.

[91] Lai Xinquan, Xue Song, Li Hai, Wang Guohua, Zheng Zhaohui, Huang Zhangxin, and Xiao Yu. A Research Report on Taiwan's Medical and Health System, Health Insurance System and Medical Price Management [J]. *Market Economy and Price*, 2014 (06): 10–16+20.

[92] Qiu Yulin, and Yuan Tao. Experience in Drug Price Management in Taiwan [J]. *China Social Security*, 2016 (11): 80–81.

[93] Wang Yanan, Guan Haijing, Liu Guoen, and Sun Lihua. Purchase Mode and Payment Price of Medical Insurance Drugs in Taiwan [J]. *China Health Policy Research*, 2015, 8 (12): 18–22.

[94] Wang Jun. Separating Medical Treatment and Drugs in Taiwan and Japan [J]. *Chinese Pharmacy*, 2011, (7): 48–49.

[95] Tzeng-Ji Chen. *Li-Fang Chou and Shinn-Jang Hwang Journal: BMC Health Services Research*, 2006.

[96] Hao Lan. Taiwan's Dilemma of the "Dual-track System" of Separating Medical Treatment and Drugs[J]. *China Drug Store*, 2008 (12): 40–42+44.

[97] Zhang Jie, Xiong Xianjun, and Li Jinghu. Taiwan Health Insurance Drug Price and Payment Management System [J]. *China Medical Insurance*, 2015 (04): 67–70.

[98] Chen Jing, Zhao Xizi, Zhao Liang, and Shi Lvwen. Experience and Enlightenment of Drug Price Regulation in Germany, Japan and Taiwan [J]. *China Drug Store*, 2017, 28 (25): 3464–3467.

[99] Shao Rong, Ren Lei, and Jiang Rong. A Study on the Price Adjustment System of Medical Insurance Drug Payment in Taiwan [J]. *Price Theory and Practice*, 2017 (04): 80–83.

[100] Cai Weizhen. Taiwan's Medical Insurance Measures to Control Drug Expenses and Their Implications [A]. Pharmaceutical Affairs Management Committee of Chinese Pharmaceutical Association. *Proceedings of the 2018 Annual Meeting of Pharmaceutical Affairs Management Committee of Chinese Pharmaceutical Association and Academic Forum* [C]. Pharmaceutical Affairs Management Committee of Chinese Pharmaceutical Association: Chinese Pharmaceutical Association, 2018: 8.

[101] Jison, Xu Zhisheng. Drug Payment System and Total Payment System: The Experience of Taiwan in China [J]. *Shaanxi Agricultural Sciences*, 2012, 58 (02): 220–222+227.

Index

Note: Page numbers in *italics* indicate figures; those in bold indicate tables.

Printed in the United States
by Baker & Taylor Publisher Services